Community Paediatrics

Community Paediatrics

Leon Polnay

MB BS, BSc, FRCP, DObst RCOG, DCH
Reader in Child Health, University of Nottingham

David Hull

BSc, MB, FRCP, DObst RCOG, DCH
Professor of Child Health, University of Nottingham

SECOND EDITION

CHURCHILL LIVINGSTONE
EDINBURGH, LONDON, MADRID, MELBOURNE, NEW YORK AND TOKYO 1993

CHURCHILL LIVINGSTONE
Medical Division of Longman Group UK Limited

Distributed in the United States of America by
Churchill Livingstone Inc., 650 Avenue of the Americas,
New York, N.Y. 10011, and by associated companies, branches
and representatives throughout the world.

First published 1985
    Reprinted 1988
    Reprinted 1990
    Reprinted 1992
Second edition 1993

ISBN 0-443-04250-0

British Library Cataloguing Data
A catalogue record for this book is available from
the British Library.

The
publisher's
policy is to use
**paper manufactured
from sustainable forests**

Produced by Longman Singapore Publishers Pte Ltd
Printed in Singapore

Preface

Community Paediatrics has changed considerably since the first edition of this book. Our knowledge of the subject has increased, the services have grown and the providers of those services have developed into a consultant-led work force, with training posts at senior house officer, registrar and senior registrar levels. We decided that we would write a completely new edition that reflected the changes in knowledge and practice and the new health service climate and culture in which we are expected to deliver these goods. Expansion of the number of contributors reflects the way that services have developed in Nottingham, not just in Child Health, but also in Child and Adolescent Psychiatry, Clinical Genetics and Mental Handicap. This new edition is an introductory text that covers the breadth of the subject and the major concepts. It has been written as a source book for the MSc course in Community Paediatrics. The references and guides to further reading should provide a good introduction to the expanding literature.

Our thanks are due to the contributors who suffered our harassment on top of that generated by health service reforms, and our families whose tolerance and patience of this endeavour is quite remarkable.

Nottingham, 1993   L. P.
                                                             D.H.

Contributors

Mitch Blair
BSc, MSc, MB BS, MRCP
Senior Lecturer in Child Health, University of Nottingham

Ann Craft
BSc, PhD
Senior Lecturer in Mental Handicap, University of Nottingham

Julia Faulconbridge
MSc, C Psychol
Consultant Clinical Psychologist, Nottingham Community Health NHS Trust,
Honorary Lecturer in Clinical Psychology, Leicester University

Ann Howard
MB BS, LRCP, MRCS, DRCOG, MFCH
Senior Clinical Medical Officer, Nottingham Community Health NHS Trust

Tom Hutchison
MB ChB, MRCP, DCH
Consultant Community Paediatrician, Bath District Health Authority

Chris Jarvis
BSc, SRD, MBDA
Chief Paediatric Dietitian, Nottingham City Hospital NHS Trust

Derek Johnston
MA, MD, FRCP, DCH
Consultant Paediatrician, University Hospital, Nottingham

Shirley Lewis
MB ChB, DPH, DObst RCOG
Consultant Community Paediatrician, Nottingham Community Health NHS Trust

Mary McKay
MB BCh, BAO, MSc, MRCP
Lecturer in Community Paediatrics, University of Nottingham

David Mellor
MD, FRCP, DCH
Consultant Paediatric Neurologist, University Hospital, Nottingham

Marian Miles
MB BS, FRCP, FRCP(E), DCH
Consultant Community Paediatrician, Parkside Health Authority, London

Colin Newton
MSc, BSc, PGCE
Senior Educational Psychologist, Nottinghamshire Educational Psychology Service

Yin Ng
MB BS, MRCP
Consultant Community Paediatrician, Nottingham Community Health NHS Trust

Jackie Nicholson
MB ChB, DCH
Senior Clinical Medical Officer, Southern Derbyshire Health Authority

John Pearce
MB BS, MPhil, M RCP, FRCPsych
Professor of Child and Adolescent Psychiatry, Nottingham University

Connie Pullan
MB MS, MD, FRCP
Consultant Community Paediatrician, Nottingham Community Health NHS Trust

Sandy Raeburn
PhD, MB ChB, FRCP
Professor of Clinical Genetics, University of Nottingham

Andrew Tandy
BSc, MB BS, MRCGP, MRCP
Lecturer in Community Paediatrics, University of Nottingham

Helen Venning
BMed Sci, BM, BS, MRCP
Consultant Community Paediatrician, Nottingham Community Health NHS Trust

Derek Wilson
MA (Psychol), MA (Child Psychol)
Educational Psychologist, Nottinghamshire Educational Psychology Service

Contents

1. Origins 1
2. Health Services 6
3. Education Services 20
4. Health Promotion and Health Education 33
5. Social Services 41
6. Benefits 57
7. The Law 66
8. Information 73
9. Surveillance 95
10. Avoiding Infection 121
11. Eating Well 141
12. Growth 167
13. Intellectual Development 185
14. Emotional Development and Disorder 205
15. Poor Homes and Families 221
16. Accidents 237
17. Avoiding Harm: Child Protection 249
18. Special Needs 277
19. Physical Handicap 290
20. Vision 310
21. Hearing 323
22. Language 335
23. Learning and Health 345
24. Learning Disability 366
25. Emotional and Behavioural Problems 386
26. Counselling 418
27. Young Adults 429
28. Genetic Counselling 441

Appendices:

A. Common Problems 457

B. Support Organisations 463

C. Sources of Information 466

Index 471

Editors' note

For ease of reading, the masculine gender is used throughout this book, except where obviously inappropriate, but the feminine is intended to be equally applicable.

Origins

"Ou venons nous, ou sommes nous, ou allons nous?"

Child Health Services in the community began in Britain 200 years ago. Their development followed a growing awareness of the inter-relationship between environment and health – Public Health – and a change in public attitude; it was no longer possible to ignore or simply accept the ill health of the poor. The industrial revolution had led to dense populations in poor housing which provided a substrate for devastating epidemics of infectious disease. A combination of social conscience, sometimes tempered with self interest in terms of fitness to work and the wish to reduce the need for charity, with scientific investigation and innovative ideas, led to a wide range of services whose primary aim was the *prevention* of disease. The main tools for prevention were regulation of the environment at home and at work and education particularly with regard to hygiene and nutrition.

LANDMARKS

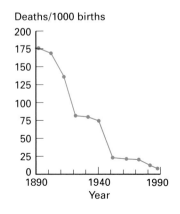

Infant mortality

Deaths/1000 births

1769. George Armstrong established a dispensary for the infant poor and home visiting in London.

1833. The Factory Act prohibited the employment of children under 9 and restricted the working day of 9–11 year olds to 9 hours a day. It established an inspectorate to judge the fitness of children to work.

1842. Edwin Chadwick. His report on the sanitary conditions of the labouring population of Great Britain recommended that expenditure on sanitation would increase longevity and reduce demand on Poor Law Relief.

1847. The first Medical Officer of Health was appointed in Liverpool.

1867. The first successful health visiting service was established by the Manchester and Salford Ladies Sanitary Reform Association to 'employ respectable working woman to go from door to door offering physical help and health advice'.

1888. Local Government Act established elected County Councils and empowered them to appoint Medical Officers of Health who were required to possess a qualification in Public Health.

1890. The first School Medical Officer was appointed by the London School Board.

1891. The first certified course for health visitors was established in Buckinghamshire.

1893 and 1899. Education Acts gave local authorities discretionary powers to provide special schooling for blind, deaf, defective and epileptic children.

1899. First centre opened in St Helens to supply free sterilised milk to infants and mothers and advice and consultation.

1904. Report of the Interdepartmental Enquiry on Physical Deterioration and the 1907 Education (Adminstrative Provisions) Act was commissioned because of the very high (40–60%) rejection of army recruits for the Boer War. Its 53 recommendations covered: an anthropometric survey, air pollution, housing and open spaces, diet and adulteration of food, physical exercise, alcoholism, juvenile smoking, sexually transmitted disease, and the medical inspection of school children. This important and far sighted report, most of whose recommendations would still apply today, laid the foundations for the school health service.

1908. The first school clinic opened in Bradford.

1916. Report on Maternity and Child Welfare and 1918 Maternity and Child Welfare Act. This Act provided free ante-natal and post-natal clinics, medical cover for births and child health services for children under 5 and led to the development of child welfare centres.

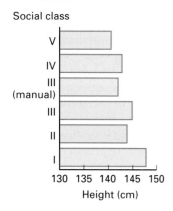

Children aged 11 years, by height and social class

Social class

Height (cm)

THE NATIONAL HEALTH SERVICE

These developments in the 19th and the first part of the 20th century laid the foundations for community paediatrics in the UK. They predate the National Health Service and the widespread development of the specialty of paediatrics practised in a hospital setting. The child health services remained part of the local authority.

1942. The Beveridge Report laid the foundations of the National Health

Service and established a social security system which provided access for everyone to comprehensive health services.

1944. Education Act required the local authority to provide free medical treatment for all school children and for parents to allow medical examination in school. School meals and milk were made available and school clinics were to provide services including treatment of minor ailments, child guidance, orthopaedics, ENT, audiology, speech therapy, orthoptics, remedial exercises and chiropody, and special investigation for rheumatism, asthma and enuresis. The Act also expanded the responsibility of the Local Authority to provide education for children with handicaps and 11 categories were established: delicate, diabetes, educationally subnormal, epileptic, maladjusted, blind, partially sighted, deaf, partially hearing, physically handicapped and speech defective.

1946. National Health Service Act was established to provide 'a comprehensive health service designed to secure improvements in the physical and mental health of the people of England and Wales and the *prevention*, diagnosis and treatment of ill health'. It established a tripartite system of general practitioner, hospital and local authority services with the community child health services in the latter.

1967. Sheldon Report recommended that child health services in the community be provided by general practitioners.

1973. NHS Reorganisation Act brought together the tripartite system into Area Health Authorities, removing the child health services from Local Authority Control.

COURT REPORT

'Fit for the Future', the report of the committee on the Child Health Services chaired by Prof Donald Court, which was published in 1976, included a comprehensive review of all health services for children and made important recommendations for change. Not all these have been implemented, but the report became a powerful catalyst for change, particularly towards an Integrated Child Health Service.

"We want to see a child and family centred service; in which skilled help is readily available and accessible; which is integrated in as much as it sees the child as a whole, and as a continuously developing person. We want to see a service which ensures that this paediatric skill and knowledge are applied in the care of every child whatever his age or disability, and wherever he lives, and we want a service that is increasingly orientated to prevention".

Among the committee's recommendations were:

- A multiprofessional team in each health district for the diagnosis, assessment and treatment of handicapped children – the District Handicap Team.
- At least one Consultant Community Paediatrician per district with special skills in developmental, educational and social paediatrics.
- A general practitioner paediatrician (GPP), with special interest and appropriate accreditation.
- A child health visitor (CHV) who combines preventive and curative responsibility for children.

Only the first two have been implemented so far.

Since the Court Report

The first Consultant Community Paediatricians were appointed in Newcastle and Nottingham shortly after the Court Report. The service has changed from one which was responsible to public health doctors to one of teams led by paediatric consultants. The grading of community health doctors as clinical medical officer (CMO) and senior clinical medical officer (SCMO), has been broadened to include training grades at senior house officer, registrar and senior registrar levels to prepare them for consultant appointments. Many committees have sat and made recomendations on the future of CMOs and SCMOs; it now seems probable that they will be fully integrated within the secondary service for children, the CMOs being staff grade appointments and SCMOs associate specialists.

Many roles have or are changing. The central task of health visitors and school nurses in child health surveillance is recognised. Family doctors are taking on many of the duties of the child health doctor, mainly in pre-school surveillance. The work in community child health is increasingly demanding higher levels of specialist training to provide a referral service for family doctors and a much closer working arrangement with other paediatricians as part of a district service.

At the interface between public health and community paediatrics is the need to establish a district-wide system to ensure that there is information about the health and health needs of the whole population as well as a clinical service for individuals. Community paediatricians need to re-discover, if indeed they have lost them, their roots in public health. Community paediatrics must be a 'health driven' service and the community paediatrician an informed advocate for the services necessary to promote the health and well-being of children.

The interfaces between community paediatrics and education and social services have been of major importance throughout the history of the service. They are being drawn closer together by the consistent emphasis on interdisciplinary working arising in major reports, policy documents and legislation. Important examples are the Court Report, the 1981 Education Act and the 1989 Children Act. Working together at local, District, Regional and national levels has always been the key to successful services.

The importance of prevention, highlighted by the first innovations 200 years ago, is reasserting itself. These goals of community paediatrics have been incorporated in district services as a whole and the separation of hospital and community services is giving way to the concept of a combined child health service.

REFERENCE

Report of the Committee on Child Health Services 1976 Chairman S D M Court, Cmnd 6684, HMSO, London

2 Health Services

Providing health care is a service industry. One way or another those who receive the service pay for it, whilst those who provide it, are paid to provide it. In this chapter the arrangements in the UK will be described.

In 1948 in the UK, the National Health Service (NHS) was introduced. The high principles on which the service is based are: that the service is comprehensive, it is free at point of delivery, there is equality of access and equality of standard of care, there is a commitment to quality and freedom of choice for patients and providers. The British Medical Association, 'the doctor's trades union', have commented on the realities of the present service in the light of these intentions in a statement called 'Leading for Health'.

The NHS enables each doctor, nurse or other health professional to give health care to a child without first establishing who will pay. In effect everyone pays and the Government collects and distributes the money. Initially the money was allocated according to arrangements in place in 1948 and then subsequently in response to bids from the Health Authorities. In 1974, to try and achieve a fairer distribution, an attempt was made to re-allocate the funds according to the size of the population served. Some argued that it would be more equitable to distribute the monies according to need, that is those health regions with poor health indices should get more money, but that was not even attempted. Even the redistribution by population was not fully accomplished before a bigger problem loomed.

The overall development of any service is constrained by the amount of the resources available. Since 1948 there have been dramatic innovations in medical care, many of which are very expensive. Over the same period, no doubt in part due to progress in information dissemination, particularly by television, the expectations of 'customers' has risen. These and other factors have led to the present position: we do not have enough money to have what we would like. The difference between what is desirable and what we can afford is increasing. This is nothing new for poorer countries or countries riven by strife but it is now the position of stable wealthy western countries as well. We are faced with the task of agreeing how the resources should be allocated. In Oregan State in the United States of America, the people were invited to place items of the health provision in a list by priority which has since

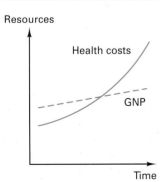

Health costs

Resources

Health costs

GNP

Time

been called the Oregan Trail. Such exercises touch on the deeper question of who should decide the priorities. However, it is clear to all that we can no longer afford expensive unproven treatment programmes.

The response of the UK Government which administers a Health Service which is more economic (cheaper?) than similar services in most wealthy countries in terms of consuming national resources, has been to make every effort to ensure that the service is as efficient and cost effective (good value for money) as is possible and to involve the public and the profession in making choices. In its wish to ensure a 'value for money' service the Government introduced a new Act (Health Service and Community Care Act 1991) which aims to devolve management decisions down to the local services level. It also introduced 'quality management'.

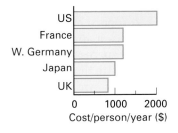

Health cost comparisons

Cost/person/year ($)

HEALTH STRATEGIES: THE HEALTH OF THE NATION

Before discussing the arrangements, we need to consider the strategy. The World Health Organization has set itself targets and has invited nation states to do likewise. The UK Government has produced a consultative document, a Green Paper called the 'Health of the Nation' (1991) which indicates what it has in mind for England and Wales. The targets set in the document specifically concerned with the services for children are weak, but many of the general recommendations would have a beneficial effect on the health of children, for example action to stop smoking. One major theme in the 'Health of the Nation' is 'variations' in health. When discussing these 'variations' it states

> 'Tempering idealism with pragmatism is especially needed in relation to the challenge presented by the variations in good health, illness and death. England like other developed countries, has wide variations between different parts of the country, different ethnic groups and different occupational and income groups...'

and goes on

> 'The reasons for these variations are complex. The Government does not believe there is any panacea – here or elsewhere in the world – either in terms of a full explanation or a single action which will eradicate the problem. But neither difficulty is a reason for inertia.'

It then asserts that progress can be made on three fronts: **first**, through the continued general pursuit of greater economic prosperity and social well-being; **second**, through trying to increase the understanding of the variations, and other action which might effectively address them; and **third**, through specific initiatives to address the health needs of particularly vulnerable groups whether geographical, ethnic, occupational, or others who need specific target help. It believes that the reformed NHS (post 1989 Act) offers significant opportunities for action on the second and third points.

The final 'White Paper' on the 'Health of the Nation' unfortunately did not address the variations in health, but identified specific disorders or services, like screening for cancer, smoking, coronary by-pass surgery, teenage pregnancies, suicides etc. At first glance it appeared that children had been overlooked again; however, to be successful most of the health promotion exercises would have to begin with the infant and child. Although paediatricians may think that is self evident, health service planners and managers need to be reminded from time to time.

AIMS AND NEEDS

The purpose of any population-based Health Industry should be to meet the health needs of the population it serves. Individual hospitals and individual practitioners are going to be more self interested. For that reason the purpose and aims of the enterprise have to be stated and agreed. The professional body of doctors working in the specialty services for children, the British Paediatric Association, have stated what they think the purpose and aims of the Health Service for Children should be, in a document called 'Towards a Combined Child Health Service'.

In individual hospitals and community units around the country, all of whom have been invited to apply for 'Trust status' within the new management arrangements, small interdisciplinary groups have met together and been invited to produce a 'mission' statement. What do we think we do? What is our vision? It is an invitation to dream, but it is uncomfortable for those of us who have to deliver the service in the face of limited resources. Nevertheless we must lift our eyes, so the BPA stated its vision:

'The purpose of the health service for children is to enable as many children as possible to reach adulthood with their potential uncompromised by illness, environmental hazard or unhealthy lifestyle.'

The aims of the service are to:
- provide a high quality health service for all children, (from before birth to adolescence and young adulthood), when and where it is most appropriate,
- support families in the care of their children,
- promote a safe and healthy environment for children.

However, something more specific is required. The Management Executive at Government direction produced a Patient's Charter which applies to the service for children as well as adults. It expects its employees in the Health Service to implement it without indicating how.

The BPA produced a list which they hope will be used as a basis for the aims of Children's Services within individually managed units and trusts. They are:

When they are well, children need a service that:
- enables their parents and families to protect them from disease and environmental hazards and to promote their good health.
- is performed by health professionals who are sensitive to the special needs of children at all ages, from before birth to adolescence and young adulthood.
- provides counselling for parents and for young people appropriate to their understanding, sensitivities, background and culture.
- acts to create a safe healthy environment.

When they are ill or thought to be ill, children need a service that:
- ensures that their parents know when to seek help and how to find it.
- provides 24 hour access in emergencies.
- supports parents in the care of their child.
- is provided by staff who are trained in the care of children of all ages and sensitive to the special needs of children because of their age and differing maturity.
- provides hospital care according to the guide 'Welfare of Children and Young People in Hospital' (DoH 1991).

So in the UK we now have a Health Service with 'high principles', a Government with 'noble intentions', management arrangements which are thought to be 'enabling' and a professional statement with 'great vision'. So if we wish to complain it will have to be with respect to the management, the funding or the work experience!

MANAGEMENT

Management – the task

The word management can be used to mean either **the task** of making the most effective use of resources or **the people** responsible for running an organisation. Management in the first sense is a subject worthy of study like geography, economics or medicine. There is an agreed body of knowledge, decorated by principles, theories and speculations. It has its founders, its teachers and its fashions. In its widest interpretation it can include almost everything involving people (Drucker 1989). When the government invites doctors to become involved in 'management' they are not inviting us to change our discipline. Nevertheless some knowledge of the kind of notions which drive the 'managers' is helpful, it increases empathy and limits irritations and that must be good for the service as well as ourselves.

Lessem (1989) in his book on 'Global management principles' describes four 'domains' of management. To characterise each domain he quotes an authority thus:

The primal domain from *A Passion for Excellence* by Peters and Austin 1985:

> 'We believe that the word management should be discarded and leadership installed in its place. Such leadership involves giving everyone in the organisation space to innovate. Listening to customers and your people, and asking both for their ideas...'

The rational domain from *The Effective Executive* by Drucker 1967:

> 'Whether he works in a business, or in a hospital, in a government or in a labour union, an executive is expected to get right things done...'

The developmental domain from *The Developing Organisation* by Leivegoed 1980:

> 'The management of the future will need to acquire two sorts of knowledge: insight into the development of the human being during the course of life so that he can handle his development in all his plans; and understanding of the development of social structures, and in particular of commercial organisations and of society in general'.

The metaphysical domain from *Real Management* by Agha Hasan Abedi:

> 'We may ask ourselves if wisdom is merely human reason and perception confined within the prison of the human ego, or is wisdom, nature its laws and its principles. We attempt to give precedence to nature.'

That gives a flavour of management as a discipline; if nothing else it illustrates that it is not a simple insensitive set of rules nor is there only one solution. Management is about people, where they work and how they live. Work is our major occupation during our effective years. Having said all this, it would appear from government papers that they have the 'rational domain' in mind with a generous grain of 'primal' market place strategies. The rational domain is about getting things done, the primal domain about inspiring activity. A more mature and sensitive culture which is expressed in the other two domains, where the emphasis moves to mutual awareness and a respect for the world in which we live, is likely to have more lasting benefit.

Some books on management confine themselves to personal management: how to order you own life to succeed in the world of work. Week-end courses where the participants play 'psychological' games with facilitators are as fashionable in the health industry as other organisations. These activities are not relevant to this chapter.

Management – the people   The people called 'the management' have the task of directing, planning, and running the enterprise. They have to formulate policies, define objectives and assess performance. As health professionals provide the service and they know what it is, it is obvious that they have to be involved in the management of the industry. The 1990 Act in the UK aims to involve doctors and other health professionals more in management but so far money has been provided to buy more 'managers' but not to release doctors and others from their duties to assist in management. It is the managers who hold the budgets so it seems that self interest will not encourage change. Enforcement of the stated objectives might lead to changes in management structure. Currently (1993) the managers in the UK are in the main managing Sickness Hotels and not a Health Service Industry.

THE ORGANISATION

The purchasers   The National Health Service has a pyramidal structure, the national Management Executive relates to the Regional Health Authorities which delegate to the District Health Authorities and Family Health Service Authorities which purchase the service.

   The overall objectives of the Health Service Management are stated to be **for patients**, better health care and greater choice of the services available and **for staff**, greater satisfaction and rewards for those working in the NHS who successfully respond to local needs and preferences. To achieve these objectives the Government requires that Regional Health Authorities and District Health Authorities ensure that the health needs of the population for which they are responsible are met. These might be called the contractural objectives and are, (1) that there are effective services for the prevention and control of diseases and the promotion of health, (2) that their population has access to a comprehensive range of high quality, value for money services and that (3) they set targets for and monitor the units for which they continue to have responsibility. These are the **'Purchasers'**; they decide how the money is spent, they draw up the contracts.

The providers   It is a mistake to think that only those who work in the Health Service provide health care. The greater part of care is provided by families, and the health provision is often needed when 'families' are not in place or are unable to provide what is required. So there are four levels of care.

   Self care. We solve for ourselves a large majority of our health problems without seeking professional help. This 'self care' is influenced by friends, relatives, informed busybodies, friendly chemists, and the views of experts and journalists in newspapers and on radio and TV.

The next three layers are within the Health Service.

Primary care. This is, in the main, provided by the primary care team working in Health Centres and homes. Exceptions are the care of the newborn, for the great majority of births are in hospitals, and the treatment of accidents and emergencies in Hospital Casualty departments. General practitioners and the primary care teams provide all children with health care within the context of the family and the home and for 24 hours a day.

This primary service includes:

- attention when a child falls ill.
- referral when a child has a problem requiring specialty care.
- shared care of children with complex problems.
- health surveillance, illness prevention and health promotion – for older children this is normally provided by the school health services.

Secondary care. If specialist services are required then they are initiated by referral from the General Practitioner. The specialist support service in child health has by tradition had two arms, the hospital and the community service. Consultants with hospital and community teams support the primary care service by providing specialty health care for children within the context of the family, home, school and hospital.

This secondary service includes:

- 24 hour hospital service for acute problems (medical, psychiatric and surgical)
- consultative service to family doctors, (medical, psychiatric and surgical)
- service to well and sick newborn infants
- service to disabled, chronically sick, and children at disadvantage
- professional advice and management on health surveillance, illness prevention and health promotion in Health Districts
- health surveillance, illness prevention and health promotion in Health Districts in those areas where these are not performed by the primary care teams. This activity should decrease as primary care teams take on this service
- professional advice and service to other local Authorities.

It is the aim of the Management Executive that the primary care and secondary care service should be integrated more closely so that patient management is more consistent and there is less duplication.

Tertiary care. This is a service which, for both professional and economic reasons, cannot be provided within every health district. Traditionally such services have been developed in teaching hospitals and usually remain on teaching hospital sites. The Government takes advice about those services which have limited distribution across the land, the 'supraregional services'. Until recently each Region also had a responsibility to develop and control regional services but that is no longer the case. Now for these conditions 'money will flow with the patients'. Clearly in paediatrics where specialist tertiary services are essential, but the work load may be small, there is a need to consider what country-wide network is required. If the Government is no longer willing or able to control this service because it no longer directly controls the funding, then the professional bodies will have to publish their views.

INITIATING AN ITEM OF SERVICE

The service is initiated in two ways. The first depends on the parents recognising that their child is ill, and wishing to have advice and being able to obtain it. It follows from this that children in poverty are disadvantaged in four ways, for they are more likely to suffer illness, their needs are less likely to be recognised, their parents are less able to seek help and less help is available. This must be one of the major reasons for 'variations'. The initial contact opens the door to the comprehensive local service. The second is a service to all children. It is more concerned

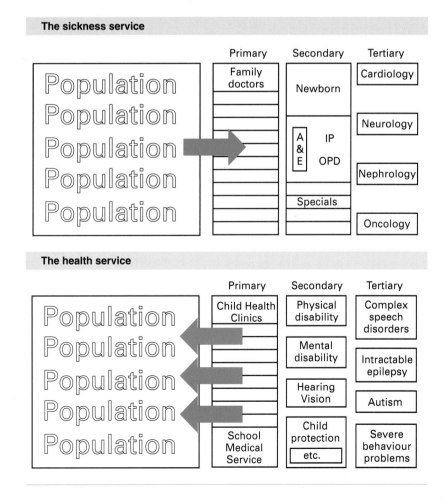

with health promotion and sickness prevention but is does recognise illness and offer treatment. Here the initiative lies with the service and not the family. It is a major social service.

These two services have developed separately from different origins but there is little advantage in keeping them apart and much to be gained by bringing them together into a single combined service that provides a secondary specialist service wherever it is required, in hospital, school, home or clinic.

The advantages of a combined service are that it would:

- make more efficient, cost effective and flexible use of the limited resources
- avoid unnecessary duplication
- centre care around the child in the family and not an institution like a hospital
- enable the support services to work more closely with the primary care team
- ensure better continuity of care between hospital and community
- encourage better communication so that everyone will know what each other is doing
- more fully recognise the wider responsibility to children than contacts initiated by the child and family
- breakdown the artificial division between prevention and treatment. Health promotion will be everybody's business
- protect long term health promotion strategies and encourage them to flourish
- more successfully address the health needs of children at social disadvantage.

Once a service industry has identified what is needed (need), that is, what it aims to supply, it can then plan service (process) and what resources, places, materials and workforce (structure), it needs to provide.

THE STRUCTURE

The BPA document gives an outline of the desired structure for a Health Service for Children. It will have two parts, one based in an Institution or Hospital, the other in a Community. The hospital-based and community-based services are closely related and interdependent.

The HOSPITAL service should be provided within a comprehensive children's department and includes:

- **Accident and Emergency Department** with facilities for children on the same hospital site as the comprehensive children's department.
- **Outpatient facilities,** preferably in a dedicated outpatient department for children, linked to the inpatient facilities and incorporating facilities for child psychiatry.
- **Day case facilities** for children.
- **Inpatient facilities for children**, providing beds for paediatric medical care (including children with infectious disease), child psychiatry, general surgical and orthopaedic care and in many health districts, ophthalmic and ENT surgery. Accommodation for the parent or carer to be resident with the child is essential. The children's wards should accommodate all children requiring hospital care irrespective of medical or surgical specialty. The number of beds provided should be sufficient to meet the fluctuating demands for admissions and for the high throughput which are the characteristics of children's wards. Young infants need a protective environment so cots in cubicles should form *at least* 40% of the total bed number. Adolescents need special accommodation.
- **Intensive care facilities** for children.
- **Neonatal services** including short term intensive care in all District Health Authorities and long term intensive neonatal care in some. The maternity service should be available on the same hospital site as the comprehensive children's department.
- **Rehabilitation department** for children.

The hospital should also provide accommodation so that the Education Authority and the Social Service Department can fulfil their responsibilities to children whilst they are in hospital. A 'Hospital School' and 'Social Service Department' are essential components of a comprehensive children's department within a hospital.

Either on the HOSPITAL site OR in the COMMUNITY there should be:

- **A Child Development Centre** for comprehensive assessment and therapy of children with learning difficulties, physical disability and chronic illness. It will provide clinical facilities and accommodation for members of the District Handicap Team and other professionals with expertise in children's care (physiotherapists, speech therapists, occupational therapists, psychologists). It should also provide a base for a peripatetic service, to encourage the increasing tendency for children to be assessed and receive care within their home or school. The care of children with special needs is a responsibility shared with Education, Social Services and other local Authority Departments as well as voluntary agencies.
- **Respite care facilities** for children with life threatening illness, severe chronic disability and multiple handicap. Provision of respite care is another shared responsibility.

The COMMUNITY services should provide:

- **Clinics** within the community, nurseries and schools.

The community service's accommodation may be located within or outside the hospital. A common base for the combined service which facilitates contact and communication between all the staff in the service has advantages of efficiency and economy, simpler record keeping and data collection, and it will be less confusing for children and their families. Steps should be taken to ensure that the development of effective community services is not compromised by inadequate funding of the acute hospital service.

THE PROCESS

It is a mistake to confuse structure with process, and all too often the process aims to 'use' the structure and not meet the health needs of children and their families. One of the purposes of audit is to try and stop such activities.

Medical care within the HOSPITAL will include:

- General inpatient and outpatient services, day care, emergency care and some specialist medical services.
- Surgical services for children (eg general, orthopaedic, ophthalmic and ENT surgery) and care in the A & E department.
- Services to all healthy newborn infants and sick or premature infants who require special care.
- Child psychiatric care including services for children with learning difficulties.
- Children's intensive care, neonatal intensive care, the specialised tertiary services.

Medical care to the COMMUNITY will include:

- Oversight of the Health District's surveillance, illness prevention and health promotion services.
- A consultation service for children with general as well as developmental problems or behavioural disorders and as a back up to the GP surveillance programme.
- Provision of the surveillance programme for school children.

- An audiology service for children.
- An ophthalmic service for children.
- A service for children with disabilities, including early recognition and intervention, comprehensive assessment, regular review, respite care and advice to Education Authorities and Social Service Departments.
- Advice to schools and statutory service obligations under the provision of the Education Act 1981.
- Input to services for children at social disadvantage.
- Advice to the Child Protection Service.
- Advice to the Adoption and Fostering agencies.
- Counselling service for adolescents.
- Advice to children undertaking employment with particular support for those with difficulties.

These services will address the responsibilities identified by the Disabled Person's Act and Children Act.

The COMBINED CHILD HEALTH SERVICE will need:

- Collection and analysis of information for identification of service need and planning.
- Service development. Establishing manuals of practice, standards, targets and assessment of outcome measures.
- Audit on clinical and resource issues.
- Professional development. Teaching and training programmes.
- Innovation. Development and research programmes.
- Joint planning with other agencies providing services for children.

Nursing

Nursing care for children is as special as the medical care and is provided in all the clinical areas identified above.

Children's nursing service in hospitals. Nurses trained to look after children are required in all inpatient units nursing sick children, medical, psychiatric and surgical. If children are cared for in a joint A&E department, or a single intensive care unit these should have 'children trained' nurses on their staff.

Children's nursing service in community. Nurses skilled in the care of children with complex problems now provide a community service which allows some children with technically demanding care to be nursed at home or at school.

Neonatal nursing services. Nursing sick or preterm newborn infants needs special skills. Such nurses are a precious and limited resource. They too provide a community service which allows some infants to leave the neonatal unit sooner than would otherwise be possible.

Health visiting service for children. Traditionally Health Visitors have overseen the care of all children particularly until the age of five. Health Visitors are central to the Child Health Surveillance programme. They play an important part in the 'primary care child health service'. But they are also integral to a number of the Community Child Health programmes, eg for social disadvantage, child protection, children with special needs. That component of their work also should be in the contract for the child health services. Health visitors' responsibility involves the whole family, including the elderly.

Liaison and specialist Health Visitor Service. Health Visitors with specialist training play a central and expanding role in some specialty services, eg diabetes, physical disability, child protection etc.

The School Nursing Service. School nurses are key health professional staff in schools where they offer continuity, surveillance and counselling.

Support services

Professions allied to medicine. Provision for speech therapy, physiotherapy, occupational therapy, play therapy, clinical psychology services and dietetics for children both in the hospital and community is required.

Medical support services. Pathology, pharmacy, radiology, genetic counselling should all have staff identified and able to provide a service for children.

Management. The Combined Child Health Services will require support staff and facilities in administration, management, personnel, finance, audit, record systems and information services.

Health service to schools

The school health service provided by the 'school doctor' and the 'school nurse' is identified in many of the functions given above. The medical services should be led by consultants who have had appropriate training. The service provided by the nurses and doctors and other health professionals within the combined child health service will for the foreseeable future contain elements of primary care, health promotion and sickness prevention as well as a specialist service for children with learning difficulties, disabilities and complex disorders attending schools. A close working relationship with the primary care services is essential.

AN ITEM OF SERVICE

A service industry provides 'items of service'. In the case of a Health Service it is an interaction between a child and a health professional. For each item of service it is helpful to construct a quality management programme according to the agreed definitions.

Quality Management: Definitions taken from the International Standard Guidelines (ISO 9000 – 9004)

- **quality policy :** the overall quality intentions and direction of the organisation and this should be formally stated by top management
- **quality management :** this will determine and implement quality policy and must have some control or influence on the planning and distribution of resources
- **quality systems :** this is the structure that identifies the service, the standards, and the resources needed to ensure quality
- **quality control :** these are routine activities aimed at monitoring the service and identifying unsatisfactory performance
- **quality assurance :** this is planned systematic action to demonstrate to the management and to the user that the service provided meets the user's requirement.

Audit

Quality assurance includes **audit**, and it is clearly an exacting task because it will involve an estimation of what is needed, of what is possible with resources available and what can be reasonably expected of the staff given their professional skills, and the benefits and risks to the patient and the service. Our efforts at audit are bound to be tentative for many reasons but it is worth attempting. The reasons include:

It is in the children's interests that we should, for the purpose of audit is to raise standards. The risk is that it will merely waste time.

It is in our interests because it will allow us, if it is effective, to use our time and energy more effectively.

It is required albeit in a very limited and not too satisfactory a form by the higher professional training bodies which are concerned with the training of consultant staff and therefore might act as a bar to obtaining accreditation. Accreditation is not a necessary requirement in paediatrics but it is in other disciplines for junior staff who work with children.

It is in itself a valuable educational tool. It allows the introduction of clinical change in a controlled manner. It demonstrates to the established and the learners how to define clinical requirements, how these might be changing, how they might be addressed and which approach is the more effective. The educational value is thought by some to be the main benefit of medical audit.

It should, linked to financial audit, make all the staff concerned and the 'users', in our situation their families, aware of the cost of the service and the commitment of the carers.

Last but not least the government 'invites' us to do it. It may become a required part of any contractural arrangements though there is no guidance on this at the present.

Audit only makes sense against the background of quality management.

STANDARDS AND OUTCOMES

Standards, policy statements, protocols, guidelines, manuals of practice are all words which are being used in an attempt to set up frameworks for quality assurance. There are difficulties with such exercises, for even timely statements produced by the most distinguished panels of experts often fail to recognise the complexity of the item of service and settle for what can be measured, which may be a measure of service (short waiting times) or a crude outcome measure like mortality rates which are influenced as much if not more by many factors which are nothing to do with the Health Provision. It seems probable that there will be much talk in the future about clinical standards, agreed outcome measures and achievable targets.

One aim of this book is to broaden the discussions beyond a narrow review of limited, measurable, hospital activities.

REFERENCES AND FURTHER READING

British Medical Association 1991 BMA agenda for health, leading to health.
    BMA, London
British Paediatric Association 1992 Towards a combined child health service.
    BPA, London
Department of Health 1991 The welfare of children and young people in Hospital.
    HMSO, London
Drucker P S 1989 The new realities in government and politics, in economy and
    business, in society, in world view. Heinemann, Oxford
Lessem R 1989 Global management principles. Prentice Hall, New York
Nottingham Health Service for Children 1991 Report. University Hospital, Nottingham
Secretary of State for Health 1991 The health of the nation. HMSO, London
Smith R (ed) 1991 The BMJ view, health of the nation. BMA, London
Townsend P, Davidson N (eds) 1988 Inequalities in health: The Black Report. Penguin,
    Harmondsworth
Whitehead M 1987 The health divide. Penguin, Harmondsworth

3 Education Services

A number of key pieces of legislation have had a bearing on the education of children in the UK including those with very significant health and educational needs. The overall trend of the last decade has been towards the inclusion of children with even the most complex needs in quality mainstream education and away from more segregated options such as special units or schools. Rights for pupils and their parents have also increased substantially over this period. This has been associated with changes in the language used to describe children and their needs away from categorical labels towards more detailed and sophisticated profiles of strengths and needs.

The changes have reflected new understandings about the rights of individuals with disabilities and changes in thinking about the most appropriate forms of education and provision. They have led to a major shift of responsibilities away from medical services to those in education for decision making and providing appropriate learning and teaching for all children. The importance of integration in a local community, the importance of parental involvement and developmental perspectives have influenced educationalists, but it is clear that the power of governmental policy and preference has been even more potent in shaping the course and pace of events especially since the late 1970s.

STRUCTURE AND FUNCTIONS OF EDUCATION SERVICES

The complex nature of Education Services in Britain in the 1990s is clearly illustrated by the fact that in the majority of English counties and Metropolitan Districts the Local Education Authority (LEA) is the largest single employer. The variety of personnel needed to carry out the duties of a LEA and the total costs of such a workforce ensure that Education Departments spend the lion's share of local authority resources – the monies raised by local taxation – as well as requiring significant funding from central government via the Department for Education (DFE). This latter source of funding is increasingly allocated in grant form with clear guidelines being given by the DFE on how it should be spent.

Significant legislation and events

This list provides a brief outline of key points of educational legislation that have had a major impact on what has happened to individual children, where and how they have been schooled, and even how they have been described.

Before 1970

1886 Act separated idiots and imbeciles from lunatics

1896 Poor Law School Committee Report notes the accumulation of 'defective and afflicted' children in schools and calls for special schools

1899 Elementary Education (Defective and Epileptic Children) Act. Local authorities urged, but not required, to make special instruction available

1907 School Medical Service set up

1913 Mental Deficiency Act. Education Authorities given duty to ascertain which children aged 7–16 were 'defective'

1921 Education Act. This enabled Education Authorities to compel parents of 'certified' children to send them to special schools

1944 Education Act. Local education authorities had a duty to provide Special Education Treatment in special schools or elsewhere for children ascertained to have 'a disability of body or mind'. The LEA now had a duty to provide free schooling from 5–15 in separate primary and secondary schools. Parents had the duty of ensuring that children of compulsory school age 'receive education suited to their age, ability and aptitude, either by regular attendance at school or otherwise'. LEAs had the duty of enforcing this.

1970s

1970 The Education (Handicapped Children) Act, brought 'severely subnormal' children into education, no longer were they considered ineducable or unsuitable for school attendance.

1974 Local Government Reorganisation. School Health services, including speech therapists, school doctors and nurses become part of the National Health Service and thus no longer the responsibility of Education Committees.

1976 Education Act, suggested duty for LEAs to provide special education in normal schools where practicable, but this section was never implemented.

1978 Warnock Committee Report. Recommended abolishing statutory categories of handicap in favour of assessments of 'special educational needs'. Children were no longer to be considered ESN but rather as having 'learning difficulties'.

1979 180 000 children in state special schools, 15 774 in non-state special education.

1980s

1980 Education Act. Parents were given the right to express preference for the school they wished their child to attend and new rights to appeal. The LEA must comply unless this prejudices efficient use of resources or efficient education. This did not include special or nursery schools.

1981 Education Act. A child has 'special educational needs' if he has a learning difficulty which calls for 'special educational provision'. When the LEA needs to formally determine this provision a formal assessment leading to a 'Statement of Special Needs' is to be carried out. Children with special educational needs are to be educated in ordinary schools, provided that account has been taken of parental views and that education in such a school is compatible with the:

1) child receiving appropriate special provision

2) the provision of efficient education for children with whom he is to be educated and

3) the efficient use of resources

1986 Disabled Persons Act. New procedures for the assessment of needs and the involvement and consultation with people with disabilities before Social Services provision is made. LEAs must formally tell Social Services whether a young person is disabled the year after their 14th birthday and let them know when they will leave school.

1987 Corporal punishment banned in all state-supported education.

1988 The Education Reform Act introduced a National Curriculum for all pupils with associated assessment and testing. The Secretary of State now prescribes attainment targets, courses of study and assessment arrangements in 10 subjects (Maths, English and Science being core) for all pupils of compulsory school age. This Act also allows schools to opt out of local authority control and for the majority to become financially managed by themselves (Local Management of Schools). By early 1992, 265 secondary schools had voted to opt out of LEA control and become grant maintained.

1989 The Children Act. A sweeping reform of child care law strikes a new balance between family autonomy and child protection. Parent duties are now 'parental responsibilities' and Education and Social Services must work more closely for children in need. Education Supervision Orders have been introduced if children are not receiving suitable full time education.

1990s

1990 The 1989 Children Act is made law.

1991 Increased segregation in special schools in 15 LEAs but significant decrease in segregation in 44 LEAs since 1982. 15 of the latter reduced placement in special schools by more than 25%.

1992 Dramatic variations across the country in the percentage of children placed in special schools. For example a child in Knowsley is four and a half times more likely to go to a special school than a child in Cornwall at this time. Funding is increasingly allocated in grant form with clear guidelines being given by the DES as to how it should be spent.

Title of Support Service	Principal functions and typical role
Advisory and Inspection Service	Monitoring, reviewing, and evaluating standards and effectiveness of schools and teachers. Appointments of senior staff within schools. Contributing to staff development and appraisal. Researching and reporting on practice in school to the Education Committee. Each school within an LEA is likely to have a named Inspector or Advisor.
Careers Service	Providing advice to pupils at the end of their school careers on further education, employment or training. Making links between the Education Service and Industry.
Curriculum Support Service (a wide range of initiatives are likely to be encountered under this heading)	Some typical areas of curriculum support are likely to be: **Library Services** • Providing books and other media materials on loan to schools • Providing advice on setting up of school's own library **Arts in Education** • Specialist equipment and advice to schools in Music, Art, Dance and Drama **Professional Development and In-Service Training Support** • Responding to schools training requests providing resources for staff development
Catering Services (now competitively tendered)	Providing school meals; maintenance of local nutritional standards
Education Welfare Service	Improving school attendance; monitoring part-time employment of pupils; advice to parents on free school meals, clothing vouchers. Each family of schools is likely to have a named Education Welfare Officer (EWO)
Educational Psychology Service	Advising schools, parents and LEA on children's learning and development needs especially where there are difficulties in learning or behaviour. Statutory assessment of children under the 1981 Act. Each school within an LEA is likely to have a named Educational Psychologist and the service is typically provided to children 0–19 years
Section II Support Services	Helps schools meet the additional needs of ethnic minority pupils and students through English language teaching and community and curriculum development work
Special Educational Needs Teaching	A range of teacher titles and roles will be found within this service. Specialist teachers of the Hearing Impaired and the Visually Impaired will be employed by most LEAs as will teachers employed to work with very young children with severe learning difficulties and their families. Portage Home Visiting Services will often be part of support offered as well as teachers employed to work in mainstream schools with individual pupils with learning or behavioural difficulties. This service will typically be involved with children 0–19 and its staff will work peripatetically.

Organisation structure

It is helpful to look at a LEA as delivering its service at two levels — a central administrative level and a local school and college level. As well as helping make sense of the structure and function of the Education Service this split between central and local levels is also enshrined in recent leglislation (Education Reform Act 1988) which limits the amount of revenue that LEAs can retain centrally to pay for administration costs and for services to schools and the amount that must be delegated directly to individual Schools and Colleges where spending decisions are the responsibility of the Governing Body. Before looking in more detail at these two levels of LEA structure and service, it is worth saying something about how the service provided by Education Departments varies with the age of the child. Most of an Education Department's expenditure will be directed at children of statutory school age, ie between 5 and 16 years. Pupils attend years 1 to 6 in their primary school and years 7 to 11 in their secondary school. Many LEAs provide education for a percentage of preschool children (aged between 3 and 5 years) within nursery schools or classes but this is not a statutory requirement and there are therefore large variations nationally in the amount of nursery provision funded by LEAs. Beyond the age of 16 (Tertiary phase of Education) many LEAs make provision via Sixth forms, Sixth Form Colleges and Further Education Colleges.

Central administration

Its role and functions. The Central Administration of a LEA is responsible for the planning and delivery of policy (both local and national) and for the allocation of resources to schools. The administrative personnel will be led by a Director of Education or Chief Education Officer supported by a team of administrative and professional officers. The administration is responsible to an Education Committee of locally elected councillors and it is at this political level that decisions are made and spending priorities decided.

The administration of a LEA is typically to be found within a Local Authority's management headquarters or County Hall. Geographically large Authorities are likely to also maintain a number of local delivery points or Area Education Offices whose 'areas' will often correspond to District Council boundaries. Such Area Education Offices will contain a range of administrative and professional staff and will be responsible for day to day support of schools in the Area on matters such as school budgets, staff appointments, pupil exclusions and so forth.

LEA at the school level

Its role and functions. Individual schools within a local education authority admit pupils from a defined neighbourhood or catchment area and children living within a school's catchment are entitled to receive their education at that school. (Education Law does not dictate that children must attend a school to receive their education, simply that they must receive an education. Some parents elect to provide this themselves for their children at home. This arrangement is often known as 'Education otherwise'.) Secondary schools typically serve a larger catchment area than primary schools and receive pupils from a number of different primaries or 'feeder' schools. A secondary school and its feeder primaries are sometimes known as a 'family of schools' and may meet together to share and agree policy and practice.

School management. The Headteacher is responsible for the day to day decision making within a school and he or she is responsible in turn to the Governing Body of the School. The Governing Body is made up of locally elected politicians, parents, representatives from the school's teaching staff and non teaching staff (eg midday supervisory assistant or school secretary) local business people and others. The responsibilities and powers of school governors have significantly increased in the last five years in line with Central Government's philosophy of progressively devolving power from LEA level to the level of the individual school. Thus major budgetary decision making, appointment of teaching staff and individual school policy and practice are now all issues which are within the Governors' decision-making powers.

Staff structure

Teaching staff. Within a primary school the organisation of the teaching staff is generally clear to an outsider. The Headteacher and the Deputy Headteacher form the senior management of the school, and have responsibilities beyond their actual teaching role. Individual teachers are typically responsible for the delivery of the curriculum to a class of children and the majority of their time is spent in contact with that class teaching across the full range of subjects covered within the National Curriculum.

Within a secondary school staff organisation is much more complex and staff will typically undertake an *academic* role via their teaching in a particular subject area and a *pastoral* role via their regular contact with their 'tutor set' or 'form group'. The pastoral work of teachers involves a responsibility for the general welfare and social development of pupils and includes issues such as attendance, friendships, bullying, health and related areas.

Non Teaching Staff: Apart from teachers a range of other adults will be found working within a school

Teaching Assistants	Sometimes known as welfare assistants, nursery nurses or support assistants. Many primary schools will employ one or more teaching assistants who will have training in child development and welfare (often the NNEB certificate) and work alongside teachers in the classroom
Midday Supervisory Assistants	Responsible for lunchtime arrangements and the welfare of pupils during the lunch break
Kitchen Staff	Responsible for the preparation and serving of lunches
Secretarial Staff	Responsible for the management of the school office, pupil records, etc.
Librarian	Many secondary schools will have a librarian or staff responsible for the upkeep of stock and often for audio-visual services to teachers and pupils
Cleaning/Caretaker Staff	Have a range of duties concerned with the maintenance of the building as a working environment

Perspectives

The medical and the educational perspective on children with disabilities are different. Understanding the differences in the types of questions asked about disability and the kind of interventions made is of more than philosophical interest: it is crucial to any effective partnership between school health personnel and staff in the teaching profession. It has only been within the last fifteen years that the educational perspective on disability has been clearly articulated. Previous to this teachers responsible for the education of disabled children borrowed heavily from the medical model of disability to make sense of their practice. Thus children diagnosed as 'educationally subnormal' (ESN) were seen as requiring 'special educational treatment' by specialised 'remedial' staff. Such terms are now rarely if ever used within educational thinking in the nineties and an understanding of the educational model that has replaced them is needed by the health service personnel working with schools. One useful way of clarifying the differences between the medical and educational approaches to disability is to consider the typical questions asked from within each perspective.

Questions asked about disabled children from a medical perspective

Diagnostic questions:	How are the typical features of the disability best described? What are the common features across individual cases? How do these features interrelate? How does the overall picture differ from that seen in other conditions and disabilities?
Epidemiological questions:	Who is affected by this disability? What is its prevalence? Is this increasing or decreasing?
Aetiological questions:	What is the cause of this condition? What is the influence of pre-, peri- and postnatal factors? What weight should we give environmental vs genetic factors?
Prognostic questions:	What is the likely course of this condition? What are the likely outcomes? Can normal functioning be restored?
Therapeutic questions:	What treatment or combination of treatments is likely to be most effective in restoring normal functioning or limiting further deterioration? Where is this treatment available?

In clear contrast, to understand a disability from an educational perspective leads us to ask a quite different set of questions about the individual child.

Questions asked about disabled children from an educational perspective

Profiling questions:	What are this child's strengths and weaknesses? What observations and in what settings will the teachers need to make to ensure a full profile is achieved?
Questions about learning history and style of learning:	In what situations does the child appear to learn most effectively? How have the skills the child already has been learned?
Questions about a child's overall needs:	What development has taken place in the child's self help skills, personal and social development? Emotional and behavioural needs and independence are of interest along with academic and language skills.
Questions about curricular priorities:	What aspects of this child's present approach to learning are acting as barriers to future learning? What types of learning experiences are priorities for this child?
Questions about curricular access:	What teaching conditions/resources/styles will need to be provided in order to maximise this child's access to the National Curriculum? What must the teacher plan to ensure that the curriculum offered has breadth, balance and provides learning experiences which are age appropriate and relevant to this child's particular situation?
Questions about future learning:	What are the next steps in development? What teaching plans can be made? What learning targets can be set?

The primary concerns of a teacher are to look at the individual child and his or her unique educational needs. Those needs will be seen as essentially *relative* and only capable of being understood in the context of the learning situation the child is in. This situation crucially includes such factors as the skills, attitudes and resources of the individual teacher as well as the overall organisation and ethos of that school itself. Thus what may be viewed as a special need or difficulty in one teaching situation may not be apparent or be much less apparent in another differently organised situation. It is for these reasons that such questions as: 'What is this child's handicap?' 'What is his IQ?', 'What are the correct treatments for his condition'? do not figure amongst the prime concerns of an educational venture. *Schools are not treatment centres* (if they were they would be organised quite differently). They are social institutions responsible for delivering a curriculum, a range of learning experiences, to their pupils regardless of their disability.

Because of these fundamental differences in the questions asked by each approach to disability and the differences in the overall aims there are as a result important differences in the way a child with a disability is viewed from each perspective.

Medical perspective	Educational perspective
Child is described in terms of his/her deficits and divergence from the norm. These deficits exist exclusively within the pupil	Child is described by unique Individual Profile of strengths and weaknesses. Needs and difficulties seen as *relative* to variety of environmental factors. Difficulties arise as a result of interaction between pupil and environment
Child is categorised by diagnostic label	Child is categorised by curricular needs and support required to meet those needs
School placement by categorical label	School placement determined by availability of resources needed for curricular access
Exceptionality defined by comparison with the norm	Individual assessment identifies teaching priorities
Specialist staff and specialised resources characterise remediative approaches	All teachers have a role and contribute to curriculum delivery
Curriculum for disabled pupils is specialised and different from regular curriculum	Curriculum is same for all but modified in level, rate and methods of delivery for disabled pupils (ie the curriculum is 'differentiated')
The exceptional needs of disabled pupils are highlighted	Needs in common of all pupils emphasised

It is clear from this table of differences in emphasis that the outcomes for disabled pupils in terms of type of provision likely to be made are also likely to differ. Broadly speaking a medical perspective will tend to highlight a need for segregated or special education and an educational perspective will tend to give rise to education being provided in an integrated setting.

Despite these differences in aims and outcomes, an understanding of the medical perspective on an individual pupil is important to the work of teachers. A knowledge of the child from this perspective is likely to provide helpful pointers as to those areas of curricular planning likely to need particular attention to ensure access to learning experiences for that pupil. This will be most obviously true for pupils with visual and auditory impairments where a medical profile of deficit will be essential to enable appropriate teaching arrangements. It will also be true for pupils with less objectively definable disabilities such as 'autism' – for a teacher to know that a child is viewed as 'autistic' from a medical perspective is very likely to mean that those aspects of the curriculum concerned with interaction and relationships will figure highly in the child's overall timetable. However knowing the diagnostic label that has been assigned to a child does not change the fundamental nature of the teacher's task which is to ensure maximum access to the curriculum. This is the teacher's task *whatever their pupils' difficulties* and it is essentially an individualised exercise that will need to be gone through for each child in turn. It will be based on a detailed understanding of that child's particular strengths and weaknesses in learning. From an educational perspective there is no 'one size fits all' treatment for any child's difficulties. However the aims of education are the same for all.

> '...to enlarge a child's knowledge, experience and imaginative understanding and thus his awareness of moral values and capability for enjoyment ...'

> 'to enable him to enter the world after formal education is over as an active participant in society and a responsible contributor to it capable of achieving as much independence as possible'
>
> Report of the Warnock Committee. DES 1978

Schools do make a difference

Educators have become increasingly convinced that the characteristics of schools are important determinants of academic achievement (Edmonds 1982).

Since the mid-1970s the impact of schools on children's learning and behaviour has become increasingly accepted following a number of substantial studies in Britain and elsewhere (Rutter et al 1979, Phi Delta Kappa 1980). It is now well accepted that children from similar home backgrounds can perform quite differently depending upon which school they attend, even if they share characteristics usually associated with lower academic and behavioural performance.

Successful schools share a number of features including:

- effective leadership
- positive atmosphere and ethos
- work oriented lessons that are understandable and clearly focused on the teaching and learning of the curriculum
- teachers working and planning together
- formal reward systems and public celebration of success
- pupils expected to share responsibility for day to day matters
- high teacher expectations of pupils
- closely monitored pupil progress
- parental involvement in the school, classroom and their children's learning

This research has given impetus to the effective schools movement and school improvement initiatives internationally. There has also been increased interest in managing schools for excellence particularly in the context of newly prevailing ideas about market forces and account-abilities (Beare et al 1989). School managers seek both to effectively lead and manage their schools in the 1990s including their budgets, admissions on the one hand and professional development of staff and the implementation of a National Curriculum on the other.

Raised expectations

This has coincided with progressive approaches to educational and intellectual assessment of children which have now soundly rejected notions of children having a 'fixed potential' or an unchanging intelligence quotient (IQ). The old faith in accurate figures to succinctly summarise a child's future academic potential has been superseded with a fresher, more optimistic approach to children's learning, viewing it as flexible and developmental. Evidence suggesting that IQ scores would be increased by sitting children on radiator pipes before an assessment on a cold day, or that by feeding teachers with false scores, attainments could be dramatically altered in either direction have added weight to this rejection. Increasingly the relativity of attainment and performance in the context of different individuals operating in varying learning situations has been acknowledged.

This removal of a fixed ceiling of expectation on pupils' progress has largely been welcomed and has led to approaches to assessment which are more descriptive, formative, criterion or curriculum referenced. Such assessment describes what a child can and cannot do, as compared with a set of expectations or criterion, and their design allows planning for future teaching and learning. Such assessments provide much more information on which to form planning and are less likely to lead to a feeling of 'So what?' which was often the response to the results of IQ tests. These are more likely to inform educational planning and teaching programme construction by suggesting next developmental steps or targets.

Progressive approaches to the leadership and management of effective schools as well as to the assessment of individual needs reflect fresh ideas about the essentially interactive nature of the thinking, action and relationships of children and adults. Development issues and problems are not seen as existing purely within the individual but instead are increasingly perceived by educationalists as existing in an active social context in which transactions are constantly occurring.

All of the above nestle into the debates surrounding nature versus nurture theories, putting tremendous weight behind the optimism of the latter position. That children's capabilities are so flexible and developmental and so influenced by the emotional and meaningful nature of their learning context seems to leave little doubt that many of our traditional ideas about children's capacities were highly blinkered and limiting. This appears as true for the education of those with the most severe and complex learning difficulties as it is for those with more exceptional gifts of learning.

Future trends in education

In the 1990s schools in Britain and elsewhere face imposed change of an unprecedented nature. In the context of the 1988 Education Reform Act, the Department of Education and Science in Britain recognised that in schools there are:

- uncertainties about the precise nature of the changes they are required to implement;
- anxieties about their ability to cope within the timescales set for implementation (DES School Management Task Force 1990).

In Britain up until the 1970s a mixed economy was favoured with a highly valued set of public services working alongside a free enterprise business and manufacturing world. Education like health care, transport and energy, was characteristic of the public services. These services had a well researched and established tradition and were supported by a set of beliefs in what was being done. There was an acceptance of the public service ethos in Britain and it was known to have its own ethic and to be well motivated by a sense of goodwill amongst its participants. Rights of individual citizens, children and adults, to such public services went unquestioned.

The arrival of a radical Conservative government in Britain and a similarly right wing government in the United States was to set the scene for much stronger moves towards a free enterprise culture where market forces could be brought to bear on public as well as private services. The idea began to be promoted and eventually to take hold that it was inefficient and unfashionable to fund public sector work or industry. The government's fiscal policies reflected the notion that there was no need to give public services and industry money just for the sake of it or because it always had been. The 1980s saw threats to many areas of public funding including health, social and educational services and moves towards focused financing and the encouragement of 'opting out' of state control. Some areas of the public sector were deliberately abandoned or starved whereas a number of private sector developments were actively rewarded. British education, a time-honoured area of substantial expenditure, was one of the most important and early targets of this change of approach. Politicians levelled serious criticism at the door of educationalists with particular reference to standards of teaching and education, lack of choice for parents, the dependency of schools on centralised local authorities, and a number of others. Legislation and focused financing were to be the tools to bring about change in schools and the advent of free market forces in the world of education.

A list of some of the key changes being addressed in schools

- implementation of a national curriculum
- assessment and testing for all pupils at ages 7, 11 and 14
- local financial management of schools
- delegated budgets to schools
- new examination syllabus and exams
- teachers' pay and conditions of service
- appraisal schemes
- records of achievement
- technical, vocational and educational initiatives
- integration of pupils with special needs
- reduction in support role of local authority
- increased parental choice of school and involvement in school government

At the same time central government has made it easier for parents to access private education and has attempted the development of new privately run and generously joint financed city technology colleges. It has also made it possible and financially rewarding for schools to opt out of local authority control and achieve grant maintained status.

Society has changed ideologically, technologically and demographically but education has not always reflected the diversity of these changes. There have been significant cultural changes to many schools' catchment areas. Individual child and family needs have changed enormously in the last twenty years with many more families breaking up. With one in three marriages ending in divorce the traditional family unit is no longer a predictable element of community life. Schools have increasingly found themselves with a much broader role within the community offering a sense of wider family and parenthood to many children and their families. These developments are reflected to some extent in curriculum developments in areas such as personal and social education. Increasingly the community is looking to local schools to meet all the needs of its children whatever their culture, creed, need or disability.

Despite the rhetoric about parental empowerment and involvement the overall picture in education is quite mixed. There have been some excellent examples of effective empowerment of parents whose children have learning difficulties or behavioural concerns, in initiatives that have involved home visiting, such as the Portage Schemes, or parent groups (McConkey 1986). Parents have been written into legislation and are involved formally in statutory assessments following the 1981 Education Act, and as governors and recipients of test and assessment data in the light of the Education Reform Act. Many primary schools and nurseries have developed parental involvement in reading (see PACT schemes for example) or in maths (IMPACT Maths scheme for example) and many discussions and conferences now involve parents as of right when discussions about their child are occurring. School records are now open to parents in most areas of the country and much has been done to overcome anxieties about professional confidentiality.

School managers have been encouraged to work in increasingly open and facilitating ways, with a collegiate style rather than traditional line management becoming the preferred approach. Managers in schools have had to take on more responsibilities, particularly financial, with the thrust of legislation encouraging maximum decentralisation of schools. Accountability has increased rather than reduced with this development, particularly towards parents and school governors who are getting increased information on school related performances and power in relation to school management.

The local education authority has and looks set to continue to lose its primary importance in leading and managing schools financially and philosophically. The school as in other countries has become the key unit. Just as hospitals have been granted trust status, schools have been given LMS status to financially manage their own affairs, or have opted out of LEA control completely. The school governors have become the key power brokers and parents have been included among their ranks via the legislation. The local authority is however being pressed by the government to operate much more corporately and this is enshrined in legislation such as The Children Act which requires the Education Department to work much more closely with Social Services.

Community based developments and initiatives which emphasise a child's right to local education whatever their needs, parallel community care initiatives that have followed the Griffiths report, by other agencies. This is epitomised by the inclusion of some children with severe learning or physical difficulties in various mainstream schools throughout the country. This can be seen as a clear indicator of the desire among many parents and educationalists to move away from segregated education. However in at least 15 LEAs the use of segregated provision has actually increased since the 1981 legislation, mentioned earlier. Still, with gradually more pupils with special needs attending ordinary schools – encouraged by the integration aims of the 1981 Act – and with special schools extending their curricular range, the principle has gained ground that all pupils:

'share the same statutory right to a broad, balanced and differentiated curriculum relevant to their needs' (National Curriculum Council 1989)

Pressure for equal opportunities has encouraged the wider acceptance of this principle and the 1988 Education Reform Act provides it with statutory recognition. A right to a share in the curriculum does not of course ensure access to it or progression within it. Some pupils will have sensory or physical difficulties which make access a challenge, while others have emotional or other kinds of learning difficulty.

Some will meet attitudes and practices in schools which do not actively encourage full participation. Achieving maximum access and subsequent progress for pupils with special educational needs will challenge the co-operation, understanding and planning skills of teachers, support agencies, parents, governors and many others (National Curriculum Council 1989).

Educational changes in the 1990s have been characterised by:

- decline in public service ethos
- increased financial independence and self management for many schools and some 'opting out' of local authority control
- the introduction of a national curriculum and related legislation
- broader roles for schools in the community and in partnership with parents
- new approaches to the leadership and management of schools
- increased inclusion and non segregation of children with severe and complex special needs in mainstream education in many parts of the country

---

What of the future?

It is likely that the 21st century will see many new developments which if we could look into a crystal ball may well include the following:

- broader role for schools, the buildings being used in many different ways during the day, at nights and weekends

- adults involved more in school based education for themselves as new forms of national educational and vocational qualification become available
- more use of information technology leading to more education being carried out at home and non school community alternatives interfacing with centralised mainframe information databases and terminals
- increased civil rights for children with severe and complex needs to local education by right
- appraisal and accountability for results becoming key forces in schools with close links to performance or competency related pay and accreditation
- increased level of involvement of parents in their own children's learning and teaching, in partnership with schools
- more educational opportunities for young people aged 16–21 and older
- increased cooperation between schools paradoxically within an increasingly competitive environment
- more opportunities for pupils to monitor and record their own achievements and to exercise more control over their own learning.

Finally, in relation to health and education services, we recognise the necessity for much closer systems of dialogue and more localised planning through the combined effect of shrinking public services and the Children Act, but perhaps more fundamentally we want to put children first.

REFERENCES AND FURTHER READING

Beare H, Caldwell B, Millikan R 1989 Creating an excellent school: Some new management techniques. Routledge, London
DES 1978 Enquiry into the education of handicapped children and young people, Warnock Report. HMSO, London
DES 1981 The 1981 Education Act. HMSO, London
DES 1987 Primary schools: Some aspects of good practice. HMSO, London
DES 1988 Education Reform Act. HMSO, London
DES and Welsh Office 1988 National Curriculum Task Group on Assessment and Testing. HMSO, London
DES School Management Task Force 1990 Developing school management, the way forward. HMSO, London
Edmonds R R 1982 Programs for school improvement: an overview. Educational Leadership, December
Frederickson N 1988 Continuing professional education: towards a framework for development. Management and the psychology of schooling. The Falmer Press, Lewes
National Curriculum Council 1989 A curriculum for all. National Curriculum Council, London
Phi Delta Kappa 1980 Why do some urban schools succeed? The Phi Delta Kappa Study of Exceptional Urban Elementary Schools. Phi Delta Kappa Press, Bloomington, Indiana
McConkey R 1986 Working with parents, for teachers and therapists. Croom Helm, London
Rutter M, Maughan B, Mortimore P, Ousten J 1979 Fifteen thousand hours: secondary schools and their effects on children. Open Books, London

4 Health Promotion and Health Education

Health promotion is an important component of Community Paediatrics alongside screening and management. To some degree it is included in every chapter of this book, but is particularly highlighted in Child Health Surveillance, Accidents, Eating Well, Children with Learning Difficulties and Young Adults. Every consultation provides opportunities for health promotion and every programme for health care should have health promotion as one of its components. Community Paediatrics must concentrate not only on the consequences of poor health, but also on the causes in terms of diet, exercise, risk taking and exposure and lifestyle.

Health of the Nation

The UK Government's aim, as expressed in the 'Health of the Nation' report is to develop a health strategy which focuses upon the prevention of ill health and the promotion of good health as much as upon the treatment and care of those who are already ill. This strategy has always been a central pillar of paediatric practice particularly within child health and school health services. Key areas, objectives and targets are identified for important health problems, which are avoidable and which are also measurable. In the consultations in the 'Green Paper', the health of pregnant women, infants and children was identified as a key area with targets for reduction in stillbirths and infant deaths; an increase in breastfeeding; and a reduction in dental caries. In the final 'White Paper' report, the key areas are coronary heart disease and stroke, mental illness, HIV/AIDS and sexual health and accident prevention.

Getting messages over

Spoken. Patients forget 50 per cent of what they are told in consultations, despite our best intentions. They will forget more if they are anxious or worried, two fairly frequent occurrences. The more people are told in terms of numbers of statements, the less they are likely to remember. Unlike our students, they will probably not take notes and we may not give them a handout (or write in the parent held record)! Parents and children start with very different levels of knowledge of general English and medical terms. We therefore need to develop habits of defining terms and checking that the information that we have given has been understood. Parents and children are often not sufficiently assertive in a medical consultation and many will leave with an incomplete understanding of what has been said rather than ask further questions or admit to their failure to understand the 'explanations' given. It is good practice to repeat information, to write down important points (legibly), and to obtain feedback from the patient on their understanding. Listening is as important as talking. A video of one of our own consultations can be an educational and sometimes a disturbing experience.

Written. The written word can be very useful in supplementing the information given in a consultation. However, a well stocked wall of pamphlets is not a substitute for face to face discussion. It is a challenge to all of us to actually read all our supply of patient information leaflets and decide just how useful they are and how consistent with our own advice. A cynic might look to see how many leaflets are found in the clinic waste baskets at the end of the day and how many chewed remnants are to be found on the clinic floor, having been used as entertainment for young children. Posters may be used as a form of interior decoration to cover the cracks in the walls or they may be used more effectively as part of a planned, professionally directed programme aimed at a particular problem. Readability is important and materials which demand advanced reading skills will be of very limited benefit.

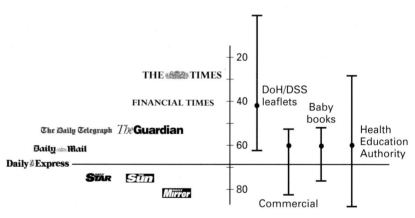

Behaviour change

Imparting knowledge is not the same as bringing about change in health related behaviour; it is only the first step in this process and for many this will not be enough. Information must be given with an understanding of the recipient's ideas and home situation. Emotional issues may block action as may approaches based upon arousal of fear. Information needs to be discussed openly and translated into small practical steps which can be measured and supported. For example, advice such as 'take more exercise' or 'you must lose weight' could be modified as 'try walking to school rather than take the bus' or 'see if you can stick to one sweet a day'. These behaviours can be recorded and the children seen and supported over a period of time. Consistent, sympathetic and repeated health promotion messages are far more likely to succeed than one off lectures. Success and appropriate behaviour change can be rewarded. Work with groups with similar needs is not only an efficient use of resources, but also provides much needed peer group support.

INFORMATION ON HEALTH RELATED BEHAVIOUR OF PARENTS AND CHILDREN IN THE UK

This information is to underline the importance of health promotion. Greater detail will be found in the chapters of this book on young adults, children with learning diculties, nutrition and surveillance as well as in the references at the end of this introduction.

Up to 25 per cent of children in inner city areas are iron deficient at the age of 12 – 15 months.

Three-quarters of all children took more than 35 per cent of their energy as fat and some children consumed 50 per cent as fat (Wenlock et al 1986).

In Northern Ireland, 20 per cent of school leavers of both sexes smoked cigarettes and drank alcohol regularly (Riddock et al 1991). The authors also showed a decline in physical activity in the late teens with 17 and 18 year olds being 50 per cent less active than 11 to 14 year olds.

One-quarter of all smokers will die prematurely through smoking related diseases.

Very low levels of physical activity were demonstrated in British school children age 11–16 (Armstrong et al 1990). 84/163 girls and 37/103 boys showed no periods of sustained exercise causing a tachycardia for more than 10 minutes over a weekday and this figure rose to 112/163 and 65/103 at the weekend.

After the age of one year, accidents are the commonest cause of death in children, 40 per cent from road traffic accidents. In an average District of 250 000 population in any one year, there will be 7 deaths, 500 admissions with 15 suffering permanent disability and 10 000 attendances in accident and emergency departments for 50 000 children (Royal College of Physicians Report on Preventive Medicine 1991).

Studies of drug and solvent misuse amongst secondary school children suggest misuse levels of about 16 per cent, of which 5 per cent represent 'hard' drugs (hallucinogens).

In 1983, 134 people died as a result of sniffing — more young people now die from solvent abuse than from 'hard' drugs.

In the mid 1960s, 2 per cent of girls and 6 per cent of boys reported that they had experienced sexual intercourse before the age of 16; whereas in a recent study the figures had risen to 35 per cent of girls and 46 per cent of boys.

The number of teenage pregnancies continues to rise. In 1990 there were over 120 000 such conceptions in England and Wales, approximately 9 000 to under 16 year olds. One-third of these ended in legal abortion.

SUPPORT FOR HEALTH PROMOTION

At national level, the Health Education Authority is the central agency which is responsible for an overview of the nation's health education programmes and produces many of the materials that are used. Other national voluntary organisations such as the Child Accident Prevention Trust have an important influence in their area of interest. In District Health Authorities, the District Health Education Unit staffed by District Health Education Officers and Senior Health Education Officers will be able to provide advice and materials to health professionals, to schools, playgroups and other organisations. In addition, the Local Authority will also be providing services to support accident prevention, in particular road safety.

SCHOOL HEALTH EDUCATION

Many mature adults will have some hazy memories of the hygiene classes they had in school. For many of us, if we had anything at all at school, it was of the 'nits, feet and the dirty bits inbetween' variety. During the 1970s there was a surge of interest in school health education. The Health Education Council and the Schools Council combined in a large scale project to develop material for children aged 5–13. This was published in 1977 in two packs – 'All About Me' for younger pupils and 'Think Well' for 9–13 year olds (SCHEP 1977). These were comprehensive programmes, employing the model of a spiral curriculum approach, so that health topics and themes were introduced, then returned to and developed at different stages as the child grew and matured. The packs were written for pupils in mainstream schools, but many teachers in what were then ESN(M) (now MLD) schools seized upon the material, welcoming its broad and wide-ranging approach. Before long, however, teachers in special schools began to ask for material which was specifically designed for their pupils so they would not have to modify and adapt the mainstream packs.

In 1979 an ESN(M) extension to the original project began, with an early change of name to 'Health Education for Slow Learners' as the new approaches to children with special educational needs, recommended by the Warnock Committee, gained currency (DES 1978). The project built upon the model used in the earlier packs and developed material specifically for children with mild and moderate learning difficulties. In 1983 the three 'Fit for Life' books were published (McNaughton 1983).

A further project, funded by the Health Education Authority, had the task of developing a health education training programme for teachers of pupils with mild and moderate learning difficulties. 'Special Health' was published in 1989 and contains five core units and four option units in a programme designed to be used by groups of teachers, either in one school, or drawn from a number of schools (Combes & Craft 1989).

The National Curriculum Council has produced two relevant guidance documents for our subject – 'Health Education' and 'Education for Citizenship' (NCC 1990). The health education document is very comprehensive and envisages the subject as a cross curricular theme which will fit into other work that pupils are doing.

> 'Essential features of health education are the promotion of quality of life and the physical, social and mental well-being of the individual. It covers the provision of information about what is good and what is harmful and involves the development of skills which will help individuals to use their knowledge effectively ...'

Health education cannot be left to chance. While health concerns such as smoking, HIV/AIDS and personal safety require individual attention, none should be dealt with in isolation. A coherent health education programme is required if pupils are to be encouraged to establish healthy patterns of behaviour, to acquire the ability to make healthy choices and to contribute to the development of a healthy population.

Nine components form a framework for health education – substance use and misuse; sex education; family life education; safety; health-related exercise; nutrition; personal hygiene; environmental aspects of health education; psychological aspects of health education. Sex education, while seen as part of health education, has a unique legal position and we shall be considering it in more detail. In summary, health education has an undoubted place within a school's curriculum and published material exists to support such teaching.

SEX EDUCATION

School sex education is likely to be seen as the most sensitive of topics within health education and it has a special position with regard to legal requirements.

Legal position

Under the 1986 Education Act school governors now have the responsibility of deciding whether or not sex education should have a place in the curriculum. If the governing body decides in favour of school sex education (and most have) a written statement of their policy with regard to content and organisation has to be produced. The relevant DES circular (DES 1987) clearly outlines the position and the responsibilities of governors, school head, teachers and the Local Education Authority. A number of LEAs have produced guidelines on health and/or sex education in schools. Members of the school medical service should be familiar with any relevant LEA policies.

Planning and organisation

While the legal requirements of school sex education give it a unique status, approaches to its planning, organisation and teaching have much in common with any other area of health education.

Whether we are considering sex education or home economics we should give consideration to:

- parents' views
- children's home background and culture
- children's social world (growing up in Britain in the 1990s)
- peer pressures
- children's changing needs as they mature and develop
- the knowledge, values, feelings, attitudes and skills that children bring with them to the classroom
- the school's hidden curriculum
- availability of suitable teaching resources

Pupils with moderate learning difficulties may have special needs in relation to the way in which sex education is given but the *content* should be very similar to that offered to any child. For a comprehensive sex education programme for older pupils with learning difficulties, Craft and members of the Nottinghamshire Sex Education for Students with Severe Learning Difficulties Project (1991) have produced material for students with severe learning difficulties, and this offers a useful overall plan and a wealth of teaching strategies.

Parental involvement

Under the 1986 Education Act parents were given opportunities for a larger say in school sex education. The number of parent governors was increased and any parent can make representations on sex education to the governors and head teacher. In addition, any parent can raise matters concerning the operation of the school at the annual parents' meeting called specifically for that purpose. Although parents do not have the legal right to withdraw their child from school sex education, in practice many LEAs would, in the last resort, allow parents to do so.

All this means that schools have to pay careful attention to the way in which parents are informed about and involved in classroom sex education. One widely used approach is to invite parents to come along to look at the teaching resources the school plans to use. If the school nurse is involved in the programme her presence is important, signalling clearly that a co-operative, team approach has been adopted. Such meetings can serve several purposes – besides putting parents in a position to be able to answer a child's questions in relation to, for example, a teaching video, the occasion can allow group or individual discussion of parental anxieties (for other approaches see Combes & Craft 1987; Craft & Cromby 1991). The school nurse or doctor can have a special role to play in offering individual advice to parents.

THE ROLE OF THE SCHOOL MEDICAL SERVICE

There are a number of ways in which members of the school medical service can make a contribution to school and individual health education.

Teacher support

Very few teachers get specific training in health education, although they may have had opportunities to attend in-service training events. Teachers may ask for advice about individual pupils and their families. They may also need to update and refresh their own knowledge about health topics. The school nurse or doctor, easily approachable on the teacher's territory of classroom or school, is likely to be the first and most important point of contact. If necessary, links can be made between the teacher and other health professionals.

In the classroom

Many school nurses and doctors take an important part in classroom teaching, usually in tandem with the class teacher. Sometimes this is confined to specific topics in sex education, for example menstruation, contraception, sexually transmitted infections, HIV/AIDS. However some schools have felt that this 'medicalises' the topics concerned in an unhelpful way and have preferred either to use members of the school medical service as supporters and providers of information outside the classroom (see section above), or to co-teach the whole of the health or sex education programme with the school nurse. Much depends on personal preferences and the amount of time available for such a regular commitment.

Individual counselling

Either at a school medical, or as the need arises, the school nurse or doctor can play an important part in counselling on individual or family health-related problems. Often the school nurse will be well-known and well trusted by the pupils. They may seek her advice on a whole range of topics, from the relatively trivial (although not to the pupil concerned) to the very serious, such as a disclosure of sexual abuse.

Link to community

As staff of the Health Authority, members of the school medical service will have ready access to people and resources which may not be so easily available to the teacher. For instance, Health Authority colleagues will include staff in family planning clinics, the HIV/AIDS Information Officer and Health Education/Promotion Officers. The Health Education/Promotion Unit will have free posters and leaflets and a collection of teaching resources for loan to schools and school medical service staff. Outside speakers and resources can enliven the school health education programme and suggestions are likely to be welcomed. Training for school medical service staff on helping with health education programmes in schools may be available locally from Health Education/Promotion Units.

REFERENCES AND FURTHER READING

Amos A 1990 Selling tobacco to children. British Medical Journal 301: 1173-4
Armstrong N, Balding J, Gentle P, Kirby B 1990 Patterns of physical activity among 11–16 year old British children. British Medical Journal 301: 203–5
Balding J W 1991 Making health education work: spiralling into some recycled ideas. Current Paediatrics 1:59–60
Blackburn C 1992 Improving health and welfare work with families in poverty. Open University Press, Buckingham
Combes G, Craft A 1987 Health education for children with special needs. In: David K, Williams T (eds) Health education in schools. Harper Education Series
Combes G, Craft A 1989 Special health: A professional development programme in health education for teachers or pupils with mild or moderate learning difficulties. Health Education Authority, London
Craft A and Members of the Nottinghamshire Sex Education for Students with Severe Learning Difficulties Project 1991 Living your life: a sex education and personal development programme for students with severe learning difficulties. LDA, Cambridge
Craft A, Cromby J 1991 Parental involvement in the sex education of students with severe learning difficulties. Dept. of Mental Handicap, University of Nottingham Medical School
Department of Education and Science 1978 Special educational needs. The Warnock Report. HMSO, London

Department of Education and Science 1987 Sex education in schools. HMSO, London

Department of Health 1992 The health of the nation. HMSO, London

Hillman M, Adams J, Whitelegg J 1990 One false move ... A study of children's independent mobility. Policy Studies Institute, London

Jervis M 1987 Across the cultural divide. Special Children 9: 20–22

Kellmer Pringle M, Butler N R, Davie R 1966 11,000 seven year olds. National Children's Bureau, London

Ley P, Bradshaw P W, Kincey J A 1971 Patients' compliance with medical advice. First annual report. Unit for Research in Doctor/Patient Communication

McNaughton J 1983 Fit for life. Levels 1, 2 and 3. Macmillan Education, Basingstoke

National Curriculum Council 1990 Health education. Curriculum Guidance Series No. 5. Education for Citizenships. Curriculum Guidance Series No. 8. National Curriculum Council, London

Riddock C, Savage J M, Murphy N, Cran G W, Borecham C 1991 Long term health implications of fitness and physical activity patterns. Archives of Disease in Childhood 66: 1426–33

Royal College of Physicians 1991 Preventive medicine. A report of a working party of the Royal College of Physicians. RCP, London

SCHEP 1977 All about me and think well. Thomas Nelson, Walton-on-Thames

Smith R 1981 Health education by children for children. British Medical Journal 283: 782–3

Spencer N J, Perkins E R 1981 The place of health education in paediatric practice. In: Hull D (ed) Recent Advances in Paediatrics. Churchill Livingstone, Edinburgh, pp. 249–59

Townsend P, Davidson N (eds) 1982 Inequalities in health: The Black Report. Penguin, Harmondsworth

Wenlock R W, Disselduff M M, Skinner R K, Knight I 1986 The diets of British school children. Department of Health, London

Wyke S, Hewison J (eds) 1991 Child health matters. Open University Press, Milton Keynes

5 Social Services

Social services by their provision develop a framework of aid, advice and supervision where an individual's or family's own resources are limited. Social work training covers 2–4 years with further post-qualifying study being available. Basic courses consist of either a degree course, for example social science, followed by a 1 year qualifying course with practical experience, or relevant experience and a 2–3 year qualifying course. The degree of professional independence and responsibility, for example decision on the personal liberty of clients, is related to the qualification and experience of the social worker. The aims of social work are to:

- identify personal and social problems and family breakdown and poverty which cause emotional and social stress
- resolve these problems and reverse their harmful effects, if possible
- or, if this is not possible, ensure that the situation does not deteriorate

Structure of social services

Local Authority

Social Service Committee

Director of Social Services

Team leader Senior Social worker Social worker Community worker Home helps, aids	Day nurseries Assessment units Children's homes Hostels Day centres	Adoption Fostering Day care Residential care Abuse Courts Handicap Health Welfare rights
Area teams	Resources	Advisors

- prevent as far as possible those conditions in which problems thrive, such as family stress, bad housing or poverty
- promote favourable conditions which encourage the personal and social enhancement of individuals, families, groups and community.

STRUCTURE OF DAY CARE FACILITIES

Great demands are being made for facilities for day care for pre-school children. Some arise from the financial need of many mothers to work, some from a lack of an extended family and some because of perceived inadequacies of the care of the child at home. In other instances handicap in the child or the parents produces special needs for the family. Because of the importance of the pre-school years for later educational progress and social interaction, the substitute care must be of high quality to provide appropriate experience and stimulation and the element of nurture and continuity of care necessary for normal emotional development. Problems arise when the approach in the 'home' and during 'day care' differs and the child is unable to understand.

Childminders

Childminders have to be legally approved and registered with social service departments. In spite of this requirement much illegal and unsatisfactory childminding still takes place with the emphasis on income for the minder rather than the needs of the child. Overcrowding, and lack of toys or stimulation may be common in such arrangements, the children leading a dull, uninteresting life. There may be frequent changes of minder and the failure of a close relationship to develop between minder and child. The provision of training courses for childminders and appropriate support services can ensure a much higher level of care. Most surveys of childminding have been very critical of this system. The child who is quiet and withdrawn is perhaps particularly vulnerable in the childminding setting, the childminder not having the skills, the 'licence' or sometimes the motivation to explore the origins of the child's problems in his natural home.

Day nurseries

These are generally run by social services departments, but others are run privately or by various voluntary organisations. They all have to obtain registration and approval by the local authority social services department. Day nurseries are staffed by nursery nurses (who have undergone a 2-year training) and have an experienced matron and deputy in charge. In general the nurseries escape many of the criticisms levelled at child minders. However, some operate on a 'custodial system' with a high standard of physical care but lacking the important individualisation of care. Others may be given the grandiose but well earned title of 'therapeutic day care centre'. In this situation, the nursery nurse acts as a proper substitute mother, providing a programme of activities special to that child's needs. Parents are involved in activities in and outside the nursery and hence continuity is established between nursery and home. Many nurseries have units for handicapped children and have additional input from physiotherapists, speech therapists, etc.

Family centres

Day nurseries, even in optimum conditions, cannot meet all the needs of severely disadvantaged children and their parents. The needs are not simply to provide an alternative to home or provide continuity with the home, but to improve the child care skills of parents and their attitude towards the family. The family centre is essentially a day care setting in which parents attend as well as their children and in which a number of programmes are set up to teach parenting skills and to increase the confidence and self-esteem of parents. The Radford Family Centre in Nottingham was staffed by a social worker, health visitor, playgroup leader, community teacher and ancillary workers and provided an early model for such care.

Stated aims of Family Centre:

- to promote practical parenting skills related to play and stimulation, day-to-day physical care, and awareness and management of health problems
- to promote better home management through a home economics programme
- to promote literacy
- to provide insight for parents into the needs of children, both in family life and in education
- to promote satisfaction for parents in parenting, to help parents to enjoy their children
- to reduce dependence on agencies for day-to-day care and acute problems.

Playgroups

These are run by trained playgroup leaders and the playgroup movement is represented by the Pre-school Playgroups Association. They also need to be approved and registered with the local authority. Attendance may be from one to five mornings a week. They provide an opportunity for children to meet, play and socialise and for parents to meet too. Playgroups may be held in church halls, community centres, private premises or attached to schools, health centres or various social work agencies. Although to some extent restricted compared to a nursery school, the value of playgroups compares very favourably with other resources for pre-school children.

Mother and toddler groups

These are for younger children. The mother is expected to stay with her child. They often 'graduate' to the playgroup. Mother and toddler groups not only provide play facilities for the child but also important support for the mother who may be lonely, isolated and harassed.

Combined nursery centres combine the merits of the day nursery which is able to provide extended whole day care for the children of working mothers with the advantage of a nursery school for that part of the day that the child would normally attend. This combination of education and social service provision is a pattern that is being implemented more frequently.

PROVIDING CARE

The thrust of the Children Act 1989 is to support families in the care of their children recognising that whenever possible children should remain with their families. Emphasis is on shared care which means better partnership with parents.

Local authorities are required to protect children from family breakdown and to enhance parental authority. In providing appropriate support and care, consideration must be given to the wishes of the child and the parents, the child's religious persuasion, racial origin, cultural and linguistic background.

Children who were previously '**in care**' are now '**looked after**' by the local authority. Children may be looked after on a voluntary basis when they are **accommodated**. These are children who were previously **received into care**. Other children are looked after because of a Care Order granted by the court.

Accommodation is provided for a child who has no one with parental responsibility to care for him, is lost or abandoned or when his carers no longer provide a suitable home or care. The parents retain full control and can remove the child from accommodation at any stage without notice. However it is expected that arrangements will be made to minimise abrupt changes for the child. Exceptionally children over 16 can be accommodated. Local authorities have discretion about requiring a contribution towards the cost of accommodation.

The child may be accommodated in a foster home, or a residential home. Arrangements for older children may provide greater independence. Necessary arrangements include consultation and the drawing up of a plan to cover the reasons for and expected length of stay and contact.

Local authorities are required to provide other services to support families. Foremost is **day care** which includes day nursery provision, play groups, childminding, out of school clubs and holiday schemes, befriending services, parent and toddler groups, toy libraries and drop-in centres.

Family centres may or may not be residential units. Some offer a therapeutic service, others have a community or self-help orientation. All are designated to promote childcare in a family setting.

Those organising daycare services need to know how to obtain advice about the health and development of the children concerned. Most day nurseries have a named child health doctor and health visitor. All children in daycare should be included in local child health surveillance programmes.

FOSTER CARE

A child may be fostered if he is being accommodated or when he is being looked after by a local authority on a Care Order. Foster care may be provided on a short term or long term basis. Long term fostering is used less frequently now since permanent substitute care is usually better contained in adoption.

Long term fostering usually involves older children who do not want to be adopted or for whom adoption is impracticable.

Short term fostering should not extend beyond six months by which time plans should have been made for the child to return home or for a move to a permanent placement. Some foster parents provide a specialist **bridging** service for disturbed or seriously disadvantaged children who need a period of stability and support in a family setting between a move from a disorganised home to an adoptive one.

Voluntary organisations can make foster placements. The local authority must ensure that the arrangements are satisfactory and that they safeguard the child and promote his welfare. The usual limit to the number of foster children is three. This does not apply to larger sibling groups. Foster parents are provided with comprehensive information about the children placed in their care including details about health and development.

The foster carers

Fostering is a skilled task and foster parents are important members of the professional team caring for the child. Foster parents are usually recruited locally and assessed by a social worker. Applicants submit a medical report and a police check is made. Foster parents may be approved for a particular child or for particular circumstances. The system for approval varies and may involve a fostering or combined fostering and adoption panel. Training and support for foster parents are essential and the National Foster Care Association (NFCA) provides a valuable service to promote and improve the quality of foster care.

Foster allowances

Allowances are paid to foster parents. The amount varies between different agencies and reflects the age and the need of the child.

Private fostering

This refers to an arrangement made between a parent and a private foster parent. The local authority is required to visit in order to ensure that the foster parent is suitable and that the arrangements are satisfactory but there is no process of approval or registration. Proposals to privately foster for a period in excess of 28 days must be notified to the local authority by the foster parent and natural parent. The usual upper limit of three children applies. Health care has to take account of all aspects of health and development with particular regard to children from minority racial groups. Good care is enhanced by sharing information about the child's medical history. This process can be facilitated by the use of personally held records. Financial arrangements are agreed between the foster parent and parent.

Health care

A positive approach to health includes attention to preventive surveillance as well as treatment of illness and accidents. A fostered child must be registered with a general medical practitioner and receive dental care. Under the Review of Children's Cases Regulations 1991, Children Act 1989, a medical examination and written health assessment should be undertaken either **before** placement or **as soon afterwards as possible**. In either case a comprehensive health and developmental assessment is recommended (using the appropriate BAAF form), in order to provide a baseline from which to monitor the child's development. Further health reviews must take place at six monthly intervals for children under the age of two years and at yearly intervals thereafter. Further assessment is recommended prior to any change of school or as indicated by the child's needs.

Health and developmental reviews may be undertaken by a general practitioner, community child health doctor or other paediatrician. Arrangements vary depending on local resources. In any case specialist paediatric advice must be available to the responsible local authority. The designated adviser may be the medical adviser to the adoption panel or a child health colleague.

To avoid fragmentation of health information, health contacts should be entered in a parent (or carer) held record. Older children enjoy making their own entries on a record, My Health Passport, published by BAAF.

Health issues

Children being looked after by the local authority have frequently received irregular or inadequate health care previously. This often reflects the pressures under which the family has lived. Some children have relatively straightforward health problems involving hearing, vision and gaps in immunisation. Others exhibit more complex conditions including multiple handicap, learning difficulties, emotional and behavioural disturbances and growth irregularities. Child abuse may have been identified or may come to light gradually as the child responds to security and feels able to share the painful information.

Issues around consent

Authority to sign consent forms in relation to medical treatment can be delegated to foster carers. A suitable card has been designed by NFCA. Children of sixteen or over can give or withhold consent to examination and give consent to treatment. Younger children, depending upon the doctor's view of their capacity to understand, have the same rights.

Other care situations

Residential care. The health care of children living in children's homes is subject to the same Regulations outlined above.

Children on a Care Order placed with parents. Such a placement may precede the discharge of a Care Order. Factors which have to be considered include contact with family members, health care needs, education, needs of siblings and support services. A police check is required and review of the health status of the carer may indicate the need for an examination.

Childminding is a form of care for children up to the age of eight years.

The recommended childminder: child ratios are

1:3 children aged under 5
1:6 children aged 5–7
1:6 children aged under 8 of whom no more than 3 are under 5
(to include childminder's own child)

Childminders work in their own homes and are required to keep records of the children. The local authority maintains a register of childminders. Supervision includes scrutiny of premises, equipment and arrangements for play out of doors. The local authority has to be satisfied that a child minder is 'fit' to care for children. This fitness is comprehensive and takes account of physical and mental health.

After care

Local authorities have a duty to prepare young people for the time when they cease to be looked after. The Children Act Regulations require that they advise, assist and befriend each child with a view to promoting his welfare. The school health service should promote an understanding of health care and how to make access to health services. Young people who have lived in an institutional setting are especially vulnerable. Many become homeless. Young women are at risk of becoming unmarried teenage mothers and some young men enter prison or become beggars.

Number of children in care (England and Wales), DoH

Year	1980	1990
Total	100 158	63 810
	Percentage by age	
Under 1 year	1.4	2.7
1–4 years	9.2	14.8
5–9 years	19.0	20.1
10–15 years	46.3	39.1
16 years and over	24.2	23.2
	Percentage by sex	
Boys	58.9	53.7
Girls	41.1	46.3

The above figures reflect changes in practice which, by providing better supporting services, have reduced the number of children admitted to care. Information as it is currently collected does not identify the turn-over of children nor the number of placements experienced. However there is some information (Bebbington & Miles 1989) which reflects how disadvantaged these children are.

Of 2500 children admitted to care

- only 25 per cent were living with both parents
- 75 per cent of the families received income support
- only one in five lived in an owner occupied house
- over 50 per cent lived in 'poor' neighbourhoods

The association between deprivation and admission to care was greater than that shown in a 1962 study.

The extent of **residential care** has been reduced with the emphasis on family placements. Increasingly it is now used for adolescents and children requiring a specialist service. Of the children in care (looked after) 75 per cent are placed equally between foster and residential homes. Foster homes cater for 77 per cent of preschool children and 65 per cent of 5–10 year olds but only 15 per cent of children at secondary school (Rowe et al 1989).

In the same study Rowe found that black children were over represented accounting for 19 per cent of admissions. Asian children were under represented in all age groups while African and Afro-Caribbean children were over represented in the preschool and 5–10 age groups. It is not clear whether the low figure for Asian children reflects the strength of the family support or that child care services are not acceptable to their parents. Children in care experience health problems and are at high risk of psychiatric ill-health (Bamford & Wolkind 1988).

Reasons include:

- loss of a health advocate sufficiently intimate with the child's history
- low priority given to medical examinations and history taking
- poor use of growth charts
- poor use of data from health records

Outcomes

Useful information about children who have been cared for by local authorities has been published by the Department of Health.

Placement breakdown is affected by:

- age: breakdown increases with increasing age at placement
- long period in care
- long period on placement waiting list
- previous placement breakdown
- previous unsuccessful attempts to rehabilitate with parents
- other children of similar age in placement household
- child ambivalent about placement
- unrealistic expectations of parent and/or caregivers
- separation from familiar background, contacts etc.

Placement involves risk taking

- with adolescents up to 50 per cent of placements terminate early or break down (Rowe et al 1989)
- in longterm foster placements (usually involving older children) breakdown rates of 20–40 per cent are reported (Rowe et al 1989, Berridge & Cleaver 1987)
- with short-term placements up to 20 per cent terminate unsatisfactorily (Berridge & Cleaver 1987)

Placements with relatives appear to be more stable despite involving older children who often have complex problems (Rowe et al 1989). With regard to **educational achievements,** Triseliotis and Russell found that adopted children succeeded better than those in residential care.

Permanence influences achievement favourably (Aldgate 1990) and this finding is supported by Garnett (1990) who found that children in settled placements, although in care, fared better than those who entered care late after a period of insecurity.

ADOPTION

Adoption as a social activity has been practised throughout history. Adoption as it is understood in this country at the present time dates from the 1926 Adoption Act. It involves the total, irrevocable transfer of parental responsibility from the child's natural parents to the adopter or adopters. This closed model which severs birth relationships and replaces them with another permanent set was originally designed to protect the illegitimate and orphaned children of the First World War and to provide legal security for them and their adopters. Adoption was socially acceptable and became a welcome solution to the twin problems of illegitimacy and infertility.

Number of adoption orders, 1974–89	
Year	Children
1974	22 502
1979	10 870
1974	8648
1989	7044
1990	6533

England and Wales, OPCS

Initially adoption was undertaken mainly by infertile couples who wanted and received healthy young babies. The process was invested with strict confidentiality which amounted to secrecy which often extended to the child himself. The adoption of older children, or those with disabilities, was considered unwise. Indeed emphasis was placed on excluding doubtfully fit children in order to avoid placing stress on the new parents. In 1973 the research study by Rowe & Lambert showed that there were many children in care and out of touch with their natural families who needed a family placement. This finding, coupled with the recognition of the frequently unsatisfactory outcome of long-term fostering (George 1970) and the demonstration that families could be found for children with special needs, resulted in a reappraisal of the adoption process.

The Children Act 1975 introduced very significant changes to adoption. The Act gave priority to the welfare of the child and recognised the need for security by facilitating adoption. Further adoption provisions of the Act were contained in the Adoption Agencies Regulations 1983 and were of particular interest to doctors concerned with child health. The Regulations introduced the statutory requirement to appoint a medical adviser to adoption work. Thus the examples of good practice, which had been developed and promoted by the various organisations which amalgamated to become the British Agency for Adoption and Fostering (BAAF) in 1980, were recognised and made mandatory.

In 1930, 4500 children were adopted. By 1940 this figure had doubled and in 1950, following the Second World War, the number rose to 14 000. The effect of social pressure resulted in a peak year in 1968 when nearly 27 000 adoption orders were granted which included 9000 babies. A subsequent change in social attitudes together with a more flexible approach to family life, better support for single parents, improved methods of birth control and the availability of abortion, resulted in a sharp decline in the number of babies being placed for adoption. In 1975 the total number of adoption orders fell to 21 000 of which only 4548 involved babies. By 1980 orders had halved and only 2599 babies were placed. Currently the number of children placed annually is around 7000 of which just over 1000 are babies.

The following trends should be noted:
- there has been an appreciable and continuous fall in the total number of adoption orders made
- there has been a gradual increase in the relative number of older children adopted.

Age at adoption with % in parentheses (England and Wales, OPCS)

Year	Age (years)					
	Under 1	1–4	5–9	10–14	15–17	All ages
1974	5172 (23)	6148 (27)	7462 (33)	3132 (14)	588 (3)	22 502
1979	2649 (24)	2183 (20)	3572 (33)	2013 (19)	453 (4)	10 870
1984	1836 (21)	1935 (22)	2605 (30)	1728 (20)	526 (6)	8648
1989	1115 (16)	1865 (27)	2244 (32)	1331 (19)	458 (7)	7044

Adoption practice

Who can arrange an adoption? Arrangements for adoption can only be made by an adoption agency except in the following circumstances:
- when the prospective adopter is a relative
- when placement follows a High Court Order

The arrangement of an adoption by an authorised agency is known as an **agency placement**. The child is placed either at the direct request of a parent or by the local authority. Usually the adopters are unknown to the child and his family.

The authorised agency may be based in the social services department (the Children Act 1975 having required all local authorities to ensure that an adoption service was available) or be an approved adoption society. Examples of the latter include the Catholic Children's Society and the National Children's Home.

Non-agency applications may be made by step-parents, other relatives who care for the child or non-relatives who might be private or local authority foster parents. Official statistics relating to the number of children adopted by relatives and step parents are incomplete. In 1975, 43.5 per cent of adoption orders were granted to adopters one of whom was a parent. Currently the figure is nearer 30 per cent and presumably reflects the move from secrecy.

An **adoption order** can be made following an agency placement or on an application by a step parent or relative provided that the child has lived with the applicants for thirteen weeks. In practice the interval is longer because of court timetables. A non-agency application by a non-relative requires a minimum 12 months interval before an adoption order can be granted. An order can be made on a child up to the age of 18 years.

Who can apply to adopt?

Adoption is considered for a variety of reasons. These include infertility, a desire to increase family size without adding to the population or a wish to care for a child with special needs. Since there are very few babies available for adoption and there are, at any one time, about 35 000 considering adoption, adopters are encouraged to consider children with special needs. Potential adopters can contact a local authority agency or a voluntary society which usually covers a wider area. The latter may offer a service for a particular religious group or specialise in the placement of children with special needs, for example Parents for Children. BAAF produce a useful guide for potential adopters, 'Adopting a Child', which is regularly updated. There are few restrictions on eligibility laid down by statute but agencies can be selective within the Regulations.

Age of applicant

By law adopters must be at least 21, or 18 when a parent is adopting a child jointly with a step parent. Agencies operate their own upper age limits. When a healthy infant is being placed the limit is usually fixed at the mid or late 30s. However, guidelines also take account of the time applicants have to wait and the possibility of a further placement. Since the mean age of first time mothers is 25 (Birth Statistics) there is a reluctance to place healthy infants with older applicants. When older children, or those with special needs or disabilities, are being placed the maturity and experience of the applicants warrant special consideration and a more flexible approach. Nevertheless, at all times, agencies need to be satisfied that adopters can expect to remain active and healthy enough to care for a child until he becomes an adult.

Health

There are no statutory health requirements but adopters have to obtain a comprehensive medical report, which includes a health history, for consideration by the agency's medical adviser. Health factors which give rise to debate include a smoking habit, obesity and excessive alcohol consumption. Some agencies take a firmer stand than others and, for example, exclude applicants who smoke.

Most agencies will only place babies with infertile couples and they require completion of fertility tests before an adoption placement can be considered. Since investigation and treatment can now last many years and take a couple into their early forties expert counselling is required to support couples having to make choices.

Marital status

A sole applicant may apply to adopt. If two people apply to adopt jointly they must be married thus complying with the European Adoption Convention. Agencies look for stability and some stipulate minimum periods for which the couple have been married or have lived together.

Services

For birth parents and relatives. Birth parents have access to information and counselling services whether they agree to adoption or not. They should be involved in making plans for their child whenever possible although this presents difficulties when they are opposed to adoption. Some agencies have moved further than others in facilitating meetings between parents and prospective adopters and encouraging parents to be involved in the selection of adopters. This practice is easier to achieve with baby placements.

Other relatives, especially grandparents, need support to cope with the pain and loss involved and may be able to contribute to adoption plans.

For adoptive parents. Prospective adopters need information about the process and the characteristics of children available for adoption. Post adoption support services are also relevant but their delivery is patchy.

For adopted people. Under Section 51 of The Children Act 1975 adopted people were given the right, on reaching the age of 18, of access to their original birth certificates. (This was always the case in Scotland.) Progressively more adoptees pursued this right and by the end of 1990 33 000 had made use of it. This does not reflect dissatisfaction with adoption but rather the need for information about origin and background which is necessary to give substance to identity. Others wish to trace birth parents and family and for this reason the **adoption contact register** was introduced in 1991 in England and Wales. The register allows birth relatives to record a wish for contact which can be pursued by the adopted person. It will not help an adopted person to learn about his relatives if they have not entered onto the register.

Adoption procedures

The Adoption Agencies Regulations 1983 defined the composition and functions of adoption panels. In some areas the panel also considers longterm fostering placements.

Composition of panel. The maximum number is 10, the minimum 7 and must include at least one man and one woman. Members include a chairman, who is usually a social worker, 2 social workers employed by the agency, a management representative, a medical adviser and 2 people independent of the agency. The latter are expected to make a special contribution and often include an adoptive parent, a representative of an ethnic group or a psychologist. A legal adviser is not required to be a member of the adoption panel but an adoption agency has to obtain legal advice about each case presented to the panel.

Adoption panel functions. The panel makes **recommendations** to the **agency** who in turn makes **decisions**. The panel is required to meet and cannot carry out business by correspondence.

The panel has to recommend for individual children:

- whether adoption is in the child's best interest and if so,
- whether the child should be freed for adoption.

Freeing is the process whereby parental responsibility (previously parental rights and duties) are transferred to the agency. It was intended for use mostly in baby adoptions where mother and agency were acting together. Its future use is under review.

Either at the same time or subsequently the panel has to recommend:

- whether prospective adopter(s) would be suitable adoptive parent(s) for a particular child.

The matching process follows the detailed assessment of prospective adoptive parents which is undertaken by a social worker. After assessment the applicants are considered by the panel for approval. Once the agency has made a decision based on the panel's recommendations:

The following procedures are undertaken by the agency:

- natural parent(s) notified
- prospective adopters notified
- prospective adopters supplied with written information (including details of history, religious and cultural background, health and developmental status) about the child before placement
- health information forwarded to general practitioner before placement
- adopters' local authority notified
- adopters' health authority notified and thereby the health visitor
- adopters' local education authority notified if:
  a) child of compulsory school age
  b) child considered to have special educational needs

In the case of a baby the proposed new name is given. This is not always practicable when older children are involved. At all times case records must be treated as confidential and securely stored for at least 75 years.

Role of medical adviser

The regulations require the agency, under the medical adviser's direction, to obtain health information about the natural parents and prospective adopters and health and developmental information about the child. This information has to be collated and presented to the panel to assist them in their tasks and the adviser needs to keep health issues to the fore when a placement is being agreed.

Some of the health information is difficult to obtain. It may be withheld or missing because, for example, the child has moved many times and had many different caregivers. The medical adviser needs time, communication skills and a good working knowledge of medical networks to facilitate information collection.

Some panels have more than one adviser, one to consider adult health issues and one to concentrate on paediatric aspects. The adviser may examine all the children himself or liaise with general practitioners, child health and other colleagues. More specialist paediatric advice may be sought for many conditions including children with multiple handicaps, genetic, chronic health, behavioural or mental health problems. The adviser has to work closely with social workers and help them to use medical information appropriately. Information is usually recorded using a selection of forms designed by BAAF since they cover all health matters required by the regulations. The advantage of using nationally agreed forms is obvious. The increasing use of parent or carer held child health records should enhance the collection of health information.

When a newborn baby is placed directly from hospital it is particularly important that the medical adviser explains to the adopters that only preliminary health and developmental screening has been possible. The implications of any risk should be identified. Although direct placements are only considered when it is expected that the mother will hold firm to her pre-birth decision about adoption she cannot give her consent to adoption until the baby is six weeks old. Maternal consent can be withdrawn up to the granting of an adoption order. Adoption allowances are subject to Regulations under the Children Act. Allowances are the exception rather than the rule and are paid by an adoption agency to adopters to meet the individual needs and circumstances of a child and his new family and to secure an adoption where there might otherwise be a financial obstacle. An allowance is not a reward. The recommendation to make an allowance is made by the adoption panel and cannot be considered after an adoption order has been made. The amount of the allowance takes account of the needs of the child and the resources of the adopters but cannot exceed a fostering allowance.

Some issues to consider

Transracial and inter-country adoption. The shortage of babies for adoption in the UK has been referred to and has important consequences. Many adopters, understandably, would prefer to adopt a baby and look to inter-country adoption as a solution. However the prevailing view is that children thrive better in families with a similar racial and ethnic background to their own. This view is challenged by some authorities and the issue is currently under review by the Department of Health.

Openness in adoption. Since most adoptions involve children over the age of five, many move to their adoptive homes with a well developed history and considerable information about their birth family. Honesty within all adoptions has long been recommended but for these children ongoing contact with some relatives has also to be considered.

Studies in the 1960s and 1970s revealed the impact of secrecy on the lives of adopted people (McWhinnie 1967; Triseliotis 1973). Later studies identified the lasting distress for mothers. More recently a group of English adoptive families, where contact with birth parents has been maintained, has been reviewed with positive results (Fratter 1989).

This then is the background to a new look for adoption.

Adoption with contact preserves useful links with birth relatives. The degree of contact varies with the child's needs.

Open adoption occurs when the birth parent is actively involved in the selection of adopters and meets with them. It usually involves infant adoption and is popular with some voluntary societies. New Zealand has practised open adoption successfully for a decade (Lambert & Streather 1980).

Semi-open adoption is a widespread practice where information is freely shared but no face-to-face meetings occur.

Promotion of openness is based on the belief that it is better for the child and birth parents. The picture is less clear for the adopters but research continues and the process is under review by the Department of Health.

HIV infection. The number of babies born to HIV positive mothers can be expected to increase. Some of these will be placed for adoption without their status being known. It is not possible to screen a baby in the absence of maternal consent without risking possible legal action. If it is necessary to establish the HIV status the consent of the court should be sought through a specific issue order under Section 8 of the Children Act 1989. Prospective adoptive parents need to be advised during assessment that it may be difficult to establish the HIV status of the baby.

Outcomes of adoption

A longitudinal study by Lambert and Streather in 1980 showed that 93 per cent of the 115 children who had been adopted as babies were living with their adoptive families at the age of 11 years. A retrospective study by Raynor (1980) found that 80 per cent of young people, who had been adopted as babies, and 85 per cent of the adopters were contented. Other studies suggest that in the teenage years adopted children show more problems than their matched peers but that the problems did not persist into adult life. Overall therefore up to 80 per cent of baby adoptions prove to be successful. For a small minority problems of identity and self-esteem are longer lasting and studies of populations attending child guidance clinics suggest that adopted children are over represented.

REFERENCES AND FURTHER READING

Aldgate J 1990 Foster children at school; success or failure? Adoption and Fostering 14 (4)
Bamford F N, Wolkind S N 1988 The physical and mental health of children in care: Research needs. ESRC
Bebbington A, Miles J 1989 The background of children who enter Local Authority care. British Journal of Social Workers 19 (5)
Berridge D, Cleaver H 1987 Foster home breakdown. Blackwell, Oxford
Birth statistics 1989 HMSO, London
Department of Health 1991 Patterns and outcome in child placement. HMSO, London
Fenyo A, Knapp M, Barnes B 1989 Foster care breakdown. Discussion paper 616. Personal Social Services Research Unit, University of Kent
Fratter J 1989 Family placements and access. Barnado's, London
Garnett L 1990 Leaving care for independence. Report to DoH. HMSO, London
George V 1970 Foster care. Routledge and Kegan Paul, London
Lambert L, Streather J 1980 Children in changing families. Macmillan, London

McWhinnie A 1967 Adopted children: how they grow up. Routledge and Kegan Paul, London
Raynor L 1980 The adopted child comes of age. Allen and Unwin, London
Rowe J, Lambert I 1973 Children who wait. ABAFA, London
Rowe J, Hundleby M, Garnett L 1989 Child care now. BAAF, Research Series 6
The Children Act 1989. HMSO, London
Triseliotis J 1973 In search of origins. Routledge and Kegan Paul, London
Triseliotis J, Russell J 1984 Hard to place: The outcome of adoption and residential care. Heinemann Educational, Oxford

Benefits

Money cannot protect children from deprivation and disadvantage, but lack of it is strongly linked to ill health and educational failure. Disability occurs in all strata of society, but poverty and disability together represent a formidable handicap. A compassionate society has an obligation to its more disadvantaged members to provide help where and when it is needed. The degree to which these needs are catered for is governed by many factors; economic, political, social, personal. There is always likely to be a debate (some would say a battle) between the benefits made available and those considered eligible to receive them. Britain has a long established but complex benefit system. It is easy to become confused by the all too frequent administrative changes. Doctors can be invaluable in pointing their patients in the right direction and supporting their claims. The benefits highlighted in this chapter are those **Social Security Benefits** effective from April 1988 and include changes in the disability benefits in April 1992. The benefits may be available to all families with children, or only to those with low income and/or to those with children with special needs. **Voluntary organisations and self help groups** are also important and their contribution is briefly discussed.

Benefits

These are assessed either with respect to the caring adult(s) or to the child. Some benefits for adults are affected if they have a dependant child, for example, retirement pension, widow's benefit and income support are increased if there is a dependant child and there are maternity benefits for women expecting a child and a one parent benefit. Once children reach sixteen years old (and in certain cases eighteen) they may be entitled to additional benefits, for example severe disablement allowance, council tax discount, housing benefit. Here we are concerned only with benefits for children.

Benefits are either 'Contributory', that is related to National Insurance contributions, or 'Non-contributory', that is given as a statutory right, provided certain criteria are fulfilled or, 'Means tested' and only awarded if the claimant's income is low enough. Unless otherwise specified claims are made via the local office of the Department of Social Security, although application leaflets are often also available in Post Offices, Libraries and Health Centres.

Social security benefits

Contributory benefits	Non-contributory benefits	Means tested benefits
Retirement pension	Child benefit	Income support
Widow's benefit	One parent benefit	Housing benefit
Unemployment benefit	Disability living allowance	Council tax discount
Sickness benefit	Invalid care allowance	Family credit
Invalidity benefit	Carer's premium	The social fund
Maternity allowance	Severe disablement allowance	
	Industrial injury benefit	
	Statutory sick pay	
	Statutory maternity pay	

(From Ennals 1990)

Benefits for all

Child Benefit. This is a non-contributory benefit which is paid for all children from birth and continues, without further claim, until the age of eighteen for children in full time secondary education. It has an almost 100 per cent uptake which is probably a result of the ease with which it is obtained and it being perceived as free from the unfavourable stigma that many people associate with claiming benefits. The child does not have to be a blood relative but in most cases must be living with the claimant. There are no special extra payments to cope with the financial burden of multiple births (eg triplets) although Home Help may be available during the first year of life.

Maternity Benefits. These include a number of benefits of which the most important is Statutory Maternity Pay. The maternity pay period lasts for 18 weeks and can be taken at the earliest 11 weeks before the expected week of delivery and at the latest 6 weeks before. If a baby is born prematurely the maternity pay period is still 18 weeks. Free prescriptions and dental treatment are available to pregnant women and those with a child under 1 year. Milk tokens which can be exchanged for 'door-step' milk or dried, formulated baby milk are available to expectant and nursing mothers on income support and to children under 5 whose families are on income support.

Benefits for low income families

Income Support. This is the main benefit for people (at least 16 years old) not in work and on low incomes. In 1988 it replaced the old supplementary benefit which, in the mid 1980s, had an uptake of 76 per cent. It is currently claimed by almost 4.5 million people. The amount varies with the age of the applicant, his or her financial circumstances and family size. It acts as a passport to other benefits (free prescriptions, dental treatment, NHS glasses) and there are additional 'premiums' for disabilities within the family. The disabled child premium is added if any child is receiving Disability Living Allowance or is registered blind. As income support is a means tested benefit, the ultimate figure awarded is then set against any other income the family receives.

Family Credit. This is intended for people bringing up children on low

Examples of benefits

Family with 13 year old child with Down's syndrome and severe learning difficulties. Help required with personal care and the large amount of supervision at school and at home, during the day. Needs only a limited amount of sleep during the night and will wander around the house. Help required in connection with incontinence. Walks at a slow pace and has poor stamina. Experiences frequent challenging behaviour when out walking, ie refuses to walk and shows socially difficult behaviour towards other people. Her parents have been unemployed for 18 months and are in receipt of Income Support.

Invalid Care Allowance	£ 32.55
Child Benefit	£ 9.65
	£ 42.20

Income Support, for couple	£ 66.60
Plus premiums for dependant child	£ 21.40
Family premium	£ 9.30
Disabled child premium	£ 17.80
Carers' premium	£ 11.55
	£126.65

Actual Income Support received (Total Income Support minus income from invalid care allowance and child benefit)	£ 84.45

N.B. *Invalid Care Allowance should be claimed whether parents are on Income Support or not because it will continue even when employment is restarted whereas Income Support will probably be lost.*

Disability Living Allowance, higher level Care Component	£ 43.35
Disability Living Allowance, higher level Mobility Component*	£ 30.30
Total for week	**£ 200.30**

* Can also apply for Road (Vehicle) Tax exemption and orange car parking badge.

Same couple, but with a healthy 13 year old child without disabilities or learning difficulties

Child Benefit	£ 9.65
Actual Income Support received (£66.60 + £21.40 + £9.30 – Child Benefit)	£ 87.65
Total for week	**£ 97.30**

Same couple, but with no children

Income Support	**Total for week** **£ 66.60**

(Money as of April 1992)

wages but is claimed by only approximately 50 per cent of all possible recipients. To be eligible the claimant must be working an average of at least 16 hours a week, be receiving child benefit for at least one dependant child and have savings of less than £8000. The benefit payable is dependant on income, the family size and the ages of the children with increasing premiums for children above the age of 11.

The Social Fund. This includes grants as of right (maternity needs, funerals and cold weather), community care grants and budgeting loans. With its introduction in 1988, the latter established a new concept in benefits, namely that of *loans* from which people could buy furniture, cookers, beds etc. Inevitably it has not been without controversy. As the loan has to be repaid out of weekly benefit some people have found that their budget is so tight that they cannot afford to repay the loan. The situation is not helped by awards being discretionary on the state of the *local* social security office's tight cash budget. When there is pressure on a local budget an application may be refused when at different times of the year or in another area the same application may have been accepted. In 1990–1 over 50 000 applications were refused on the grounds of such 'insufficient priority'.

Benefits for families with special needs

The financial impact of caring for a disabled child at home is well documented (Baldwin 1985). The statutory allowances outlined below ease the burden, but rarely meet the full costs. Aids and appliances are obvious expenses, but clothes and footwear, travel and holidays, baby-sitting and child care can all cost more when there is a disabled child in the family. There is help available in some of these areas but it is often discretionary. There are also 'hidden' costs. Many parents, usually mothers, curtail their careers or stop working in order to care for their child. A disabled child limits family mobility; employment opportunities and chances of promotion may be lost or the family may move, at great cost, to try and provide more suitable accommodation or better schooling and services for their child. It can be argued that mothers in all families may have to give up their jobs to care for their children and that families often move house so that their children can go to better schools, but most families can look forward to their children becoming independent in time and the easing of financial burdens. In contrast the families of severely disabled children often see the future as a time of increasing financial stress as they struggle to make provision for their child into adulthood.

Disability Living Allowance (DLA). Introduced in April 1992 this combines the benefits previously covered by the Attendance allowance and the Mobility allowance, which it replaced. It has extended the scope of these previous allowances to cover less severe disabilities. The DLA has two parts; a **care component** giving help for similar reasons to the Attendance allowance and a **mobility component**, similar to the old Mobility allowance. It is a non-contributory benefit which is especially valuable as it acts as a passport to additional payments (income support, housing benefit, invalid care allowance), it is not set against other income in any means test for additional benefits and is tax free.

Care Component. This a vitally important benefit for disabled people who need attention or supervision from other people, who may or may not be related to them. It is paid regardless of whether the disabled person actually receives that attention or not. It is paid at three levels according to the degree of care required.

Levels of care

The **higher level** is paid when constant attention or help is needed both day *and* night.
The **medium level** is paid when help is needed only in the day *or* at night.
The **lower level** is for people who require a small amount of care for example help at the beginning and end of the day.

The lower level is an extension of the benefit previously provided by the old Attendance allowance and will help the families of children with less severe learning disabilities. The conditions of care must be satisfied continually for three months, although this time limit is relaxed for terminally ill patients. The disabled person can be any age, including 6 month old infants, although for children under 16 the mother should normally claim, unless she is not living with the child. 'Disability' is a broad term and encompasses many medical conditions including, in children, problems with breathing, eating, dressing, toileting etc. Unlike the old Attendance allowance there is less need for an examining doctor to visit the home, for greater importance is given to the information given by the claimant and the opinion of the claimant's doctor as to the degree of the disability and there is a space in the claim pack for this.

Many claims under the old Attendance allowance system were initially met with rejection. Should this again be the case, an appeal can ultimately be made through the independent Disability Appeal Tribunal. In 1988 over 80 per cent of people claiming Attendance allowance who sought a review after initial refusal, subsequently received an award. It is important to realise that like Attendance allowance, the DLA care component is forfeited if the claimant lives in any public funded institution, eg hospital or respite care, for 28 days or more. If two or more periods of less than 28 days in care are separated by 28 days or less they will be counted together. Whenever the 'threshold' of 28 days is accumulated, recipients should plan to spend a clear 29 days at home so as not to affect their benefit. The DLA care component can be awarded for life, but in the case of a child a renewal claim must be made on their 16th birthday.

Mobility Component. This provides help for people who have mobility difficulties, however, unlike the old Mobility allowance, it is not restricted to people with *physical* disablement. Under the conditions of the DLA mobility component people with learning disabilities who are often physically able to walk but, due to their *mental* impairment, have severe behavioural problems can now claim providing this behaviour grossly restricts their mobility, for example, children severely affected by autism. The mobility component is paid at two levels depending on the degree of restriction to walking.

The **higher level** is for those people whose walking ability is so restricted that the claimant could have qualified for the old Mobility allowance, i.e. he is virtually unable to walk because his problems cause restrictions on the distance he can walk, the speed he can walk, the length of time he can walk for, the manner in which he walks, and whether he experiences severe discomfort while walking. Only a minority of people with learning disabilities have severe enough mental impairment to qualify them for the higher level of payment.

Most people with learning disabilities will be more able to benefit from the **lower level**, which is for people who are able to walk but need someone to supervise them when they are out of doors, eg crossing roads, likely to fall, likely to get into danger or wander off due to a lack of awareness or behavioural problems. The DLA mobility component can be claimed by anyone aged from 5 to 65, but to get the lower rate, children must need more guidance or supervision than another child of the same age. This still means that parents who have children below the age of 5 cannot receive any financial help with their child's mobility problems, although they can be exempt from road (vehicle) tax provided the child receives the care component of the DLA. Just as with the old mobility allowance, families who receive the higher level mobility component for a child also qualify for a local authority run 'orange car parking badge' allowing them to park more easily. The DLA mobility component is not normally affected by a stay in hospital, provided the patient is still mobile.

Invalid Care Allowance. People caring for patients who receive the DLA care component at the medium or the high rate may claim for invalid care allowance if they are not in full time work. To qualify, at least 35 hours each week must be spent looking after this person. Invalid care allowance will usually stop after the patient has been in hospital for 12 weeks. However, if a child goes into hospital any additional benefit paid is usually unaffected as the parents are regarded as continuing to incur expenditure by visiting or buying the child presents. It is not tax free and, although not strictly means tested, it is taken into account when claiming other benefits. If a person receiving income support is also in receipt of invalid care allowance or is disqualified from the latter because of other benefits they receive, they may claim a Carer's Premium.

VOLUNTARY ORGANISATIONS AND SELF HELP GROUPS

Voluntary and charitable organisations have a long history of helping families to receive benefits. The importance of their role has long been recognised (DHSS 1976) and is likely to increase as restrictions in public spending on social services become greater. The priorities of such organisations vary considerably.

Some, such as the **Citizen's Advice Bureaux,** provide, as part of their service, general information and advice to families trying to negotiate the maze of social security benefits. **The Child Poverty Action Group**, as well as giving advice, plays a role in training other helping agencies and even local authority staff in these areas. It also researches the extent of poverty in the UK and campaigns for a fairer future for families with children. **The Family Fund** is a government sponsored charity that helps families who are caring for a very severely handicapped child at home.It gives grants for items directly related to the needs posed by caring for such a child, such as washing machines, furniture or taxi fares. The Fund will help when the family cannot meet the cost themselves and are not covered by existing services. **Barnardo's**, a charity dating from the nineteenth century, helps and supports children and families facing social and emotional stress. It funds and runs a huge range of projects throughout the country.

More recently many organisations have been founded to meet specific needs, for example One Parent Families, The Spastics Society and MENCAP. There is now a self help group for almost every serious disease of childhood and even one, Share a Care, whose objective is to put individuals and families with rare diseases in touch with others with the same or similar problems.These organisations help families in a variety of ways. Most importantly they provide information. Many produce publications giving detailed advice about rights and benefits available to families with specific problems. The Disability Alliance has published a book called *Disability Rights Handbook* which is a useful guide to rights, benefits and services for all people with disabilities and their families. Another excellent source of help is Contact a Family which supports families who care for children with special needs and publish *The CaF Directory* of specific conditions and rare symptoms.

Voluntary groups also provide a forum where parents can meet and exchange experiences. Information obtained in this way is often more relevant and more easily understood. Most also offer advice with individual cases, helping parents to fill out applications for appeal decisions.

Charitable organisations are often involved in providing more direct welfare benefits.The supply of aids and equipment, the provision of respite care or holidays are some examples. An important aspect of this work is that it allows families to help each other, rather than always to be on the receiving end. Lastly, these organisations represent a powerful lobby and often fund and initiate the research to back their demands.

WHO BENEFITS?

Anyone working in a caring profession has at some time or other found themselves puzzled by the workings of the social security system. Sometimes it seems that those in most need have greatest difficulty in getting help. People hold opposing views about how the system should be administered. Many believe that it should be 'user friendly', that benefits should be well advertised and that applying for them should be as simple as possible. The opposing view is that the system is already too open to abuse and that any changes that make it easier to obtain benefit will lead to the system being overwhelmed by demand, much of it fraudulant. Striking a balance between these views is not easy.

The take-up levels for individual benefits vary widely. Family credit is claimed by only about half of those estimated to be entitled to it, whereas child benefit has almost 100 per cent take-up. There are many factors which influence take-up levels. Clearly the first step in claiming any benefit is knowing that it exists. Most of us know about child benefit and establishing one's entitlement is fairly simple. But would you know how to claim for family credit and what the rules are? In general terms the more complicated the process of application and establishing entitlement the lower the take-up level. Benefits that are means tested and those where there is a discretionary element, such as the Disability Living Allowance, are the most complex. Yet it is often the very people most in need of these benefits who are least equipped to negotiate the maze.

For even the simplest benefit there are quite detailed forms to be completed. Most carry a written warning about the consequences of making false or misleading statements and this can be very worrying to people who are unsure of their rights or who find it hard to state their case clearly. Imagine the difficulties faced by someone who cannot read or write well, or someone who speaks little English. Problems in filling out the form may deter some from making an application at all, and the administrative hassle does not end with the completion of the form. Much correspondence may be generated by even a straightforward application for child benefit and where there is a need to check facts or appeal decisions a wealth of paper soon accumulates. Even when entitlement is agreed there may be errors or delays in payment. The bureaucracy may be second nature to those who administer the system but is often totally bewildering to the rest of us.

For many people there is still a stigma attached to claiming for social security benefits. This is gradually changing but the general appearance of most social security offices does little to hasten the change. Furniture screwed to the floor, grills over the desks and lengthy queues do not make for a welcoming atmosphere. Maybe they are not meant to. For some benefits, claimants have to undergo a lengthy interview. People may find this both embarrassing and intimidating, and often worry that they may prejudice their case by their answers. Recent changes in legislation, that require single mothers claiming one parent benefit to reveal who is the father of their child, do nothing to allay a sense of stigma and may in fact deter some of those most in need of support from claiming it.

Ironically receiving benefit can sometimes be a mixed blessing. Individuals may be reluctant to take low paid jobs because they fear by doing so they will end up materially worse off. The benefit system is designed to try and avoid this 'unemployment trap' but some people will find the uncertainties of giving up the relative security of state support for low paid employment too great a risk to take. Even for the employed there are complex problems. Such is the interaction between family credit and housing benefit that for many families there is little point in claiming family credit because of the serious negative effect on housing benefit. There are several examples of similar 'poverty traps' in the system and these situations also have the additional adverse effect of deterring people from applying for other entitlements.

An even more worrying anomaly can occur in families caring for a disabled child. Quite rightly such families often receive considerable financial support in the form of Disability Living Allowance. For some families this may be their main source of income, as parents may no longer be able to remain in employment because of the burden of care. But there is a large discretionary element in many of these benefits, and whether they are paid and how much is paid is dependent on the degree of handicap. All this seems very fair but can lead to problems in practice. For example a family with a child who has spina bifida may work hard over the years to help that child attain continence, only to find that achieving that goal can result in considerable loss of income. Most families would not be deterred from doing their best for their child by such considerations but some families may be torn between helping a child work towards independence and fears for the solvency of the family unit.

How then to improve the system? There are no easy answers to many of the problems, but simplification of the process would help. Recent moves to advertise benefits more widely are a welcome change and hopefully The Citizen's Charter will promote an atmosphere of helpfulness and availability among those who administer the system. Welfare rights officers play an important role in helping people. Charitable organisations and self help groups represent powerful lobbies for their members. More money helps solve most problems but is unlikely to be forthcoming. At the end of the day all workers in caring professions must see it as part of their job to help children in need and their families receive whatever they are entitled to.

A list of some of the many organisations that exist to help children and their families is given in Appendix B.

REFERENCES

Baldwin S 1985 The cost of caring: Families with disabled children.
    Routledge and Kegan Paul, London
Department of Health and Social Security 1976 'Priorities for health and personal social
    services in England, HMSO, London. p.72
Ennals S 1990 Doctors and benefits. British Medical Journal 301: 1321
Ennals S (ed) 1991 Understanding benefits. BMJ, London.

7   The Law

Although three different legal systems operate within the United Kingdom, relating to England and Wales, Scotland and Northern Ireland respectively, all support parents to bring up their children while providing state protection when the level of care is unacceptable.

Child care law in England and Wales was significantly changed by the introduction of the Children Act 1989 which came into force in October 1991. The Act has simplified the law and brought together private law, which applied to children affected by disputes such as divorce, and public law which affected children in need of help from a local authority. Legislation affecting children is currently under review in Scotland and Northern Ireland. Although implementation of the Act is the responsibility of social services departments, there are important implications for health professionals. One is contained in Section 27 which states that if a health authority or NHS Trust receives a request for help from a local authority it must comply provided that the request is compatible with statutory and other duties. Health authorities and NHS Trusts also have a duty to inform the appropriate social services department when accommodation is provided for a child for a consecutive period of at least three months, and when the accommodation is terminated. At all times interagency co-operation is essential together with greater collaboration with parents and other carers.

PARENTAL RESPONSIBILITY

The Act is based upon the belief that most children are best looked after within the family without unwarranted interference. This is reflected in the new concept of parental responsibility which replaces parental rights and duties.

Who has it?

Parents who are married both have parental responsibility. They retain it if separated or divorced and only loose it by an adoption order. An unmarried father can acquire it if the mother agrees or if a court order is made in his favour. Other people can acquire it, for example, a local authority or a guardian. Parental responsibility carries the right to determine where a child lives, how he is educated together with the duty to care for the child.

Getting the best

Welfare and rights An overriding principle of the Children Act is to ensure the welfare of the child. Under Section 1 the courts are required to give paramount consideration to welfare when reaching any decision while recognising that welfare can be prejudiced by delay. The Act supplies a checklist of factors to be regarded by the court when making an order. The court is prohibited from making an order unless so doing is better than making no order at all (the presumption of no order).

> **The checklist is not exhaustive and most of the factors are not new**
>
> The items to be borne in mind are as follows:
> - the ascertainable wishes and feelings of the child (considered in the light of age and understanding)
> - the child's physical, emotional and educational needs
> - the likely effect on the child of any changes in circumstances
> - the child's age, sex, background and any characteristics which the court considers relevant
> - any harm which the child has suffered or is at risk of suffering
> - how capable each of the parents, and any other person in relation to whom the court considers the question to be relevant, is of meeting the child's needs
> - the range of powers available to the court under the Act

Until recently children were seen as chattels of their parents. Now children who are looked after by local authorities must be consulted before decisions are made about matters which affect them. In addition to promoting their welfare, regard must be given to religion, race, culture and language. Contact with family and friends must be promoted unless it is inconsistent with their welfare.

Children in need

The law makes local authorities responsible for provision of services for children in need. They are also requested to take reasonable steps to identify the proportion of such children in their area.

Each local authority must publish information about the services provided, ensure that the information is appropriately available and develop a system whereby complaints can be made. Authorities are given discretion to decide what services they consider appropriate. Essential services include daycare, accommodation and family aides.

Under the Act a child (someone under the age of 18 years) is considered **to be in need** if:

- he is unlikely to achieve or maintain, or to have the opportunity of achieving or maintaining, a reasonable standard of health or development without the provision of services (Part III Section 17);
- his health or development is likely to be significantly impaired, or further impaired, without the provision of such services; or
- he is disabled

- health is defined to mean physical or mental health and development to mean physical, intellectual, emotional, social or behavioural development.

Health professionals will play an essential role in the identification of the children since many of them will be found through surveillance programmes. However some of the children may be chronic non-attenders or members of homeless or travelling families and particular vigilance is necessary to ensure that they do not 'fall through the net'! Children on child protection registers form one discrete group of children in need. Arrangements have to be made at local level to determine how information from health agencies is shared with the local authority.

Children with disabilities   The Act states that a child is disabled

> *'If he is blind, deaf or dumb or suffers from a mental disorder of any kind or is substantially and permanently handicapped by illness, injury or congenital deformity or such other disability as may be prescribed.'*

The definition of disabled is the one used in the National Assistance Act 1948. By the nature of their disabilities children will be known to child development teams and at other paediatric specialist centres. Local authorities are required to provide services which are designed to minimise the effect of the disabilities and to enable the children to lead lives which are as normal as possible. They are also required to keep a register of disabled children to assist in planning and anticipation of service need. Parents, and children, when it is appropriate, have to agree to registration although delivery of services does not depend upon it. It is important that parents and others are clearly informed about the difference between the disability register and the child protection register.

COURT ORDERS

Section 8 orders   These replace the custody and access orders. Each order is designed to provide a practical solution to a problem, can be made until the child's eighteenth birthday and is for a specified period. There are four orders.

A residence order which sets out the arrangements defining with whom a child is to live and confirms parental responsibility.

A contact order which requires the person with whom the child lives to allow contact with the person named in the order.

A specific issue order gives directions whereby a particular question can be answered, eg directing a parent to allow the child medical investigation or treatment.

A prohibited steps order prevents a step that would normally be covered by parental responsibility from being taken.

The first two are perhaps the most important. A residence order can only be made when a child is subject to a care order and a local authority cannot apply for a residence or contact order.

Education

Education Supervision Order (ESO). This places a child of compulsory school age under the supervision of a local education authority if the court decides that school attendance is unsatisfactory. The intention is to ensure proper education and the wishes and feelings of the child and parents must be taken into account. An ESO lasts for one year and can be extended for three years.

Child protection

Local authorities have a statutory responsibility to investigate when it is suspected that a child needs protection. Support can be offered under Part III of the Children Act but it may be necessary for the local authority or NSPCC to apply for a care or supervision order.

Care and Supervision Orders. These orders are made under Section 31 of the Children Act. The former places the child in the care of the local authority and confers parental responsibility. The latter places the child under the supervision of a local authority or a probation officer and may impose conditions such as a medical or psychiatric examination. The orders are mutually exclusive and similar to orders made under the Children and Young Persons Act 1969. A care order, unless it is discharged, lasts until a child is eighteen: a supervision order remains in force for one year initially.

Neither order can be made unless the court is satisfied:

• that the child concerned is suffering, or is likely to suffer, significant harm; and
• that the harm, or likelihood of harm is attributable to
  a) the care given to the child, or likely to be given if the order were not made, not being what it would be reasonable to expect a parent to give to him; or
  b) the child being beyond parental control.

Harm in this context includes both ill-treatment (which includes all forms of abuse) and the impairment of health or development. Confirming that the harm is significant requires a comprehensive understanding of child health and development and calls for the services of a senior and appropriately trained paediatrician.

Emergency Protection Order (EPO). This order replaces the **Place of Safety Order.** It is short term and can be applied for by anyone although in practice the local authority or NSPCC is usually involved. The order lasts for eight days, can be renewed for a further seven days and gives the applicant **parental responsibility.** An EPO can be made by a court when there is reasonable cause to believe that the child will suffer significant harm unless he is made safe. This may involve **removal from a dangerous situation** or the **prevention** of removal from a hospital or fosterhome to a harmful situation. After 72 hours the child or parent can apply for discharge of the order. While in force the court can direct that a medical or psychiatric examination shall take place and by whom. It can also direct that **no** examination is undertaken. When an examination or assessment is recommended it is important that the maximum information is obtained and that joint examinations are arranged, when appropriate, in order to avoid unnecessary repetition. The doctors concerned need to be fully aware of the directions of the court and be able to respond promptly.

Child Assessment Order (CAO). This is an entirely new order which is granted in non-urgent cases where the local authority or NSPCC suspects that a child is suffering, or likely to suffer, significant harm, but where the investigation to establish the facts requires assessment which is refused by the parents or carers. The order requires the production of the child and lasts for seven days. When applying for the order, a plan of assessment should be presented to the court. Contributing health professionals will have to ensure that an appropriate medical or psychiatric assessment can be undertaken during the time scale allowed. Since the assessment is expected to be multi-disciplinary, precise arrangements are necessary. The results of the assessment may be used subsequently in seeking a care or supervision order.

Apart from the Children Act, assessment of need can be undertaken under the Chronically Sick and Disabled Persons Act 1970, the Education Act 1981 or the Disabled Persons Act 1986.

Guardian ad Litem (GAL)   A guardian ad litem is an independent social worker who is appointed to safeguard the child's interests. One must be appointed, unless the court decides otherwise, in certain proceedings. These include care and supervision orders, emergency protection and child assessment orders. The guardian can instruct a solicitor and makes a report to the court. The guardian has a legal right of access to records held by the social services department and any health records they contain. Guardians provide important links between children, the court and the other agencies involved.

CONSENT AND OTHER CONSIDERATIONS

Before examining or assessing a child certain questions should be considered with regard to whether you have permission to do so.

A question of consent

- Who has the right to consent to the examination or assessment?
- What are the views of the child?
- Is the child the subject of a court order?
- Who has parental responsibility?
- Will the assessment be used in proceedings?
- Has a guardian ad litem been appointed?
- Is there a communication problem requiring special arrangements?

A young person of 16, in the absence of mental incapacity, and a younger child who, in the doctors view is of sufficient understanding to make an informed decision, can refuse to submit to any examination, assessment or treatment. Decisions of the court do not override the rights of these children. In the absence of freely given consent the doctor may be held in law to be guilty of assault. Valid consent includes an understanding of possible consequences.

For younger children, not able to give consent, consent should be obtained from parents. When consent is withheld by child or parents the facts should be reported to the court which gave directions. In some cases a specific issue order can be sought.

COURT STRUCTURE AND PROCEEDINGS

Public law cases are usually heard by specially trained magistrates drawn from Family Panels in a Family Proceedings Court. Magistrates are not legally qualified and are advised by a legally qualified clerk who administers the court. Magistrates are addressed as 'Sir', 'Madam', or 'Your Worship'. More complex cases are heard in a County or High Court, designated as a family hearing centre, under the direction of specially trained judges. In the County Court a circuit judge, His or Her Honour Judge X, is addressed as 'Your Honour'. In the High Court, Mr, Miss or Mrs Justice X is addressed as 'My Lord' or 'My Lady'.

Giving evidence

When writing a report it is essential to set out the facts relating to health and development clearly. Views and opinions should be identifiable as such.

Documentary evidence is admissible in proceedings under the Children Act but statement writers should be prepared to give oral evidence and to face cross examination on matters under dispute. A witness first takes the oath or makes an affirmation. He is first questioned by the lawyer acting on behalf of the party who called him to give evidence, then by those representing the other party or parties and possibly by the bench. Answers should be directed to the bench and expressed simply. Notes can be referred to after seeking the court's permission. They should be contemporaneous to the events being described. Once referred to, the notes may become evidence. Suitably qualified professionals may give an expert opinion in addition to evidence of facts.

When a doctor has evidence relevant to the case but is unwilling to appear voluntarily a subpoena may be issued by the court summoning the doctor to appear with appropriate records. Failure to comply constitutes contempt of court. More advice about courts and giving evidence is contained in the BMJ publication *ABC of Child Abuse*.

EMPLOYMENT OF CHILDREN

Law relating to child employment is contained in the Children and Young Persons Acts 1933 and 1963.

Children under 13 can only be employed except by their parents to undertake light agricultural or horticultural work. Subject to certain conditions licences may be granted to individual children to take part in performances.

Children aged 13–16 may not be employed
- before the close of school on school days,
- before 7.00 a.m. or after 7.00 p.m. on any day,
- for more than two hours on Sunday,
- to lift, carry or move anything heavy enough to injure them.

There are local byelaw modifications which include employment for up to one hour before school and requiring employers to notify the authority about children employed.

Some byelaws require the child to obtain a medical certificate from the Department of Public Health. Other statutes prohibit or limit the employment of children in dangerous or morally harmful occupations, for example in mines or on licensed premises. There are also restrictions on the types and conditions of work for 16–18 year olds.

REFERENCES AND FURTHER READING

Meadow R 1989 ABC of child abuse. British Medical Journal, London
The Children Act 1989. HMSO, London

Information

Epidemiology (Gr. *epi*-upon/*demos*-people) is the study of the distribution and determinants of diseases and injuries in human populations. Epidemiology with statistics make up the basic sciences of public health medicine. This work is often multidisciplinary and the process is dependent on good sources of information and efficient information systems. Community paediatricians as part of their duties need to monitor the health programmes for **populations** of children they serve. There are several distinct types of population to consider when referring to a population of children within a specified geographical area like a District Health Authority.

Types of population

Resident (and non-resident). This refers to all those children who are known to be resident within the area and includes children who may have moved into the area who were born in another area, that is non-resident children. These are an important group to identify when considering who is using the health services within a certain district or area.

Target. If you aim to effect an intervention programme like immunisation or examine services affecting part of a population it is referred to as the 'target' population

'At risk'. This refers to a population at specific risk of disease and there-

The population

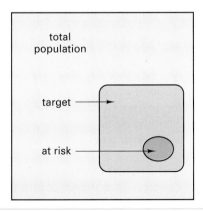

This diagram might refer to the distraction hearing test:

the **'population'** being that within the Health District;

the **'target'** group children being 7 – 9 months old; and

the **'at risk'** being those with a family history of deafness or those born prematurely.

fore in need of certain services, for example, children with a strong family history of congenital hip dislocation or congenital hearing loss, extremely premature infants, or children from a violent abusing family.

THE USES OF EPIDEMIOLOGY

Epidemiology has many uses. Basically it enables us to determine **what** conditions exist in a given population, **who** has the disease or condition, **where** the cases are located and **why** do they get the condition.

Description of disease

Description of the natural history of conditions enables useful information to be obtained about prognosis and causation.

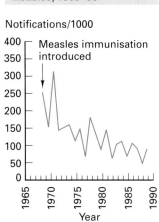

Measles, 1965–90

Notifications/1000

Measles immunisation introduced

Year

(Source: OPCS communicable disease reports 1987 – 88)

Prognosis. For example it is known from the 1970 National Child Development Study that the majority of asthmatic children under the age of 7 years do not require treatment for this condition by the time they reach 16 years (Butler & Golding 1986). When considering febrile convulsions, a knowledge of the family history and natural history of this condition helps determine treatment options and reassure parents. Children are unlikely to suffer from this condition after the age of 5 years and only 3% of those affected will go on to have true epilepsy.

Causation. Detailed cross-sectional studies describing environmental and nutritional variables have enabled hypotheses to be postulated about the causes of several diseases, for example, cot deaths and sleeping position, spina bifida and vitamin deficiency, leukaemia and the clustering of cases around nuclear power stations. Case-control studies have enabled the most influential of risk factors to be determined, for example, the link between multiple congenital abnormalities and maternal rubella, damp housing and asthma, smoking and glue ear, and HIV and immunosuppression.

Needs and planning

A knowledge of the prevalence of deafness, mental retardation and physical handicap in a population enables the planning of services for these groups of clients, such as the provision of specialist support teachers in school or the adaptation of public premises to enable access by the disabled. As sickle cell disease became more prevalent in certain communities there arose a need to provide specialist services like screening mothers at risk antenatally, the provision of a specialist counsellor and the education of hospital and community health staff about the implications for treatment and follow up. The difficulties of non-English speaking families in accessing health services provided by the NHS has led to the development of interpreter and link worker services in some Districts.

There are different forms of need depending on the perspective of the observer; perceived or felt need, professionally defined need and unmet need. In the present NHS structure the 'purchaser' is responsible for ascertaining the health needs of the local population and will have to consider all the above perspectives.

Preventative measures

When the aetiological agent or agents are known, then measures can be taken to prevent disease. The best known example of this is immunisation. Epidemiology can be used to assess the effectiveness. Primary prevention of dental caries by the fluoridation of the drinking water supplies and the prevention of rickets by dietary supplementation of Vitamin D to high risk groups (e.g. Asians) are two such programmes which have been shown to have successfully reduced the prevalence of these diseases.

Assess risk

Epidemiology is used to assess the risk of disease occurring in a community, e.g. lead poisoning in school children exposed to different volumes of carbon monoxide emission from nearby roads, the differential risks of serious road traffic accidents at different sites or the health risks associated with various forms of substance abuse. A knowledge of the different degrees of risk involved informs preventive measures such as legislative action or health education and health promotion programmes.

Effectiveness and efficiency

Once an intervention or screening test has been proved efficacious under study conditions, it is necessary to test its effectiveness when introduced into a programme within the community. Brown et al did this for the distraction test of hearing. The test carried out at about 7 months of age was shown to be effective in picking up only a small proportion of the total number of children with sensorineural hearing loss in a study within an inner city population. The authors concluded that the programme could be made more effective if the test was carried out following refresher training of the involved professionals and parental awareness heightened by the introduction of a hearing 'check' list. Efficiency could be improved if the highest risk groups were identified and tested soon after birth and the administration system was updated (Brown et al 1989).

The outcome of applying the distraction test hearing screening programme to a defined population, P = passed, > = referred to, and A = full audiological assessment. The flow chart illustrates the wider consequences of screening programmes for children, parents and the Health Services

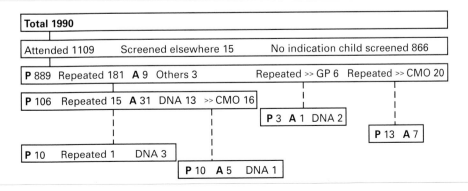

'Cost'

Cost efficiency. This means how much it costs to achieve the desired outcome in real circumstances. Immunisation programmes can be compromised by poor storage conditions of the vaccine although the vaccine might approach 100% **efficacy** under ideal conditions.

A cost effective service is one that provides the greatest effectiveness at the lowest cost. This type of analysis is particularly useful when comparing different models of service provision, e.g. intensive health visiting with a neighbourhood befriending scheme. The maintenance of breastfeeding or differential uptake of immunisation might be an outcome measure of such a service.

Cost benefit analysis is an economic analysis in which the costs of medical care and the loss of net earnings due to death or disability are considered. When a screening programme is being planned, cost-benefit analysis is applied and may determine who is going to be screened; for example, the maternal age cut off (35–40 years, depending on District) for Down's syndrome screening. The new lower cost 'triple test' can be applied to the entire ante-natal population and therefore reaches a larger at risk population not just those at highest risk (Wald et al 1988).

STRUCTURE OF INFORMATION

To use information correctly its structure has to be appreciated. There is a distinction between data and information. **Data** is the raw pieces of fact and **information** is the use of those facts for some specific purpose.

Rates

A rate is a measure of the frequency of a phenomenon. In epidemiology, a rate is an expression of the frequency with which an event occurs in a defined population; the use of rates rather than raw numbers is essential

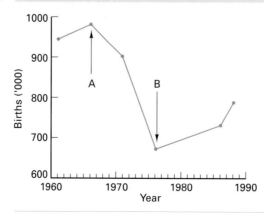

The differences in rates at two different times when the number of cases or events is identical but the denominator changes

If there were 2000 new cases of condition X, noted at both points A and B, the incidence rates of X in the population would be approximately 2 per 1000 and and 3 per 1000 respectively.

for comparison of experience between populations at different times, different places , or among different classes of people. The components of a rate are the numerator (above the line), the denominator (below the line), the specified time in which the events occur, and usually a multiplier, a power of 10, which converts the rate from an awkward fraction or decimal number to a whole number:

$$\text{Rate} = \frac{\text{Number of events in specified period}}{\text{Average population during the period}} \times 10^{n}$$

(Last)

Different sorts of rates

Prevalence: the number of persons affected at a specific point in time (numerator) as a proportion of the total number of persons in the population at that time. Prevalence may be measured at a point in time over a period of time (period prevalence).

Incidence: the number of **new** cases occurring during a specified time, (usually a year) as a proportion of the total population *at risk* of developing the condition.

Prevalence measures a combination of new and 'old' cases whereas incidence measures new occurrences only. The prevalence of a condition is a measure of the 'burden' of the condition on the community and is used in planning manpower and service facilities. It is often used to monitor chronic conditions like diabetes, asthma, rheumatoid arthritis etc. and is useful in monitoring the effect of intervention on the chronicity of illness, for example changing a swimming pool antiseptic solution may result in a measurable fall in the severity of eczema or asthma or providing skilled home nursing 'home care' may reduce the number of admissions to hospital with diabetes in adolescents.

In contrast, incidence is often used to monitor acute conditions and is a measure of the risk of disease to an individual (c.f. a population) and differences in incidence rates between communities may give valuable clues about the possible aetiology of a condition, like head injury differences between two schools with different playground surfaces or dental caries rates between two towns.

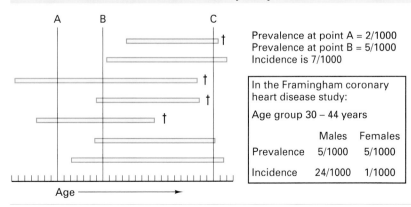

Prevalence and incidence rates in coronary artery disease

Prevalence at point A = 2/1000
Prevalence at point B = 5/1000
Incidence is 7/1000

In the Framingham coronary heart disease study:

Age group 30 – 44 years

	Males	Females
Prevalence	5/1000	5/1000
Incidence	24/1000	1/1000

Age ⟶

COMMONLY MEASURED RATES IN CHILD HEALTH

Stillbirth rate: babies born dead with a gestational age of at least 28 weeks per 1000 *total* births. There are international variations in the definitions used for stillbirths. Sweden uses fetal length (35 cm) and Denmark uses weight (under 1000 g) in addition to gestation to define stillbirths.

Perinatal mortality rate: Stillbirths and babies dying in the first 7 days of life per 1000 *total* births.

Neonatal mortality rate: babies dying in the first 28 days of life per 1000 *live* births.

Infant mortality rate: Infants dying in the first 12 months of life per 1000 live births.

Post-neonatal mortality rate: Infants dying between the ages of 1 month and 1 year per 1000 live births.

Why distinguish between the different time based mortality rates? The determinants of perinatal mortality and post-neonatal mortality differ greatly with the former reflecting antenatal and early postnatal care and the latter reflecting more social and environmental factors.

Perinatal mortality rate by DHA

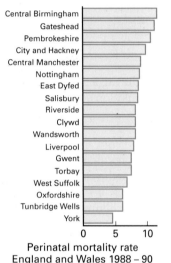

Perinatal mortality rate
England and Wales 1988 – 90

Time period of mortality rates

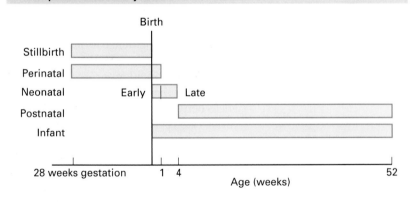

(Source: OPCS monitor DH3 91/2)

SOURCES OF DATA

Data about child health comes from a wide variety of sources and is held in a variety of forms of varying accessibility but basically it falls into two main categories: routine and special surveys.

Routine

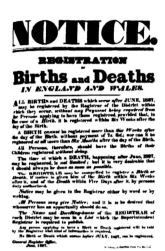

Census. This is a regular survey of the population, carried out every 10 years. The Doomsday Book is often considered to be the first national survey of this kind in the UK. Completion of the census form has been a statutory requirement since the Census Act of 1920. The answers given are treated in the strictest confidence and the results are published in an anonymous form. It is designed to count the population and its various attributes including data on the household, the numbers living in that household, amenities (bathroom, central heating etc.), marital status, occupation, country of birth, patterns of personal and public transport. The last census was in 1991 and for the first time collected data on 'long-term' illness and more detailed data on self perceived ethnicity. Analysis is available at levels down to individual electoral wards.

Births records are kept of all births within the UK. The midwife or doctor attending the delivery of an infant has to make a notification to the District Medical Officer (Director of Public Health) and the parents have to obtain a birth certificate, within six weeks, from the Registrar of births, marriages and deaths. Originally these records were kept by local parishes but now OPCS collates the data from around the country and publishes detailed analyses in quarterly and annual reports. All abortions carried out legally are registered as to the cause, as are congenital malformations ascertained within the first 7 days postnatally. The birth rate is beginning to climb again as the postwar children are coming of child bearing age.

> **Mortality data**
>
> Mortality statistics in childhood are published by the Office of Population Censuses and Surveys (OPCS) and are analysed by age, sex, cause and social class. Data is available on individual Regional and District Health Authority differences in mortality rates.

Morbidity data

GP consultation rate

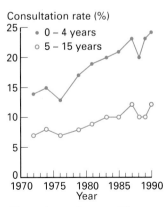

Chronic and acute illness

Infectious disease. Certain infectious diseases are notifiable (see chapter on infections) and the data is published on a weekly and quarterly basis (OPCS). In addition, data is collected from hospital and other microbiology laboratories (eg Communicable Disease Surveillance Centre).

GP consultations. There have been two national studies of morbidity statistics in general practice: 1971/2 and 1981/2. The latter involved 48 different practices of all types and 332 270 patients. Just over 71% of persons at risk consulted their GPs during the study year. The consultation rate varied with the age of the patient – the highest rate was for the under fives, 98%. Commonest reasons for GP consultation in this age group were respiratory tract and infectious disease. Increasingly, there are more consultations for preventative measures like immunisation and other aspects of child health surveillance.

General Household Survey. This is an annual survey of a sample of 12 000 households nationally and gives useful data about home accidents, acute and chronic illnesses and domestic amenities. Further details on the type of injury and accident is available from the Department of

Hospital discharge and death rates, 1979–85

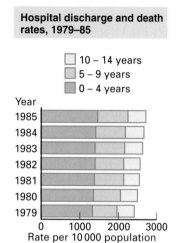

- 10 – 14 years
- 5 – 9 years
- 0 – 4 years

Year
1985
1984
1983
1982
1981
1980
1979

0   1000   2000   3000
Rate per 10 000 population

Trade and Industry Home Accidents Surveillance Scheme. A proxy measure of morbidity is obtained from analysis of sickness benefit claims (Health and Personal Social Services statistics).

Hospital episodes. Data about hospital admissions and discharges has been collected annually for over 30 years as part of the Hospital In-Patient Enquiry (HIPE) . This is a 1 in 10 sample of all admissions and discharges. It is a service-orientated statistic and therefore individual children who require multiple hospital admissions have a greater likelihood of being counted more than once. Data on hospital episodes are now collected as part of the Korner returns (see later). This type of data is useful in examining trends of hospital usage by children. The episodes are coded by ward staff using the International Classification of Diseases (ICD-9).There is a tendency for greater numbers of admissions of children for shorter time periods.

Hospital admissions

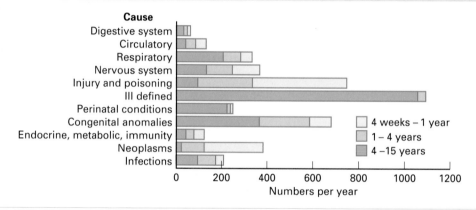

Cause

Digestive system
Circulatory
Respiratory
Nervous system
Injury and poisoning
Ill defined
Perinatal conditions
Congenital anomalies
Endocrine, metabolic, immunity
Neoplasms
Infections

- 4 weeks – 1 year
- 1 – 4 years
- 4 –15 years

0   200   400   600   800   1000   1200
Numbers per year

(Source: OPCS 8/91 DH 91/92)

Mental health. Since 1959, data has been collected on admissions to mental illness, mental handicap hospitals and Units for children aged 0–9 and 10–14. Numbers, sex and diagnostic groups are collected (Mental Health Enquiry).

Registers. There are many registers of individual diseases affecting children including: cancer, physical disability, hearing , speech and visual impairments.

Other

There are several other sources of routinely collected data about children which are useful.

Anthropometry. The St. Thomas' survey of height and growth is an annual, continuous study providing means and distributions of height and weight of children aged 5 to 9 years obtained from a large sample of school children followed up through primary school (Chinn et al 1989).

Infant feeding. There are 5-yearly surveys of infant feeding practice up to the age of 9 months giving data on the proportions of babies breast and/or bottle fed at different ages by age of the mother, social class based on parents' occupation, education and region.

Smoking and substance abuse. There are biennial and annual surveys to measure the prevalence of these behaviours among school children.

Data on Education and Manpower (health) is available from the General Household Survey (GHS) and Health and Personal Social Services statistics respectively.

Office of Population Census and Surveys (OPCS) is a central government department which collects and collates data about health and other demographic variables (see references). Many of the sources above will be available in the medical school or library.

Special surveys

The other main source of child health data are ad hoc surveys and independent epidemiological studies. There are three main types of non-experimental (descriptive) epidemiological studies: cohort, cross-sectional and case-control.

An outline of some of the better known cohort studies from which a wealth of data about the natural history of many childhood diseases has been obtained is also given with the references.

The Child Health and Education Study is a example of a **cohort study.** It included an examination of the prevalence of squint and other visual defects in 5 year olds. 973 of the 13 005 children for whom information was available were said to have had a squint at some time. Of the 7.5% of the children who had had a squint, by the age of 5, only 3.8% still had a problem. It also found that those children with squints were more likely to be of low birthweight, have had a shorter duration of breastfeeding, greater numbers of moves of household, mothers who smoked and came from larger families.

The British Paediatric Surveillance Units findings on Reye syndrome (a rare and serious childhood encephalopathy) is an example of a **case-control** study. The parents of 106 children who had had Reye syndrome and those of 185 children who had febrile illnesses were interviewed in order to compare anti-pyretic drug exposure prior to admission. 59% of the cases compared with only 26% of the controls had taken aspirin. Significantly more control children had taken paracetamol compared to the cases. The authors concluded that there was a strong association between Reye syndrome and pre-admission aspirin (Hall et al 1988). The routine use of aspirin in children under 12 years has been discouraged since 1986.

An example of a **specific enquiry** is one completed recently which examined the health, lifestyle, physical measurements and the response to antismoking advice given to adolescent smokers in a general practice

The essential differences between these studies

Cross-sectional study

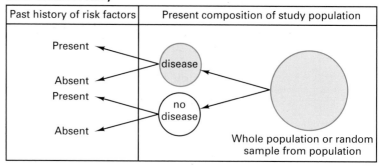

Case-control study

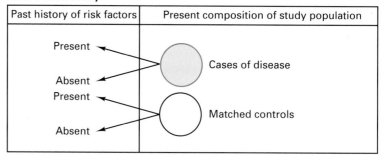

Cohort study

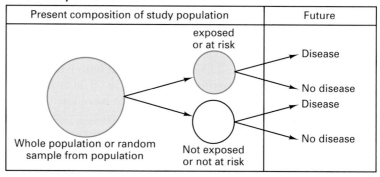

setting. The prevalence of smoking was 28% at 17 years, 11% at 15, and 3% at 13. Regular smokers were found to be heavier, drank more alcohol, took less exercise and didn't sleep as long as their non-smoking peers. The study then went on to measure the response to specific anti-smoking advice and health promotion (Townsend et al 1991).

It is quite common for different types of study to be combined, for example, a case-control study might be 'nested' within a cohort study. The first part of the study described above is a **cross-sectional** type and the second part of the study would be considered an 'intervention' study. It is also possible to pool the results of many smaller randomized controlled trials – a technique known as **'meta-analysis'**.

INTERPRETATION OF DATA

For data to be an effective source of information, its limitations must be appreciated and the following questions might be asked of it.

Is the data accurate, is it a valid reflection of the activity that is being recorded? An example of this might be the accuracy of diagnosis coding made by ward clerks interpreting doctors' case records following discharge of children from hospital.

Is the population size adequate and representative of the population you might wish to apply the data to? A study of the poor success rate of a hospital based enuretic clinic may reflect a bias in the selection of patients if applied to a community setting where a different population of children is likely to be seen.

Is it timely? An apparent trend in the decreasing number of children being admitted to mental hospital might reflect the policy of health authorities, in more recent years, to contain cases in the community as opposed to a true decrease in the prevalence of these disorders. Care has to be taken in interpreting data collected historically.

Are there alternative explanations for a particular finding? Is the association of asthma deaths to inhaler use in the 1960s due to a direct causal link with the aerosol content or related to a coincidental increase in an environmental pollutant?

An appreciation of the 'structure of data' enables the investigator to systematically analyse the various likely sources of error.

SOURCES OF ERROR IN DATA

Numerator error

Diagnostic inaccuracy is a source of error especially in considering morbidity and mortality statistics. The cause(s) of death are written onto a death certificate by the certifying physician and vary in their accuracy depending on the skills, training, interest and diagnostic acumen of the individual or the institution where that person died as well as the knowledge available within the medical community as a whole. Criteria for diagnosis may change and this may affect the magnitude of the numerator, for example, change in the use of the term 'wheezy bronchitis' to asthma.

Incomplete identification (ascertainment) of cases. An example of this is in the ascertainment of congenital malformations. OPCS ensure that all the identifying centres (all District Health Authorities) limit the identification period to within the first seven days post-natally. A sub-

Age of detection of congenital abnormalities

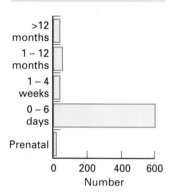

stantial number of congenital malformations are discovered after this period, especially the less obvious cardiac and urogenital anomalies. There are many factors which determine whether a patient seeks help from the health services including cultural and social factors and the availability of and accessibility to services. The effect of variations in illness behaviour is most marked in mild, non-fatal and self-limiting conditions. The vast majority of childhood illness is treated by parents and relatives within the family. It is estimated that less than 3% of a child's illness experience is within a hospital setting. This obviously limits the value of routinely collected morbidity statistics if one is applying this to estimating the child's *total* illness experience.

Recording systems. Amongst the reasons for variation in the completeness and comparability of different sources of data are:
* the doctor's view of the value of the records
* the simplicity and efficiency of a records system
* changes in the conventions for coding and classification of disease and the rules for selecting priorities among multiple diagnoses.

Denominator error

There are several sources of denominator error which can affect the accuracy of rates.

Parent Held Record: a source of valuable information

---

6 WEEK REVIEW

Name	D.O.B.- / - / -
Sticky label	
(with bar code or OMR)	I.D. No.

Date of review:- / - / -   Age: _____ Weeks
Weight _____ (Kgs.) ____ th.   Centile Head Circumference: __ . __ cms. __ th.   Centile

Risk factors for vision or hearing problems: Yes/No
Risk factors for hip dislocation: Yes/No
Feeding (Breast/bottle/mixed)
Any parental concerns?

Comments

Physical examination   Comments

Fontanelles ☐
Eyes/visual behaviour ☐
Hearing ☐
Heart/pulses ☐
Hips ☐
Spine ☐
General tone ☐
Movement ☐
Skin ☐
Testes/genitalia ☐   **Action**: none/follow up/refer comm. paed/refer hosp/other
Other ☐

☑	A	S
Normal	Abnormal	Suspect

Examiner's Name: Signature
Staff I.D. No. _____ Date:- /- /-
Where done: G.P. surgery/health auth. clinic/home/other

Population size. The size of the population is estimated at the time of the census and may vary in between because of migration into or out of the community. Estimates are made on inter-census population size which are based on previous and projected patterns of migration. It is important to be aware of changes in population size when carrying out prevalence studies at wide time intervals.

Population structure. Age, sex, changing fertility patterns, occupational distribution, housing and industrial decay or development all influence the structure of a population and the accuracy of the denominator.

Population boundaries. The local authority, social services, education and health services may have different geographical boundaries and this will influence the area within which a population is being counted. The value of co-terminosity is being appreciated in relation to health services and inter-sectoral planning like accident prevention strategies.

Errors can be reduced to a degree by the use of standard coding systems (e.g. ICD 9, READ), use of standard recording and registration procedures and the use of denominator populations derived from similar sources using comparable methods.

HEALTH INFORMATION SYSTEMS

The actual means of obtaining and analysing data can be considered parts of an 'information system'. This need not necessarily be a computer system although when dealing with large quantities of data this is obviously an advantage. As medical and clinical audit are becoming part of the work of the doctor in both hospital and community practice, considerable interest has developed in this area.

Records are a system of recording data on patients and are numerous in their structure and appearance. Clearly structured notes enable data to be collected relatively easily about a large number of children. Not all records are in the professional domain. The parent held child health record is a booklet of A5 size which contains valuable health education and promotion data as well as places for the parent to record contacts with health service and other staff. In addition, some Districts have incorporated carbonless copy sheets into the record which have been placed in the sections of the booklet relating to different stages of the child health surveillance programme, onto which midwives, health visitors, GPs, community and hospital paediatricians can write details, e.g. findings of the 6 week check or results of the 7 month hearing test (see next chapter). Both the parents and the professionals then have copies of the same data.

Much of the data collected and held on computer, e.g. staff activity analysis has been for the use of managers and administrators and therefore is structured in such a way as not to be particularly of use to the clinician. This leads to poor motivation of health workers in collecting the data, often with duplication of effort, and the relative inflexibility of much of the software means that little in the way of useful data can be extracted from the system.

In 1980, the Secretary of State for Health and Social Services appointed a working party (Korner Committee) to review the existing health service information systems and recommend changes and developments. The main recommendations were that all the health districts should have computer based integrated information systems covering all aspects of health service activity which were *patient* based and that management (and epidemiological) data would be captured automatically as the normal patient management, laboratory and scientific tasks are being performed (in contrast to a separate system of activity recording). The Committee recommended 'minimum data sets' for each area of health service activity in order that a common core of data from each district could be collated centrally for comparison. A common patient numbering system has been introduced in many districts (Korner number) in order that records might be linked. It remains to be seen how far these recommendations have been put into place and what advantages will be gained by the professionals themselves by using these district information systems (DIS).

USES OF COMPUTERS IN CHILD HEALTH

Below are given some of the present and potential uses of computer systems in child health.

Surveillance

The largest child health orientated computer system in England and Wales is the National Child Health System (NCHS) which is used in approximately two thirds of the health districts in the UK. It records data on pre-school and school health surveillance, immunisation and in some districts children with 'special needs'. Other surveillance systems are cancer registration and congenital malformation systems.

> **Ideally, a good system can:**
>
> - facilitate the early recognition of disease patterns
> - identify changes in environmental and host factors that may lead to an increase in the frequency of disease and
> - monitor the safety and effectiveness of preventive and control measures.

Individual patient care

By linking laboratory requests and results (e.g. haematology, biochemistry and microbiology) to a computer terminal on the ward or in the community, clinical decision making can be facilitated. Audiology and paramedical links could be made which would be a great advantage for the community paediatrician trying to liaise with a range of different professionals. Individual treatment protocols or screening programmes can be audited, e.g. a child who has failed to attend the clinic for a hearing test can have his record automatically highlighted so that when he is seen on another occasion this can be brought to the parents' attention.

Health Service administration

Computers can be used to schedule screening of high risk groups or the detection of regular defaulters. If it became apparent that there were a group of infants living in a specific area who were regularly defaulting on immunisation clinics, it may be more appropriate to bring the services to them, for example a mobile health visitor immunisation service for a particular housing estate. Computers can allow these groups to be more readily identified.

Research

Epidemiological research: routine statistical analysis and survey data tabulation, searching data for statistically significant correlations etc. and health care provision research, e.g. looking at trends in need for services and their resource implications are made much easier to interpret using data held in computer form and results displayed in alternative ways.

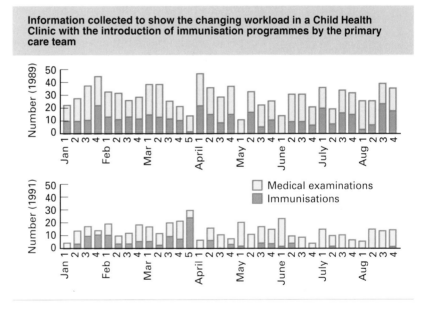

Information collected to show the changing workload in a Child Health Clinic with the introduction of immunisation programmes by the primary care team

Record linkage

An interesting development is the use of record linkage: health records of an individual patient collated from different sources in order to give a more detailed history of health events throughout that person's life. This technique has been used to study the relationships between antenatal events in mothers and the later development of disease in their infants (vaginal cancer and antenatal oestrogen treatment) or the relationship between birthweight and later cardiovascular disease in middle age discovered by linking health visitor and GP records. Most record linkage studies are done on an ad hoc basis. The use of computers enables record linkage to be done on a routine basis (Oxford Record Linkage Project). The tracking of illnesses in different members of a family and their collation can lead to a better understanding of genetic influences on disease patterns.

Data protection and confidentiality

It is essential that health workers respect the confidentiality of records and this is particularly important when considering data held on computers. The Data Protection Act 1987 has helped to set standards of good practice when dealing with data held on patients. Patients are now allowed access to their medical records on request and the 1990 Access to Health Records Act ensures that these rights are upheld. A parent can obtain access to a child's records only if the child gives consent (and is capable of giving consent).

SCREENING

Screening was defined in 1951 by the US Commission on Chronic Illness as, 'The presumptive identification of unrecognized disease or defect by the application of tests, examinations or other procedures which can be applied rapidly. Screening tests sort out apparently well persons who probably have the disease from those who probably do not. A screening test is not intended to be diagnostic.' Once a person has been found to have positive or suspicious findings further tests are necessary in order to make the definitive diagnosis.

Screening is just one component of preventative child health care and is a form of **secondary prevention** of disease. This is the prevention of an impairment from progressing or its complete removal (or cure). The recognition of a raised TSH in the neonatal period following the heel-prick screening test enables definitive investigation and diagnosis of congenital hypothyroidism and subsequent thyroid hormone replacement therapy to be administered. **Primary prevention** occurs when the impairment is completely prevented from affecting the person, e.g. immunisation to prevent infectious diseases or wearing seat belts to prevent injury in a road traffic accident. **Tertiary prevention** is the minimising of handicap, once an impairment is well established and cannot be reversed or cured.

Screening is often confused with surveillance. Surveillance is the *ongoing* scrutiny of disease; in epidemiological terms, its main purpose is to detect changes in trend or distribution in order to initiate investigative or control methods. Child health surveillance is thus a combination of activities not just the application of specific screening tests.

Surveillance includes

- early detection of disease
- health education and promotion
- arranging appropriate intervention where necessary
- monitoring the growth and development of the child
- monitoring the general well-being of the child and family (non-specific oversight)

A screening procedure should fulfil the following criteria (WHO, Wilson & Jungner 1968)

- the condition sought should be an important public health problem
- the natural history of the condition, including its development from latent to declared disease should be adequately understood
- there should be a recognised latent or early symptomatic phase
- there should be a suitable test or examination
- the test should be relatively simple and should be acceptable to the population being tested
- facilities for diagnosis and treatment should be available
- there should be an accepted treatment for patients with recognised disease
- there should be an agreed policy on whom to treat as patients
- the cost of case finding (including diagnosis and subsequent treatment of patients) should be economically balanced in relation to the possible expenditure on medical care as a whole
- case finding should be a continuing process and not a 'once for all' project.

RELIABILITY

The reliability of the test refers to the degree to which the results obtained by a measurement procedure can be replicated. The test must give consistent results when performed more than once on the same individual. There are three main sources of variation.

Variation caused by the observer – this may be due to differences between observers (inter-) or variation in the performance of the same observer (intra-), for example in the recording positive and negative responses of infants to screening test sounds.

Variation within the subject – the child's response to test sounds depends upon his level of interest and arousal. A hearing loss may fluctuate from day to day. Most physiological measurements: height, weight, blood sugar, blood pressure, vary in this way.

Variation in the method itself. The equipment may be faulty or incorrectly calibrated. Test conditions such as levels of background noise during hearing tests may vary.

All these variations can be reduced or eliminated by standardisation of equipment and procedures and intensive training and evaluation of observers.

SENSITIVITY AND SPECIFICITY

Sensitivity is the ability of the test to identify correctly those who have the disease.

Specificity is the ability of a test to identify correctly those who do not have the disease.

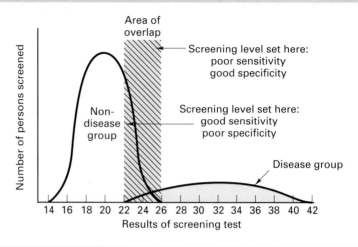

An ideal test would reach 100% sensitivity and 100% specificity. In practice, this combination is virtually unobtainable. An improvement in one criterion is often associated with a deterioration of the other. Sensitivity and specificity vary according to the level which is chosen to separate normal from abnormal results. This is shown in the diagram plotting the frequency distribution of the attribute and the results obtained when the cut-off point between 'normal and abnormal' is changed. Sensitivity and specificity are not of equal value. A test which is 40% sensitive and 90% specific could not be compared with a test which is 90% sensitive and 40% specific. In the first case 60% of those with the disease would not be detected. In the second case 10% of the diseased group would be missed, but 60% false positives would be generated. Specificity is made with the reference to the non-diseased group only, sensitivity with reference to the diseased group only.

Calculating sensitivity and specificity

REFERENCE STANDARD

TEST	True positives **a**	False positives **b**
	False negatives **c**	True negatives **d**

SENSITIVITY = (a/a+c) The ability of the test to give a positive result in those individuals who have the disease

SPECIFICITY = (d/b+d) The ability of the test to give a negative result in those individuals who do not have the disease

PREDICTIVE VALUE This is a measure of the degree to which a positive test result predicts the presence of disease (may be positive or negative) (a/a+b or c/c+d respectively)

Condition sought	Test to be applied	Agreed treatment	Justification for screening
Antenatal screening: examples			
Spinal bifida, anencephaly, hydrocephaly	Serum α-fetoprotein Detailed antenatal ultrasonagraphy	Rarely fetal surgery (insertion of shunt)	Prevention of severe handicap
Down's syndrome	Antenatal maternal serum levels of HCG Unconjugated oestriol and α-fetoprotein ('triple test')	Termination of pregnancy if agreed after counselling	Prevention of severe on mental handicap
Duchenne muscular dystrophy	Chromosomal analysis of amniotic fluid	Counselling and termination offered	50% chance of an affected male infant
Neonatal screening: examples			
Phenylketonuria	Guthrie test — heel prick blood	Low phenylalanine diet	Prevention of mental handicap
Hypothyroidism	Blood T4/TSH — heel prick blood	Thyroxine	Prevention of mental handicap
Cystic fibrosis	Immunoreactive trypsin	Pancreatic enzymes, physiotherapy	Prevent early lung damage, genetic counselling
Sensorineural hearing loss	Programmed otoacoustic emission	Early counselling and speech therapy intervention	Diminish handicap of late speech communication development
Congenital dislocation of the hip	Barlow's and Ortolani's test. Hip must abduct fully and is non-dislocatable	Splinting and observation	Poor results and need for surgery in late diagnosed cases
Undescended testes	Clinical examination	Orchidopexy	Risk of infertility, malignancy, psychological problems
Hypospadias	Clinical examination	Surgery	Psychological effects of untreated condition
Cleft palate	Clinical examination	Referral to plastic surgeon	Development of normal speech
Talipes	Clinical examination	Orthopaedic referral	Prevention of handicap
Hydrocephalus	Measurement of head circumference	Insertion of ventriculo-atrial/peritoneal shunt	Prevention of handicap
Congenital heart disease	Clinical examination	Paediatric or paediatric cardiology clinic	Correction of defect. Prevention of SBE
Pre-school screening: examples			
Squint	Cover test	Patching, orthoptic exercises or surgery	Prevention of amblyopia
Visual handicap	Detection of abnormal visual behaviour in infant — standardised test usually matching letters (STYCAR) from age 2½ – 3 years. Video-Photorefraction (not yet in widespread use)	Correction of refractive error — educational and developmental guidance	Early intervention to reduce effect of possible handicap
Deafness	Distraction test Cooperation test Performance test or speech discrimination test Sweep test Tympanometry	To audiological centre — depends on severity and cause	Minimise handicap and promote normal language development
Growth disorders	Accurate measurement of length/height	Referral to a specialist growth clinic	Discovery of conditions where treatment is available, e.g. growth hormone deficiency, coeliac disease, hypothyroidism
Child abuse or potential abuse situations	History (PMH, FH or SH) Clinical examination	Agreed procedures generally laid down at local level	Prevention of injury. Help for parents and child
Dental caries	Clinical examination	Dental treatment and health education	Prevention of pain and need for dental extraction
School age screening: examples			
Scoliosis (11 – 14 years) (not in natural programme)	Clinical examination	Orthopaedic clinic	Prevention of severe deformity
Colour blindness	Ishihara colour test	Discussion of possible career limitations. No treatment	Minimal
Infestation	Clinical examination by school nurse	School treatment centre or GP	Prevent spread
Depression	Interview. The quiet, isolated, withdrawn child is frequently missed	Discussion and referral	? Prevention of adult psychopathology

Predictive value

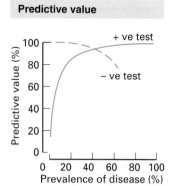

In screening and diagnostic tests, the probability that a person with a positive test is a true positive (the person does have the disease) is referred to as the 'predictive value of a positive test'. The predictive value of a negative test is the probability that a person with a negative test does not have the disease. Obviously, high predictive values are desirable. The value of the positive predictive value of a test is a/a+b and the value of a negative test is d/c+d. The diagram shows the relationship between predictive value and prevalence when the test used has a high sensitivity 95% and a high specificity 95%. Even with a screening test which has a high sensitivity and specificity, the predictive value will be low if the condition is rare.

Yield

The yield of a screening test is the number or proportion of cases of a condition accurately identified by the test (= a/a+b+c+d).

The yield of a test can be improved by:

- improving the test characteristics, i.e. increasing the sensitivity e.g. by intensive staff training
- screening at the optimum time – this requires a knowledge of the natural history of the disease. For example, screening for 'glue ear' at school entry as opposed to the final year of primary school gives a higher yield of cases because of the tendency for this condition to spontaneously resolve with increasing age.
- repeat screening – testing for colour blindness is undertaken on a once only basis around 11 years whereas measurement of visual acuity needs to be repeated at intervals since changes occur with age: the yield of the test will be greater during puberty than in the early junior school years.
- selection of high risk groups or individuals – the prevalence of disease is higher in these categories so that hearing screening of very low birthweight babies using oto-acoustic emissions will yield a group of 6% of all babies born which will contain 60% of all sensorineural hearing losses. Similarly selective screening of disadvantaged children for language problems will yield much higher numbers than in the general population of children as a whole.

Other issues

Cost. Screening for disease within a community has its costs, not only in financial terms but also in emotional ones too. For example , if a test has a sensitivity of 90% (high by most standards) and a specificity of 98% and the true prevalence of the condition is 10% of the population (n=1000), then at best the screen will pick up 90 patients. However, for every 5 'true' patients identified there is one who will have a false positive result and will be referred on for further investigation. This will mean not only additional costs of definitive tests, transport to the clinic, loss of employment but also more worryingly the additional concern and anxiety produced in a family because of the possibility of the patient having the disease itself. Similarly, if a person has the disease and the test is negative for that disease (10 of the total 100 patients will have such a result in the example given), then the costs of not obtaining early treatment may be very great, e.g. a false negative PKU or hypothyroidism test could have serious consequences in terms of late replacement therapy.

Any screening programme is only as good as the people who participate in it. One of the main issues around the **adequacy of cover** of many programmes is that the very people at highest risk are the ones who are not coming up to be screened. The prevalence of language and other developmental disorders is higher in the more deprived sections of our society and yet the services are not reaching them. There may be many reasons for this including: transport difficulties, financial restraints, organisational (the isolated single mother having to cope with four children under five years of age), and the value placed on the programme by the community. There is a significant advantage in being able to identify screening defaulters so that alternative approaches can be used, e.g. language stimulation programmes in day nurseries or 'captive' testing, i.e. the sweep hearing test or dental screening carried out for all school children soon after entry within the school itself (as opposed to a special clinic setting).

A distinction has to be made between screening tests and **case finding**. In the former, the screening test, if positive for a specific condition, is followed by more definitive tests. A McCormick toy discrimination test may be followed by free field audiometry in a controlled soundproofed room within an audiology clinic; or, a positive Guthrie test will be followed by a full blood amino acid electrophoretic laboratory analysis. In the case of detecting testicular maldescent, the test used, careful physical examination of the groin, is diagnostic in itself and need not be followed by any other definitive tests in order to make a decision for the surgeon to treat.

Who is responsible for carrying out the procedure on any individual? Neglect of this essential aspect may cause a child not to be seen at all or result in chaotic overlap and waste of effort between groups such as health visitors, school nurses, community paediatricians and family practitioners. Confusion can result from different decisions on future management. A combination of better communication between practitioners and the application of routine clinical audit to this aspect of programme management will hopefully reduce the uncertainties in this area.

A list of sources of information is given in Appendix C.

The next chapter describes the various components of the child health surveillance programme in greater detail.

Summary of Korner Report Working Group D on Community Health Services, January 1983

'For some parts of Community Health Services, wholly clerical systems would be adequate. But for others, such as the child immunisation, screening and surveillance programmes, the very active administration required and the need to co-ordinate the different programmes argue for computer-based systems justified on service-delivery grounds. For patient care services, planning considerations – the need to view District services as a whole – argue for a computer-based system. And the need to make the best possible use of highly trained nursing staff suggests that, in general, data collection and collation by nurses should be minimised.'

The basic component in respect of which data are collected is the patient or client consultation. In respect of each consultation there are nine separate areas that require collection:

- the programme within which the contact occurred
- the location at which it occurred
- the age, or age group, of the patient or client
- its content (eg the type of intervention carried out)
- the management unit to which the member of staff carrying out the work was attached
- the discipline and grade of that member of staff
- additional categorisation of the patient
- the source of referral of the patient
- subsequent action

Some examples from within the recommended data set are:

Health care programmes:

Vaccination and immunisation
Professional advice and support
Screening
School health services
Other health promotional activities

Location:

Patient/client's home
Hospital
GP premises
Other clinic premises

Age of patient:

Pre-school
School health

Content of consultation:

Technical tests and assessments, e.g. taking samples and measurements for examinations
Technical procedures, e.g. injections, syringing and related procedures
Nursing care: General nursing care
　　　　　　　 Social help
　　　　　　　 Home assessment, delivery of aids, etc.
Provision of advice, support and education in relation to health and in relation to social problems

Source of referral:

GP or hospital discharge
Other source of referral

Subsequent action:

Surveillance: Number requesting further action sub-divided by
　　　　　　 – further investigation
　　　　　　 – recall for further surveillance
Screening: Number of positive results
Number of positive results subsequently confirmed
School health programme:
– Number of children for multi-disciplinary assessment
– Number of children formally identified as requiring continuing school health service report

REFERENCES AND FURTHER READING

Barker D J P, Winter P D, Osmond C, Margetts B, Simmonds S J 1989 Weight in infancy and death from ischaemic heart disease. Lancet ii: 577–80
Brown J, Watson E, Alberman E 1989 Screening for hearing loss. Archives of Disease of Childhood 64: 1488–95
Butler J R 1989 Child health surveillance in primary care. A critical review. HMSO, London
Butler N R, Golding J 1986 From birth to five – A study of the health and behaviour of Britain's five year olds. Pergamon Press, Oxford
Chinn S, Price C E, Rona R J 1989 Need for new reference curves for height. Archives of Disease in Childhood 64: 1545–53
Hall S M, Plaster P A, Glasgow J F T, Hancock P 1988 Pre-admission antipyretics in Reye's syndrome. Archives of Disease of Childhood 63: 857–66
Last J M 1988 A dictionary of epidemiology. Oxford University Press, Oxford
Royal College of General Practitioners and OPCS 1986 Morbidity statistics from general practice 1981–1982. 3rd National Study. RCGP, London
Steering Group on Health Services Information (Chairman: E Korner) 1983 A report from working group D, Community Health Services. HMSO, London
Steering Group on Health Services Information (Chairman: E Korner) 1984 6th report to the Secretary of State. HMSO, London
Townsend J, Wilkes H, Haines A, Jarvis M 1991 Adolescent smokers seen in general practice. Health, life-style, physical measurements, and response to anti-smoking advice. British Medical Journal 303: 947–50
Wald N J, Cuckle H S, Densem J W et al 1988 Maternal serum screening for Down's syndrome in early pregnancy. British Medical Journal 297: 883–7
Wilson J M G, Jungner G 1968 Principles and practice of screening for disease. Public health papers No. 34. World Health Organization, Geneva

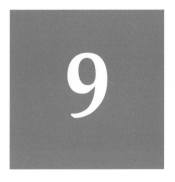

9 Surveillance

Child health surveillance is a programme that is offered to all children with the aims of preventing ill health and promoting optimum development through immunisation and education, and of ensuring the early detection of abnormalities by facilitating early recognition and referral by parents and through the application of screening tests by professionals.

> **Butler (1989) divided the preventive health care for children into:**
>
> **Primary prevention** activities: dental prophylaxis, immunisation, prevention of accidents, prevention of child abuse, health education for the child, education, advice and support to parents and health promotion;
> **Secondary prevention**: individual sceening tests and examinations, and non-specific oversight of health and
> **Tertiary prevention**: for the child with recognised special needs.

The service also includes **liaison functions** to education and social service departments. Non-specific oversight is an important concept which takes on board the importance of 'seeing whether anything is wrong' rather than confining the consultation to a search for named conditions. It implies that a vigilant and experienced person will identify a much wider spectrum of problems and needs than they would by adding further items to the list of individual screening tests.

Surveillance is the cornerstone of paediatric practice. A successful programme should result in low levels of preventable disorders, and reduce the acute load and long term disability arising from these problems. Likewise referrals will be appropriate and timely. In a poor system many referrals will be inappropriate and too late. The secondary and tertiary care systems can only function effectively and efficiently if there is a successful child health surveillance programme.

Success depends upon specific sensitive screening tests, the skills of the professionals involved and the efficiency of the system designed to deliver the programme. The content of Child Health Surveillance in the UK is summarised in *Health for all Children* (Hall 1991). This presents the evidence for the various elements of each check and recommends a core programme that has the support of all the professional bodies involved. The core programme is slim in comparison to earlier protocols because only the items of proven effectiveness are included. This means that not only will the procedures identify a child in need of help, with few false

Prevention is better than cure

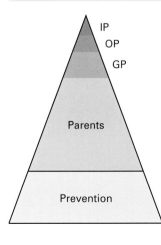

Health service contacts in the first year of life in 110 infants (Nottingham 1984)

	GP surgery	GP home visit	A & E	Hospital OPD + IP	Child Health Clinic	Total
Mean number of visits	6.5	0.5	0.3	0.8	12.9	21.1
Total	715	59	39	92	1414	2322

Top ten reasons for attending:

GP surgery

Cold	147
Cough	97
Immunisation	72
Gastroenteritis	60
Nappy rash	57
Feeding problem	52
General worry	43
Eye problem	31
Thrush	22
Stool problem	21

GP home visit

Cold	22
Gastroenteritis	14
Feeding problem	10
Ear infection	3
Cough	2
Croup	2
Pharyngitis	1
Inguinal hernia	1
Immunisation reaction	1
Balanitis	1

A & E

Minor head injury	8
Gastroenteritis	5
Cold	4
Bruising and fracture	3
Non-accidental injury	2
Inguinal hernia	2
No diagnosis	2
Feeding problem	1
General worry	1
Stool problem	1

Out-/in-patient

Gestation/SCBU	20
Cleft palate	10 (1 infant)
Pulmonary stenosis	6 (1 infant)
Gastroenteritis	6
Hypospadias	5
Inguinal hernia	5
Ear infection	3
Asthma	3
Cold	3
Umbilical granuloma	3

Child health clinic

Routine weight	736
Immunisation	204
Feeding problem	119
Six week check	78
Nappy rash	57
Cold	39
Teething	36
Eight month check	28
Eye problem	26
General worry	25

All

Routine weight	736
Immunisation	276
Colds	215
Feeding problem	182
Nappy rash	114
Cough	107
6 week check	97
Gastroenteritis	91
'General worry'	71
Eye problem	55

positives and false negatives, but also that there are interventions available that will improve outcomes. The authors place great emphasis on parental recognition of health and developmental problems and the role of health education in enhancing these skills. Child health surveillance may cost as much as £40 million per year to deliver, so it is not surprising that questions are asked about its effectiveness.

Principles of child health surveillance

- Child health surveillance is carried out in partnership with parents. The programme acknowledges the parents as the most important and effective identifiers of health, developmental and behavioural problems in their children

- The process of child health surveillance is a learning experience for parents, for children and for the health professionals. It involves an exchange of information and provides opportunities for guidance on important child health issues such as behaviour, nutrition, accident prevention, immunisation and the use of services for children

- It should be a positive experience with opportunities to reassure, build confidence, relieve anxiety and promote good health

- The process should be continuous and flexible, taking advantage of every consultation on an opportunistic basis as well as the fixed age components of the programme

- History taking and observation are the main tools for child health surveillance, complemented by clinical examination and screening tests

- A high standard of child health surveillance depends upon team work and good communication between all those involved. This includes education and social services as well as the health services

- The provision of the programme is a form of shared care between the primary health care teams and the child health services provided by community paediatricians

- The health visitor is the major health professional engaged in child health surveillance for pre-school children with close working links with the rest of the primary health care team and the district child health services. Child health surveillance by the health visitor is part of a wider family health assessment

- The school nurse is the key person for children of school age

---

STRUCTURE OF INDIVIDUAL CHECKS

Review

Consultations are not self contained. Their content is highly dependent upon information from previous checks and records. It is therefore necessary to review previously identified problems and parental concerns and to check on progress following earlier advice or referrals. Good clear notes with a summary or problem list are an important aid in this process. Important examples of this process would be checking that there is a re-examination and if necessary referral for an undescended testis discovered at the six week check; interpretation of minor injuries or poor growth in the light of social information or reports of earlier injuries; parental concerns about sleep and the effectiveness of advice given; have immunisations been given?

History

This is taken from the parents, but essential information may be provided by other sources such as other health professionals (especially the health visitor and school nurse), nursery staff and teachers. Community paediatrics often demands the collection of information from a whole variety of sources in order to build up a complete picture of each child. The child himself is an important source of history and, depending upon age and understanding, I would obtain as much history as possible directly from the child. The child should not be a passive recipient of a process in which he is talked about and examined upon, but actively involved throughout. History taking is usually the most important part of a consultation: time and a relaxed atmosphere are important ingredients for success.

The quality of history taking is frequently poor. We should recognise our own strengths and weaknesses and the way that we use different types of questions.

Asking questions

Closed Does he drink from a cup?........... Answer can only be yes or no.

Open How is he getting on with feeding?...........This enables a parent to give a wide variety of answers.

Leading He is drinking from a cup isn't he?........... This type of question presumes the answer is 'yes' and it is easy to plough mechanically onto the next question on the list without even listening to the answer!

Probing Tell me more about that........... This enables more detail to be obtained.

Multiple I see that last time you came there were problems with bed wetting, hearing, his speech and some really terrible temper tantrums. How are all these coming along? .... Most parents in the 'heat' of the consultation will be totally flattened by this barrage.

Observation

Observation during the consultation and at other opportunities, for example in the home, nursery or classroom, may provide valuable information that may be missed by history and examination alone. What is the demeanour of the child? How does he react to the new situation of the consultation? How do parent and child interact? What is his behaviour and temperament like? How does he mix with other children? What are his movements like? For example difficulty with doing up buttons, problems in climbing onto the couch or holding objects close to the eyes may provide important clues to clinical conditions.

Examination

The details of each examination will be discussed under each individual check, however, there are a number of important general points. Consider handling and responsiveness as well as the individual clinical items of examination. Even young children can be modest about being exposed to the gaze of strangers: children are entitled to the same level of privacy and modesty as are accorded to adults. During the examination explain what you are doing and what your findings are to the child and parents rather than leaving a long silence throughout as you go through 'the routine'. Talk to the parent and the child, let them participate and 'help' in the examination.

Record keeping

A contemporaneous record needs to be made of the history and findings. The record needs to be of sufficient quality (and legibility), that in the unfortunate event of the untimely death of the writer, his successor has full information on findings, the interpretation of those findings, information and discussion with parents, and further actions such as investigation, referral or follow up. The findings should be recorded in the parent held record and copies retained for the clinic, surgery or health authority records.

Interpretation of findings

Conclusions need to be drawn from the findings of the consultation about normal and abnormal features. It is important to define areas of doubt as these are, in practice, more common than clear cut 'answers'. Examples where consultations may produce valid results but lack interpretation may include records of height and weight that are not plotted on centile charts or compared with previous findings; cardiac murmurs recorded in the notes with no view of their significance; records of a detailed neurological examination (box tick syndrome), but without a view on what the whole examination means.

Discussion with parents

The findings and their significance need to be discussed with parents as well as recorded in the parent held record. Results must also be explained to the child. Time, repetition of information, opportunity to ask further questions and to check that your explanations or advice have been understood are all required. A consultation is only successful if this step is achieved.

If there is a need to discuss the findings with other people, for example the class teacher, then permission needs to be obtained from the parent for this. Confidentiality must be respected and trust will be lost when parents become aware of the dissemination of information without their knowledge or permission.

> **Next contact**
>
> - **no problems**: see at next routine check or earlier at parents' request. Congratulate everyone on progress rather than express disappointment at yet another normal check
>
> - **new problem**: review before next routine check, but no further action; request investigations or reports; provide treatment or advice; refer to another practitioner.

Information transfer

Information on the outcome of the check will be needed by the District Health Authority for local information systems and by others for individual clinical use, eg health visitor, family doctor. The parent held record is also a vehicle for the transmission of information to relevant third parties.

PITFALLS

Child health surveillance is riddled with opportunities for incorrect conclusions. Here are some of the ways that this commonly comes about.

Putting professional over parental judgement. Parents are continuous rather than episodic observers of their children. If they are concerned, their fears should be taken seriously and should not be overridden by professional judgement. Parents are likely to identify problems with vision and hearing far in advance of the surveillance programme. In the EEC study of deafness, 90% of parents had suspected a hearing loss in the first year of life, but only 10% had been found by routine testing. Hall & Hall (1988), found that among 219 children with severe vision defects only three were discovered by routine testing at a child health clinic. Parents were the major source for identification.

Initial impressions may be wrong. Impressions about a child's development made in a situation which is unfamiliar for the child may be misleading. The child's developmental abilities may be obscured by unwillingness, fear, shyness, fatigue, illness, just not liking you or perhaps simply thinking about something else. Under these circumstances, history from parents will be more valuable than observation.

Failure to make allowance for prematurity. Developmental information must be interpreted in the light of gestation. This correction needs to be made at a minimum until 2 years of age (Elliman et al 1985). For a baby born at 28 weeks gestation, 12 weeks must be subtracted from chronological age for interpretation of developmental data.

Developmental testing is not the best means of detecting developmental delay. Developmental testing has, in the past, been widely adopted as a means for early detection of children with developmental delay. They may, however, actually contribute towards a delay in recognition by false reassurance as there are frequent false negatives. The predictive value is low and many children with 'developmental delay' turn out to be perfectly normal on follow up. Greer et al (1989) found that the Denver Developmental Screening Test failed to identify 80% of children who were later found to have a poor outcome. Largo et al (1990) compared IQ at seven years with developmental quotients at 9 and 24 months showing large shifts in individual children. Children with severe problems will be picked up without testing as they differ markedly from the normal population; however, the tests are too crude to identify children with lesser problems, where observation and attention to parental concerns would be more useful (Sonnander 1987). The information on development recorded in the parent held record and the areas of concern highlighted by parents, form a basis not only for identification and assessment but also for explanation and advice. Observation of the quality of performance, for example in the fine motor area, will provide much more useful information than a count of the number of bricks piled up. Routine and repetitive tests can become

Development quotient of children aged 7 years, scored 0–1 SD when 2

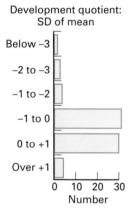

Developmental quotients of individual children can vary markedly at different ages

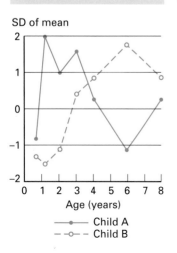

'reflex' actions for the examiner who fails to perceive individual variation and individuality.

Checks out of social context. Information about child health, development or behaviour cannot properly be understood without an understanding of social, cultural, environmental and family factors. 'Causes' may be misunderstood and advice unrealistic in terms of the resources available to the family or their traditions. These interpretations which are out of tune with the family discredit the service as a source of realistic understanding or advice. A home visit and questions to the family about their formulation of the problem may be more successful than imposing our own understanding. It is often wiser to listen carefully than to talk.

Beware the bilingual consultation! Good communication is essential as child health surveillance is essentially an educational activity. Where the family speak no English, it is easy to identify the need for an interpreter. Where English is a second language, misunderstandings are to be anticipated unless precautions are taken. History may be inaccurate or incomplete; 'explanations' may indeed be received as misinformation. For example, 'sick' may mean 'vomit' or 'generally unwell', 'fit' may mean 'healthy' or a convulsion. Advice may be only partially received because the recipient has only just translated the first part of the sentence, whilst the speaker has got to the end. In this circumstance, a mother was advised to give half strength feeds for 24 hours only, but missed the end of the sentence. As a consequence, the child continued long term on half strength feeds and was admitted malnourished.

Checking that each individual point has been understood may guard against these risks. An interpreter, if used, needs to be a person who is acceptable to the family. Sex and culture may be important factors. It is necessary to check the language skills of the interpreter as it is quite possible for this person to have translation skills that are little better than the parent. This will add errors of translation to an already confused picture. The interpreter may also add views of his own or at least colour the information in a way that was not intended by the originator.

Beware the uncooperative child. Notes may record a child as 'uncooperative' in an examination or test. Further explanation is required. An uncooperative child may well have a significant behaviour problem that requires paediatric advice. He may also be unable to do the test, eg measurement of visual acuity, when he has a visual impairment or he is developmentally delayed so that he is unable to understand the task. Ounsted et al (1983) found that 18% of 4 year olds did not cooperate fully in assessment and at follow up at 7 1/2 years, this group performed at a poorer level in all areas than those who had cooperated fully.

Ask the child. A history from a parent in the 'does he take sugar?' scenario may be frustrating for the child and also lead to important information or views being missed. The child's understanding of his illness and its cause may be quite different from that of the parent because of his stage of development or because the parent has incomplete information, inaccurate information or applies different interpretations to that genuinely held by the child.

Check measurements of growth. Measurement of growth is a part of the child health surveillance programme and the ritual of child health clinic attendence. Important errors occur at all levels. Equipment may be faulty: height measuring equipment with a difference between a standard 1 m rule and measured height of up to 8 cm was found in the Wessex Growth Study. Davies (1983), found poor techniques of weighing, inadequate use of growth charts and poor interpretation of growth patterns. Poor attention to quality of equipment, calibration, measurement techniques, calculation of age, plotting and interpretation can result in unnecessary anxiety and investigation or a failure to identify important problems.

THE CHILD HEALTH CLINIC

The Child Health Clinic is the central part of the delivery system for child health surveillance. 'Clinic' is probably not a very good descriptive term as it is in many ways unlike the traditional medical model of a clinic as it has educational, social and supportive functions and is usually open access. It would usually be held as part of the services provided by the primary health care team, though some clinics are still run by the the District Health Authority Child Health Services. In the UK, the Family Health Services Authority (FHSA) maintains a list of suitably qualified general practitioners who are on their Child Health Surveillance list and who receive extra payment for providing this service.

Staffing

The core staff of the Child Health Clinic are the Health Visitor, Doctor and receptionist. A busy clinic will often require two or more health visitors; this is particularly true in the District Health Authority clinic which may well serve several practices. The receptionist is required for records and appointments and is often involved in the sale of welfare milks and vitamins at the clinic. Additional staff are often present: the practice or clinic nurse to give immunisations; an auxiliary nurse or sometimes a specially trained volunteer to help with weighing; a playgroup leader to organise the waiting area; an interpreter or link worker where there are language problems; and a pram park attendant! Other services such as a social worker, toy library, mobile book library and various parents' groups can, with advantage, be linked to the running of the child health clinic.

Premises

Easy access to prams and pushchairs is clearly essential – ground floor premises or a lift are needed. Sufficient secure place to 'park' prams and pushchairs can present problems. The clinic should be warm, well lit and have seating and toilets suitable for adult and child use. The reception area needs to be clearly identified to avoid the difficulty of parents waiting whilst the clinic staff are not aware that they have arrived. The waiting area should be large, comfortable and well supplied with safe toys appropriate to the age range of pre-school children. Additional useful facilities in the waiting area are the ability to display and distribute health education materials and to set aside an area for a particular health education activity (parents' group, video or other activity). Consultation rooms are required for health visitor and doctor; these must provide comfort and privacy. For hearing testing, a quiet room is required. A fridge for vaccine storage is needed. Space to feed and change babies is useful in a quiet area away from the main waiting room. Safety is an important issue in clinic premises. They need to be externally secure so that children cannot escape and internally safe with special attention to stairs, doors, 'sharps' and other dangerous objects. Accident prevention programmes in the child health clinic certainly lack authority if the premises themselves present a hazard to young children.

Timing

The child health clinic is usually held on an afternoon, though morning clinics can also be successful. The total length of the session depends, quite obviously, on the number of children served, though an hour and a half is a minimum with some lasting up to three hours. Parents often need to collect older children from school at 3–4 pm so that early afternoon is easier for attendance. Some have experimented with clinics at other times, particularly where there is a high proportion of working mothers who will often find traditional clinic times difficult. Clinics may be early evening, (after work), and can be linked to late shopping days or a Saturday morning.

Equipment

The Child Health Clinic should be well equipped and it should be remembered that equipment should be maintained and some items, particularly toys, require fairly frequent replacement.

The equipment needed:

- For assessment of growth: reliable scales with a standard weight to check calibration; measures for height and length; tape measure and growth charts.
- General medical equipment: includes ophthalmoscope, auriscope.
- Equipment for tests of hearing and vision: Manchester rattle; McCormick Toy Test; sound level meter; Meg warbler: visual acuity charts (preferably linear) for use with older children. (See specific chapters on vision and hearing).
- Toys that aid observation of development: books eg Ladybird 'Talkabout' books, symbolic toys, (small dolls, chairs, animals, 'cooking set', cars, posting box, crayons and paper, bricks). (Beware of the danger of inhalation of small objects.)
- Health Education Equipment.
- Reference material: this book, Manual of Community Paediatrics (Polnay), Immunisation against Infectious Disease (DoH)
- Local resource information: playgroups, mother and toddler groups etc.

Appointments /attendances

The people attending the child health clinic are coming for a variety of reasons: some for specific checks, some for immunisation, some as a follow up, some on an open access basis to discuss problems or progress or to ask for advice from the health visitor or doctor. Some of the attenders can therefore be anticipated, but total attendances can fluctuate quite widely because of variation in the open access figures. Consequently staffing may be inadequate if clinics are unexpectedly busy. Attendance figures by year of birth and reason for attendance (check, immunisation, follow up, open access attendance), give a measure of workload. Figures, however, can be difficult to interpret: high figures are not necessarily good or low figures bad. More detailed assessment by category of problem may be needed and clinic protocols discussed.

Appointment letters for specific checks and follow ups should be friendly in style, easy to read and attractive in presentation. They need to be sent in good time, stating clearly when, where and reason for the appointments. Further explanations or health educational material relevant to the appointment may also be sent. If specific information is required, eg test results or reports, it is useful to check that these have arrived.

Conduct of a session

The Child Health Clinic takes place in protected time, which means, that as far as is humanly possible, there are no outside distractions. The telephone can be a major obstacle in achieving this aim.

The Child Health Clinic houses a wide variety of related activities

- Immunisation
- Specific screening tests
- Health education and accident prevention
- Management of problems jointly identified by parents and professionals through child health surveillance
- Sale of welfare milk and vitamins
- Play and recreation

On arrival at the clinic, parents come to reception and any clinic records are found. Attendances and outcomes are, however, recorded in the parent held record, with the non carbonated copy and possibly additional more detailed notes on individual clinical problems being retained at the clinic or surgery. The reason for attendance is ascertained from the above list and the parents directed to the doctor, health visitor or immunisation room. It is usual in most clinics for all parents to see the health visitor first as not all will be willing to tell the receptionist the reason for their visit; considerable expertise would be required by the reception staff in this as many parents come for more than one reason, eg immunisation + check + follow up of problem identified from the notes. Weighing at every attendance is unnecessary in most cases and standards of measuring, recording and plotting can easily drop (Davies & Williams 1983). It has been suggested that parents should be able to weigh their babies themselves if they so wish. It is easy to focus too much attention on weighing, but the activity can provide an opportunity to observe the whole child undressed, when abnormalities of posture and movement and injuries can be more easily seen.

Because most child health clinics do operate without appointment times, the waiting time can be longer than in other types of clinic. Use of the waiting area for play activities and health education can make this time profitable. Specific play staff and health staff are needed.

Teamwork

A meeting of the doctor and health visitor at the beginning and end of the clinic for general discussion is most useful.

Through the home

Child health surveillance through home visiting is central to the history and philosophy of health visiting. Not all parents find it easy or possible to attend child health clinics and non-attenders may have more problems than those who come – the inverse care law (Zinkin & Cox 1976). Some children may behave very differently in the unfamiliar circumstances of the clinic. Others may be dressed up in their best clothes for the visit to the clinic and problems of poverty not considered when seen out of the context of their home. Home visits draw attention to environmental limitations and hazards and show the real world and its population with whom the child lives. Many parents may feel more secure to identify and discuss problems from the security of their own home.

The 18–24 month check and the 36–42 month check are often carried out at home as are other opportunistic and follow up visits. A service that did not include home visiting as a major component would be grossly deficient.

Home visiting and local knowledge become much more effective when the area covered by the primary health care team is limited to a well defined community.

SURVEILLANCE AT SCHOOL

The Child Health Surveillance Programme moves at school entry from a clinic and home focus to one that is based in the school, but is still supplemented by home visits and some clinic attendances. In the past this has consisted of repeated examinations by the school doctor. Historically this could be justified by the high incidence of important acquired disease, eg rheumatic heart disease. Nowadays, this programme has become selective with some health authorities retaining only an entrant medical examination and an increasing number being selective at school entry also. The case for selective entrant medical examinations is strong with most problems having been identified by school nurses, parents or teachers. (O'Callaghan & Colver 1987, Smith et al 1990, Tuke 1990, Richman & Miles 1990). An effective pre-school child health surveillance programme is essential before selection at school entry can take place.

The school doctor is a paediatrician with special training and experience in the interrelationship between education and paediatrics and is well placed to build up a good working relationship with both schools and general practitioners. In most areas a school population would be

Selective school entrant examinations from a review of the notes of 1000 children (Smith et al 1990)

School nurses identified 205 problems (77 were new)
School doctors identified 345 problems (78 were new)

Only 17 new problems requiring treatment were detected by the doctor:

Speech	10
Behaviour/development	3
Undescended testes	3
Phimosis	1

Parental questionnaire or interview, discussion with teachers and improvements in pre-school surveillance should also have identified these children.

covered by quite a large number of family doctors, making liaison over individual children very difficult for them in practice.

School based surveillance programmes depend upon good communication between parents, teachers and the school health team – the school nurse and school doctor. The key person is the school nurse whose health appraisal programme is the centre piece. The school nurse and doctor must be accepted and trusted by all as a part of the school. The summary table indicates the importance of health education and health promotion as part of the programme. This is aimed at the children themselves and takes place as much in the classroom as in the medical room. Children are not only given information, but encouraged to make decisions of their own in relation to their health and to initiate referrals. For example secondary school health questionnaires are sent to the parent and pupil to fill out jointly rather than to the parents alone.

To operate an effective school health service, there should be:

- a named school nurse and doctor for every school (with specific training)
- an understanding by parents and teachers of the role of the nurse and doctor and their names
- an easy means of finding the members of the school health team
- a comfortable, private and well equipped base from which to work in school
- an information system that enables children to be identified by the school which they attend and to transfer important medical information to the school health team

UPTAKE AND ATTENDANCE

In providing a child health surveillance programme, it is necessary not only to establish clinics and other sessions, but also to determine its uptake to find out whether it reaches those who are the intended beneficiaries. Attendance figures provide a means of recording workload and allocating resources.

Examples of data that may be collected are:

$$\text{Uptake} = \frac{\text{Number of children receiving check}}{\text{Number of children eligible for check}}$$

within defined period of time eg six week checks completed by age three months

District target = 100%

Attendance = Number seen in clinic session
Often divided by: age band
seen by doctor/nurse/both
reason – check/imm/advice/FU

Interpretation of uptake and attendance figures can be difficult and comparisons unfair.

Factors which decrease or increase uptake

Increase uptake	Decrease uptake
Easy access	Difficult access
Convenient times	Inconvenient time
Good appointments/invitations	Poor appointment system
Parent understands what service is for	Poor communication about reason for appointment
Friendly staff	Unfriendly staff
Comfortable environment	Uncomfortable setting
Avoiding long waiting times	Long waiting times
Good communication with parents	Poor communication with parents
Effective programme that delivers results	Poor programme where positive outcomes cannot be demonstrated

BIRTH CHECK (NEONATAL EXAMINATION)

This would usually be carried out by hospital paediatric staff, but may also take place at home when there is very early discharge from hospital or where there is a home delivery.

The examination should always be carried out in the presence of parents and should include review, examination and discussion.

Review

- Pregnancy and delivery
- Mother's current state of health. How does she feel?
- Parental concerns and history since birth (feeding, passage of urine and meconium)
- Family history (parents, siblings, inherited disorders).
- A family tree that is kept up to date is a valuable part of the child's record.
- Social history (conditions and support at home, recorded concern about care and handling of baby or older children)

The need for services after discharge from hospital depend as much upon this background information as any findings from the medical examination.

Examination

This is a complete physical examination which includes the following important elements which must be recorded in the child health record. This is an important examination: 1:40 newborns will be found to have a congenital malformation and many 'common' abnormalities will be detected including congenital dislocation of the hip, undescended testes, heart disease, corneal and lens opacities, sensorineural hearing loss (selective testing), and biochemical abnormalities (phenylketonuria and hypothyroidism).

Examination

- Weight and centile
- Head circumference and centile
- Observation of alertness or irritability, posture, symmetry of movements, mother-child interaction
- Jaundice appearing within 24 hours requires urgent investigation
- Presence of dysmorphic features
- Inspection of the eyes: movements, fixation, presence of red reflex, discharge. Suspicion of poor vision or profuse purulent discharge (possible gonococcal infection) require urgent action
- Examination of the mouth, palpating for cleft palate
- Examination of the cardiovascular system. Soft ejection systolic murmurs are common and usually benign, but important signs include tachypnoea, central cyanosis, absent femoral pulses, thrills and enlarged liver
- Examination of the abdomen, looking for distension, organomegaly, single umbilical artery, inguinal hernia
- Examination of the genitalia to exclude hypo- and epi-spadias, undescended or incompletely descended testes; ambiguous genitalia
- Examination of the hips by Barlow modification of Ortolani test to identify dislocated or dislocatable hips, which both require orthopaedic referral
- Examination of spine for abnormalities and feet for talipes
- Hearing testing is not routinely done at this age, but the Clues List for hearing may be discussed. Tests may be carried out on high risk groups which include children with major neonatal problems and those with strong family histories of sensorineural hearing losses. The techniques available include Otoacoustic emissions, brainstem evoked responses and the auditory response cradle

---

Biochemical screening in the first week of life includes tests for phenylketonuria and hypothyroidism (carried out by the midwife from heel prick blood which is sent to a central laboratory). In some centres this also includes a screen for cystic fibrosis. Haemoglobinopathy screening is also carried out for sickle cell anaemia and thalassaemias in many centres. All these programmes require efficient and rapid communication of results and responsive treatment and counselling services.

Outcomes and discussion

This should be recorded in the parent held record and explained and discussed fully with parents. Information needs to be transferred to the family doctor and health visitor via the birth notification or other means. Referrals, investigation or special follow up arrangements should be clearly recorded. Major child care problems for discussion with parents include uncertainty about infant feeding particularly for first babies.

TEN DAYS

This is done by the health visitor at home at the time that she takes over responsibility from the midwife. Many family doctors will also do a home visit at this time to check on mother and baby.

Discussion

The following topics are usually covered on this important visit: explanation of her job and information about the surveillance programme, parent held records and immunisation; maternal concerns about her baby, herself, other children or home conditions; discussion of infant feeding, accident prevention, any worries about vision or hearing.

Examination

The hips are re-examined for CDH and most health visitors would generally inspect and observe the baby, looking at alertness and interactions, skin, eyes, umbilicus and cord.

Examination of hips for congenital dislocation

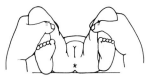

hips flexed 90°   knees flexed

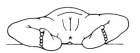

clunk+

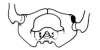

Repeat examinations reduce the risk of late diagnosis.

SIX TO EIGHT WEEKS

This check will be carried out by the doctor and is often combined with the first immunisation or the mother's post-natal check.

Review

- Information from parent held record and check lists of parental concerns. Feeding, sleeping and crying are concerns frequently expressed.
- Ask about any other concerns that are not recorded in the parent held record particularly with regard to vision and hearing, (clues list for parents), development
- How are parents and siblings adjusting to the birth of the new baby? Open questions on how the family are getting along may identify large problems.

Examination

This is a second complete physical examination undertaken with parents and accompanied by explanations of each item as it is done. Results of individual screening tests are recorded in the parent held record.

Examination

- Observation: alertness and interest; response to handling and interaction with mother; adequacy of clothing and cleanliness; dysmorphic features; posture and symmetry of movements

- Growth: plot weight, head circumference and, where necessary, length on centile chart. Upward or downward drift may indicate physiological adjustment, disease or an inappropriate intake. Careful monitoring, investigation or dietary assessment may be needed.
- Inspect eyes : manifest squint, abnormal movements, failure of fixation, structural abnormalities
- Ears: abnormality of face and pinna may be associated with deafness
- Hips: for CDH
- Genitalia: ambiguous genitalia, hypo- and epi-spadias, undescended testes
- General examination: skin; mouth; cardiovascular system; abdomen; tone

Outcomes and discussion   All findings must be discussed with parents and parents congratulated on the progress of their baby. Minor or borderline problems need explanation and review at or before the next routine check. Parental concerns whether or not they are supported by clinical findings should also be reviewed. Major problems, particularly suspicion of hearing or vision problems, suspected CDH or serious concerns about failure to thrive should be referred immediately. Topics for discussion often include immunisation, feeding (time for weaning), home safety, sleeping, crying, recognition of illness.

TWO, THREE AND FOUR MONTHS

First three immunisations against diphtheria, tetanus, pertussis, Hib and polio. Hips can be checked to detect limited abduction (CDH).

SIX TO NINE MONTHS

This check is carried out by the health visitor. Its more important components are discussion of parental concerns and the distraction test of hearing which acts as a safety net for those congenital and acquired hearing losses that have not been identified by parents or neonatal screening.

Review

- Past medical history and past and present parental concerns from parent held record
- Other concerns not recorded in the parent held record, particularly vision, hearing, general health and development
- Check that three immunisations have been given
- Enquire about changes in household, address, return to work
- Important life events, social and medical

Examination

- Hearing Test: requires two trained staff and good acoustic conditions. One re-test only permitted within one month, after which all should be referred for expert assessment
- Growth: check weight and compare with previous records on centile chart
- Observe alertness, interest, interaction with mother and strangers, general care (cleanliness and clothing), play and general development
- Eyes: observe visual behaviour and refer if there is manifest squint or parental concerns
- Hips: check for CDH by looking for limited abduction
- Genitalia: check again for undescended testes. Arrange to refer before the age of one year if still undescended

Outcomes and discussion Refer if there are concerns about hearing or vision; obvious delay in development or regression; limited hip abduction; undescended testes; persistent downward drift of growth on centile chart. Topics for discussion may include: safety (particularly in the context of increasing mobility), diet, care of teeth, play and stimulation.

FIFTEEN MONTHS

Immunisation with mumps, measles and rubella (MMR) vaccine.

EIGHTEEN TO TWENTY-FOUR MONTHS

This review is often carried out by the health visitor at home. Its content and comprehensiveness may vary widely depending upon the health visitor's assessment of family need and deprivation and the requirement to follow up previously identified concerns in health, growth or development.

Review

- Past medical history from parent held record and check lists of past and present parental concerns from the record
- Enquire about parental concerns that may not be listed in the record, particularly with regard to hearing, vision, talking, walking, behaviour and eating.
- Update family tree, and record any major changes in the household
- Record major life events

Examination

- Growth: check weight (and length if appropriate and child co-operative)
- If poor diet, poor growth, pale or high risk of iron deficiency, Hb and ferritin estimation
- Walking: observation that child is walking with a normal gait. Non-walkers at 18 months have a significant incidence of problems and should have further assessment (Chaplais 1984), eg general delay, cerebral palsy, muscular dystrophy
- Check that four immunisations have been given
- Heart and testes should be re-checked between eight months and five years of age. This can be done opportunistically or linked to a specific check.

Outcome and discussion Refer for assessment: non-walking children; concerns about vision and hearing: concerns that expressive language or comprehension are not appropriate for age. Topics for discussion may include: behaviour, safety, diet, play, mixing with other children.

THIRTY-SIX TO FORTY-EIGHT MONTHS

The aim of this review is to look ahead to full time schooling, to identify any potential special educational needs and arrange for referral and assessment where this is needed. This may be carried out by the health visitor alone or jointly with the doctor when it may include examination of the heart and testes.

Review

- Past medical history and past and present parental concerns from checklist in parent held record
- Any other parental concerns not listed in the parent held record, enquiring specifically about vision, hearing, language, behaviour and understanding
- Additional information may be available from playgroup or nursery
- Immunisation
- Changes in household: family tree; address; employment
- Important life events, social and medical

Examination

- Growth: height and weight centiles
- Observation: demeanour, play, communication
- Heart and testes if not checked since eight months of age
- Further physical examination if indicated from parental concerns

Outcome and discussion   Any children with known or suspected special educational needs should be referred to the educational psychologist usually via the community paediatrician. Topics for discussion include accidents (especially road safety, water, fire), selection and preparation for school, dental care and checks, diet. Health visitor and school nurse will need to liaise. Sometimes this review is carried out jointly.

SCHOOL ENTRANT REVIEW (54–66 MONTHS)

This takes place in the first year of full time schooling. In the past all children have been seen for health appraisal by the school nurse and for examination by the school doctor. There is very strong evidence that this is no longer necessary (O'Callaghan & Colver 1987, Smith et al 1990, Tuke 1990, Richman & Miles 1990), providing that there is a good quality of pre-school surveillance with complete medical records, ideally in the parent held records.

At school entry, all children should be seen by the school nurse for the surveillance procedures listed below. It is good practice to invite parents to this health appraisal so that they can meet the school nurse, receive information about the school health service, discuss their own concerns and very importantly be with their child during the appraisal and understand its findings.

Children may be selected to see the school doctor on the basis of previously identified problems, incomplete pre-school surveillance or lack of documentation, concerns of parents, school nurse or teachers.

Review and history – School nurse health appraisal

- Past medical history from parent held record, and past and present parental concerns from checklists
- Any parental concerns not recorded in the record, particularly about vision, hearing, speech, behaviour, general health
- Immunisation
- Changes in household: family tree; address; employment
- Important life events
- Enquire about teacher concerns

Examination

- Observation: general demeanour and appearance; general development; interaction with parents; hair; skin; teeth; posture
- Growth: height and weight centiles
- Visual acuity using Snellen chart
- Hearing: 'sweep' test at 20 dB at 500 Hz, 1 , 2, 4 MHz

Outcome and discussion

Topics for discussion include: school health services; adjustment to school; health education programme in school including aspects such as road safety and 'stranger danger'. 10–20% of children will have a problem requiring follow up by the school health team. Referral may be needed to the family doctor, speech therapist, school clinic, eye clinic, or other clinics. Findings and referrals should be explained to the parents and always discussed with the family doctor. Permission should be sought to explain relevant medical findings to the class teacher and parents encouraged to do the same.

PRIMARY SCHOOL

Following the school entrant review, a selected group of children with special needs will be followed up by the school nurse and doctor, supplemented by children seen because of teacher's concerns, parental concerns, or from information received through other channels such as copies of hospital discharge summaries or out-patient letters.

The school nurse health appraisal, which is carried out on all children every two to three years, becomes an opportunity for individual health education rather than screening, apart from visual acuity tests at 8, 11, and 14 years of age.

Review

- Past medical history recorded at entrant review
- Concerns of parents and teachers
- New information from other sources

Examination

- Observation: general demeanour and appearance; general development; interaction with parents; hair; skin; teeth; posture
- Growth: height and weight centiles
- Visual acuity using Snellen chart

Measurement of visual acuity

- Test must be carried out at a *measured* 6 m
- Illumination of the chart must be good
- Children should not be given the opportunity to memorise the letters

---

Outcome and discussion   Topics for discussion include, diet, dental care, hygiene. Referral may be made to the family doctor, dentist, eye clinic or community paediatrician.

The following children would need further consultation with the school health team:

- persistent ill health giving rise to poor attendance or performance
- academic failure, where potential medical factors have not been investigated
- children with behaviour problems
- marked incompetence in gross or fine motor activities
- concern about neglect or abuse

SECONDARY SCHOOL

In the secondary school, child health surveillance consists of the school nurse health appraisal at transfer (age 11), and at age 14 .

Review at age 11 will ensure that relevant problems are discussed with the new staff in the secondary school and that new issues related to the broader curriculum, with a larger number of teachers and classroom settings are considered. The structure of the health appraisal is broadly the same as that applied to younger children. Individual health education linked to the findings of health appraisal and the health education programme for the school as a whole are the dominant feature of health appraisal. Measurement of visual acuity using the Snellen chart and colour vision in both boys and girls using the Ishihara plates is carried out as part of the appraisal. Children with impaired colour vision will need a quantitative test such as the City University Plates which gives a measure of severity as well as diagnostic information on the nature of colour confusion.

Colour vision tests

- Ishihara is highly sensitive, but identifies very minor difficulties
- City University Plates are diagnostic for type of defect and quantitative, permitting better career guidance
- Validity of tests rests upon them being carried out under correct natural illumination

---

Review at age 14 years is to ensure that the future school leaver and his parents fully understand the significance of present and past medical problems with regard to future employment. The school nurse health appraisal remains the backbone of child health surveillance with the main emphasis on health education and counselling. In the secondary school, self referral is added to the other routes of referral because of parental or teacher concerns. The teenager should be encouraged to identify and act upon their own concerns about health and personal problems. Visual acuity is checked again at this appraisal.

Summary of screening procedures, by age

Age	Screening procedure	Immunisation	Health education	Accident prevention
Neonate	Weight, HC Full physical examination Hips Eyes – red reflex Hearing? ARC or OAE	BCG (high risk) Hepatitis B (if mother a carrier)	Feeding Recognition of illness Immunisation Services for children	Bathing Falls off table Car transport
10 days	Hips			
6–8 weeks	Weight, HC Full examination Hips Eyes – red reflex Hearing checklist		Early development – social behaviour – vision, hearing Family problems Depression Contraception	
2 months		DT Per/polio Hib	Immunisation	Stairgate Fireguard
3 months	Hips	DT Per/polio Hib	Early language and social development	Scalds Glass doors Window catches Car seats Bath safety
4 months		DT Per/polio Hib		
6–9 months	Weight Hips, testes Hearing test			
12–15 months	? Heart, testes	MMR	Diet, anaemia Dentist	Ponds and pools Medicines Chemicals Scalds Windows
18–24 months	Observe gait ? Heart, testes		Nursery, playgroup Behaviour problems Language and play	
36–48 months	Height ? Heart, testes ? Vision ? Hearing		School readiness Special educational needs Learning Language development Play Behaviour problems Nutrition, teeth	Gardens gates Ponds and pools Road safety Car seats Fires
5 years	School entrant review Height ? Heart, testes Visual acuity Hearing (sweep test) Selective follow up of children with special needs	DT Per/polio	Immunisation Adjustment to school	Road safety Stranger
8 years	School nurse health appraisal			Road safety
11 years	School nurse health appraisal Visual acuity Colour vision	Rubella (girls if no MMR) BCG	Health education in school as part of National Curriculum Teenage counselling	
14 years	School nurse health appraisal Visual acuity		Careers advice Self referrals to school doctor or nurse	
16 years		T/polio		

ARC = Auditory Responce Cradle, OAE = Otoacoustic emissions
Heart & testes should be re-checked on one occasion after the age of 8 months. This can be done opportunistically or at any of the subsequent checks
Health education is the major role of the health visitor and school nurse. It can be targetted into high, medium and low intervention, with extra help provided for first time parents, the disadvantaged and 'families' in need in general.

INFORMATION

Information is required about the uptake and performance of the Child Health Surveillance Programme at several levels. Individual practitioners will require information about there own practice or caseload for operational reasons and for internal audit. The Director of Public Health of the District Health Authority will require information on the health of the population and have an overview of service delivery. This information may also be wanted to monitor contracts. Regional Health Authorities and the Department of Health will wish to compile regional and national statistics. Academic departments may wish to critically examine components of the child health surveillance programme or to carry out longitudinal studies on a population.

It is therefore necessary to have a common database on the programme's overall performance, its results for the individual child and in relation to pockets of population or the work of individuals or of teams. The data on each child is that collected from the parent held record. From these record forms the following information can be assembled at any of the levels given above:

Uptake

- of check
- of components of check

Age carried out versus target age

Outcomes

- for total check (normal/abnormal)
- specified individual screening tests (normal/abnormal/referrals)

Linkage of district information systems will enable us to obtain data on sensitivity and specificity for some of the items in the District Child Health Surveillance Programme, for example how many of the children referred have their diagnoses confirmed and how many children are eventually identified by other routes (false negatives). This information, fed back into the system, should have a powerful effect upon the structure of the programme and its delivery.

Roles and responsibility, working relationships. The District Child Health Surveillance Programme is a very large undertaking with parental and professional input. The content of the programme has been defined in this chapter. The delivery system needs to define the roles of each of the professional staff involved so that the programme as a whole is delivered and so those involved in the programme are aware of the entire programme and not only the parts in which they are personally involved. In the same way the parents and the children who are receiving the programme should be aware of the varying professional roles in its delivery.

Records

Parent held child health records . These have been in use on a limited scale in the UK since the late 1970s. In developing countries, they have been much more widely and very successfully used. There is excellent evidence from the many sources (Saffin & Macfarlane 1988, Lakhani 1984, Miller 1990, Macfarlane & Saffin 1990, Polnay & Roberts 1989) that parents do not loose these records and that they provide an excellent means for communication of information between parents and professionals. The main advantages of the record as summarised in the Report of the Joint Working Party on Professional and Parent Held Records in 1990 are: that it is available wherever the child is seen; it is available immediately when the family move from place to place; confidentiality rests with the parents and most importantly, it involves the parents centrally in the child health surveillance programme. For each of the checks there is a section for parents to record their own observations and concerns. This is essential in terms of the parents acknowledged superiority to professionals in identifying developmental problems. Use is made of materials from the Clues List for hearing, (Hitchings & Haggard 1983), and other sources.

The UK record is of loose leaf format and A5 size. It is presented in a red plastic cover. It consists of a record of child health surveillance checks (with non-carbonated copies for health service staff to keep and for district information systems), including growth charts, parental observations, a record of primary care, dental and hospital visits and important health education information. Local or other information can be added as needed and it has been translated into several other languages including Hindi, Punjabi and Gujarati. The record is illustrated and is presented to the mother either in hospital or at the health visitor's birth visit.

The record is also used as a source of important health education material which is immediately available to the whole population and which has the endorsement of the medical and nursing professions. Material covered includes the management of common health problems, when to call the doctor (recognition of ill health which can be enhanced by the use of check lists such as baby check), advice on feeding at different age groups and information on accident prevention.

The presentation of information is in a simple format that provides easy readability (reading age 12.6 years), whilst being presented in a suitable form for adults. This information can be looked at independently by parents or used by health workers to reinforce explanations that they have given. The success of the parent held record is determined by the importance health workers and parents attach to referring to the health information in it, referring to parental checklists as well as professionally recorded records and asking for and writing in the record at each consultation.

Research on parent held records in the UK has shown that most parents would like to hold the record of their child's health and development; the records are rarely lost; most health visitors and family doctors find it a better system than clinic held records; working class mothers with less access to other sources of information make good use of the record; clinic attendances for checks may be improved; and the system is of particular value with highly mobile families such as those from the armed forces (Lakhani 1984, Saffin & Macfarlane 1988, Polnay & Roberts 1989, Miller 1990, Macfarlane & Saffin 1990).

Parents's record

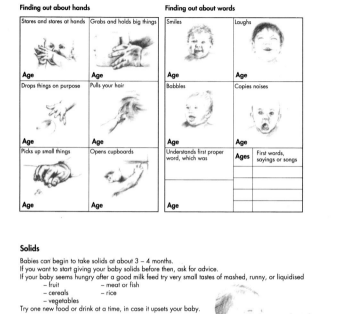

Finding out about hands

Stares and stares at hands	Grabs and holds big things
Age	Age
Drops things on purpose	Pulls your hair
Age	Age
Picks up small things	Opens cupboards
Age	Age

Finding out about words

Smiles	Laughs
Age	Age
Babbles	Copies noises
Age	Age
Understands first proper word, which was	Ages	First words, sayings or songs
Age		

Health education

Solids

Babies can begin to take solids at about 3 – 4 months.
If you want to start giving your baby solids before then, ask for advice.
If your baby seems hungry after a good milk feed try very small tastes of mashed, runny, or liquidised
– fruit   – meat or fish
– cereals   – rice
– vegetables
Try one new food or drink at a time, in case it upsets your baby.

Don't add salt.
Babies kidneys can't cope with too much salt and they get thirsty.

As your baby gets older, give more food that is less runny.
Then your baby will need less milk, but give other drinks like
– cool boiled water
– tap water from 6 – 7 months
– very dilute fruit juice
– fresh, pasturised milk from 12 months (not skimmed or semi-skimmed).
Give finger foods but watch your baby – babies can choke on crumbly food.

You can try
– brown bread or toast
– peeled, sliced apples, pears, carrots
– small sandwiches
– thin slices of cheese.
– chapati

Other records. The parent held record has clear advantages for health authorities in that it greatly simplifies problems related to storage, access, communication and confidentiality. However, there are also needs for professional records for additional reasons. General practitioners are required by their conditions of service to keep individual records on their patients. Health visitors will also need to keep individual records which will contain the summaries of child health surveillance data and extra information on clinical contacts and discussions and correspondence. Child health doctors will need detailed records of their consultation work arising from the child health surveillance programme and other referrals. There are rapid moves towards computer-based systems which are particularly effective for child health surveillance.

Patients already have access to computer based information on them. From 1st November 1991, they also have access, with some safeguards, to other medical records on them that are written from that date. The accuracy, quality , style and 'tone' of records are clearly most important. Many practitioners already give their patients open access to records.

Birth details

BIRTH REVIEW	Name D.O.B.- / - / - *Sticky label* *(with bar code or OMR)* I.D. No.

Comments on pregnancy and birth

Place of birth:
Type of delivery:
Birth weight: _____ . _____ Kgs. (_____ Lbs. _____ ozs.)
Head Circumference: _____ . _____ cms. . _____ th. Centile
Heelprick test: date – / – / –
Repeat (if done) – / – / –
Sickle test (if done) – / – / –
B.C.G. immunization (if done) – / – / –
Hip examination:
Feeding (Breast/Bottle)
Weight at
_____ Days; _____ . _____ Kgs. (_____ Lbs. _____ ozs.)
Comments:

10 – 14 DAY REVIEW

Date of Examination – / – / – Age: _____ Days
Head Circumference: _____ . _____ cms. _____ th. Centile
Hip Examination:
General Examination:

Feeding (Breast/Bottle)

Comments:

Action:

Action:

Which   ☐ All or Not to have ⬚
Immunisations?   Reason _____

By whom?   ☐ GP or H.A. Clinic ⬚

Name: Signature:
Staff I.D. No. _____ Date: - / - / -

Name: Signature:
Staff I.D. No. _____ Date: - / - / -

Hopefully with parent held records and open access the temptation to write comments such as 'getting uglier and uglier' will be a thing of the past.

Registers of special needs (District). Many districts will keep registers of children with special needs. These are in addition to other child health records and enable a track to be kept of referral and review, to anticipate needs and to audit the service. Information may be kept on identity of child, professional caseloads within which he falls, nature and severity of special needs, resources currently deployed and dates for further reviews.

Information on caseload. Individuals will also want to use the data from child health surveillance to produce a profile of their own workload and population. Information may be collected about the children by age and sex, about the geography of the population, uptake and outcomes of the surveillance programme, including numbers with special needs.

REFERENCES AND FURTHER READING

British Paediatric Association 1990a Community child health services, an information base for purchasers. BPA, London

British Paediatric Association 1990b Report of the Joint Working Party on Professional and Parent Held Records used in Child Health Surveillance. BPA, London

Butler J 1989 Child health surveillance in primary care. HMSO, London

Chaplais J den Z 1984 The late walking child. In: Macfarlane J A (ed) Progress in child health, vol 1. Churchill Livingstone, Edinburgh

Colver A F 1990 Health surveillance of preschool children: four years' experience. British Medical Journal 300: 1246–8

Commission of the EEC 1979 Childhood deafness in the European Community. EEC, Brussels

Davies D P, Williams T 1983 Is weighing babies in clinics worth while? British Medical Journal 286: 860–3

Dearlove J, Kearney D 1990 How good is general practitioner developmental screening? British Medical Journal 300: 1177–80

Elliman A M, Bryan E M, Elliman A D, Palmer P, Dubowitz L 1985 Denver developmental screening test and preterm infants. Archives of Disease in Childhood 60: 22–4

Greer S, Bauchner H, Zuckerman B 1989 The Denver developmental screening test: how good is its predictive validity? Developmental Medicine and Child Neurology 31: 774–81

Hall D M B (ed) 1991 Health for all children. Oxford University Press, Oxford

Hall D M B, Hall S M 1988 Early detection of vision defects in infancy. British Medical Journal 296: 823–4

Hitchings V, Haggard M P 1983 Incorporation of parental suspicions in screening of infants. British Journal of Audiology 17: 652–3

Johnson A, Goddard O, Ashurst H 1990 Is late walking a marker of morbidity? Archives of Disease in Childhood 66: 486–8

Lakhani K 1984 The evaluation of a home based health record book. Archives of Disease in Childhood 60: 1076–82

Largo R H, Graf S, Kundu S, Hunziker U, Molinari L 1990 Predicting developmental outcome at school age from infant tests of normal, at risk and retarded infants. Developmental Medicine and Child Neurology 32: 30–45

McCormick B 1988 Screening for hearing impairment in young children. Croome Helm

Macfarlane A, Saffin K 1990 Do general practitioners and health visitors like parent held records? British Journal of General Practice 40: 106–8

Miller S A St J 1990 A trial of parent held records in the armed forces. British Medical Journal 300: 1046

Morley C J, Thornton A J, Cole T J, Hewson P H, Fowler M A 1991 Baby check: a scoring system to grade the severity of acute illness in babies under six months old. Archives of Disease in Childhood 66: 100–6

Nicoll A 1984 The value of selective pre-school medical in an inner city area. Public Health 98: 68–72

Nicoll A 1985 Written materials concerning health for parents and children. In: Macfarlane A (ed) Progress in child health. Churchill Livingstone, Edinburgh

O'Callaghan E M, Colver A F 1987 Selective medical examinations on starting school. Archives of Disease in Childhood 62: 1041–3

Ounsted M, Cockburn F, Moar V A 1983 Developmental assessment at four years: are there any differences between children who do, or do not, cooperate? Archives of Disease in Childhood 58: 286–9

Polnay L 1990 Child health surveillance policy. Nottingham Health Authority, Nottingham

Polnay L, Roberts H 1989 Evaluation of an easy to read parent held information and record book of child health. Children & Society 3: 225–60

Richman S, Miles M 1990 Selective medical examinations for school entrants: the way forward. Archives of Disease in Childhood 65: 1177–81

Saffin K, Macfarlane A 1988 Parent held child health and development records. Maternal & Child Health 13: 288–91

Sonnander K 1987 Parental development assessment of 18 month old children: reliability and predictive value. Developmental Medicine and Child Neurology 29: 351–62

Smith G C, Powell A, Reynolds K et al 1990 The five year school medical – time for a change. Archives of Disease in Childhood 65: 225–7

Tuke J W 1990 Screening and surveillance of school age children. British Medical Journal 300: 1180–2

Zinkin P M, Cox C A 1976 Child health clinics and inverse care laws; evidence from longitudinal study of 1878 preschool children. British Medical Journal ii: 411–3

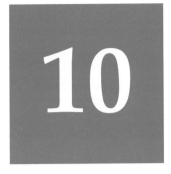

10 Avoiding Infection

Infectious diseases are still a major cause of illness. Falling mortality rates in the Western World have taken much of the fear out of epidemics, but it would be a mistake to become complacent. Problems remain. If one assumes that most of those designated on the death certificate as 'respiratory' are due to infections, then in the UK, infections are still the commonest cause of death in the post-neonatal period. In some countries, infections like pneumonia, gastroenteritis, tuberculosis, whooping cough, measles, malaria, tetanus, and diphtheria, remain collectively by far the most important causes of death in all age groups. Of 14 million child deaths a year, about 12 million are due to infection. Poor nutrition and lack of adequate facilities for treatment are important contributory factors. In the UK, infections are the commonest reason for children of all ages being seen by family doctors. Children under the age of 9 years can be expected to have 6 to 8 upper respiratory tract infections each year, of which 3 will be accompanied by constitutional symptoms.

Recording infection

In the UK detailed information on the epidemiology of infections is available from a variety of sources. There are however many inherent sources of error in these assessments. The information on death certificates may be inaccurate or incomplete. In some the cause of death will be uncertain. Statutory notification of some infectious diseases, although a legal responsibility of doctors, is also an incomplete exercise. Until recently a fee of only 25p was payable for each notification; this has now been increased to £2. Nevertheless the data do provide a basis for local and national monitoring. The Communicable Disease Report from the

---

Notifiable infectious diseases, UK

AIDS	Measles	Scarlet fever
Acute encephalitis	Meningitis	Smallpox
Acute poliomyelitis	Meningococcal septicaemia	Tetanus
Anthrax	Mumps	Tuberculosis
Cholera	Ophthalmia neonatorum	Typhoid fever
Diphtheria	Paratyphoid fever	Typhus fever
Dysentery	Plague	Viral haemorrhagic fever
Food poisoning	Rabies	Viral hepatitis
Leprosy	Rubella	Whooping cough
Leptospirosis	Relapsing fever	Yellow fever
Malaria		

PHLS Communicable Disease Surveillance Centre at Collindale provides regular information on notified diseases and laboratory reports of infections.

Mortality due to the main infectious diseases (England and Wales 1988, OPCS)

Cause	Age (years)			
	0–1	1–4	5–9	10–14
Deaths from all causes	5808	1078	612	563
Pneumonia and influenza	103	25	5	3
Acute bronchitis/bronchiolitis	102	50	4	—
Acute laryngitis/tracheitis	5	16	3	—
Acute epiglotitis	—	12	2	—
Gastroenteritis	42	4	—	1
Meningococcol infection	52	65	10	15
Septicaemia	24	13	4	2
Chicken pox	1	1	1	1
Measles	—	2	—	—

The Royal College of General Practitioners produces weekly data from a sample of practices (sentinel practices) which is particularly helpful for following infections like chicken pox and influenza, which are not notifiable and would not otherwise be recorded.

Morbidity statistics from General Practice, Third National Study, 1981–82

Cause	Childhood consultation rates/1000 at risk	
	0–4 years	5–14 years
Upper respiratory infection, non febrile	593.0	164.4
Upper respiratory infection, febrile	214.1	82.9
Acute otitis media	317.0	86.5
Tonsillitis	167.2	142.0
Laryngitis/tracheitis	44.1	14.2
Bronchitis/bronchiolitis	247.5	71.1
Influenza	15.3	14.5
Pneumonia	11.0	6.1
Whooping cough	53.3	10.1
Intestinal infection, presumed or proven	191.1	32.5
Measles	40.5	8.8
Mumps	32.0	21.8
Rubella	24.2	9.3
Chicken pox	16.9	13.1

Susceptibility to infection

Children are not all equally susceptible to infection. Although a certain element of infection is 'bad luck', other factors can be identified.

Genetic. Certain children are more prone to infection; for instance, children with Down's syndrome are more likely to develop upper respiratory tract infections. Mild and severe immune deficiency states run in families.

Environmental. Environmental factors are important with respect to the spread of infection. Good housing, clean water supplies and adequate sanitation contribute enormously to the control of infectious diseases like tuberculosis. Likewise, poor environment is a factor in the continual high prevalence of infectious disease in inner city areas. New infections introduced into isolated communities where there is little herd immunity may be devastating, for example, measles in Eskimos.

Age. The prevalence and severity of certain infectious diseases relates strongly to age. Thus the prevalence and severity of whooping cough and bronchiolitis is greatest in very young children whilst tuberculosis peaks in the pre-school child and in adolescence and early adult life. Mumps tends to be more severe in adults.

Geographical. Many infectious diseases are largely confined to certain climates or areas of the world. However rapid international travel means that children can travel far in the incubation period.

Background nutrition is of paramount importance in the susceptibility and reaction to infection. In the malnourished the death rate due to measles or whooping cough can be very high. Children with any chronic illness are also more susceptible to infection, particularly if the disorder or its treatment results in undernutrition or immunosuppression.

Immunisation history is of obvious importance in determining individual susceptibility to particular infections.

Improving the conditions under which people live, for example by ensuring clean water supplies, adequate sanitation, adequate food supplies and storage, has a major impact on the incidence, spread and severity of infectious disease. Improved housing with adequate light, heating, ventilation and abolition of overcrowding had been shown to reduce the incidence and spread of infection.

For some infectious diseases isolation of infected persons and efficient contact tracing can be a very effective means of control as in tuberculosis. Day nurseries have a constant dilemma when they have an outbreak of diarrhoea which can readily spread in this environment. Sometimes it is necessary to close the nursery for a short time, but since many of the children are in nursery because of anxieties about their welfare or development this should be carefully thought through. Outbreaks of diarrhoea should be reported to the Environmental Health Officer who will investigate the cause.

Health education has an important part to play in the prevention of infectious diseases such as Hepatitis B and HIV. Their association with unprotected sexual activity and drug abuse are important messages for adolescents to understand, but education may need to start earlier.

Immunisation has had a dramatic effect on diseases like smallpox, diphtheria and poliomyelitis; smallpox has been erradicated, indigenous polio is now not seen in many countries, and diphtheria is rare.

Agencies involved

Prevention
Government policy
Family doctor
Health visitor
Child Health Service

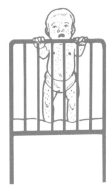

Control
Community physician
Environmental Health Officer
Microbiologists
Public health laboratories
Isolation units

Prevention of infection

Immunity is more than vaccination

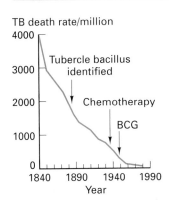

IMMUNISATION

The aim of immunisation is to produce a specific immunological defence against infection without significant risks to the recipient. The first recorded evidence of immunisation was in the 6th century BC in China when dried smallpox crusts were introduced intra-nasally. Modern developments in immunisations start with Jenner who in 1796 demonstrated experimentally the protective effect of cowpox extracts against smallpox.

Theoretical basis of immunity

During an infection both B and T cell lymphocytes are sensitised. The B cells will then produce specific antibodies against the organism which act to neutralise the toxin (antitoxin antibody) or enhance phagocytosis (opsonic activity). The sensitised T cells multiply on exposure to specific antigens and release chemicals such as lymphokines which attack the organism and invoke a local inflammatory reaction. This specific memory is usually life long. The aim of immunisation is to sensitise the system whilst avoiding the unpleasant features of the natural illness. This may be achieved by using attenuated live organisms (e.g. oral polio, BCG) killed organisms or parts of them (e.g. pertussis, typhoid) or modified toxins (e.g. diphtheria, tetanus). With live vaccines the very low grade infection from a single dose provides a prolonged stimulus and long lasting protection. With killed vaccines or toxins the stimulus is short lived and more than one dose needs to be given to give satisfactory immunity. Some vaccines are now being manufactured by a recombinant DNA technique which has the potential for a very wide range of vaccines.

Reaction to vaccination

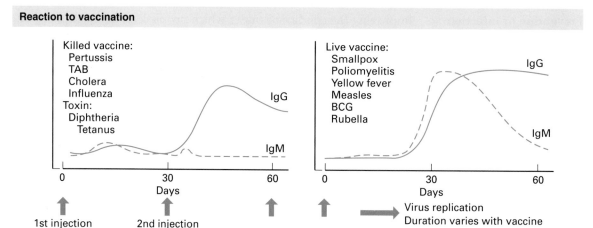

Categories of vaccine

Toxoids	Diphtheria, tetanus
Inactivated bacterial	Pertussis, typhoid, cholera, Hib
Live bacterial	Tuberculosis (BCG)
Inactivated viral	Poliomyelitis (Salk), influenza, rabies, hepatitis B
Live viral	Smallpox, polio (Sabin), yellow fever, measles, mumps, rubella

Temporary defence can be given by passive immunisation. Immuno-globulins must be given by injection; they may be given as pooled human immunoglobulin which contains a mixture of antibodies against the infections prevalent in the blood donors, or specific immunoglobulin prepared from blood taken from patients in the convalescent phase after a natural infection or immunisation. Protection against hepatitis A is pooled immunoglobulin; specific varicella/zoster (VZ) immunoglobulin is used to give temporary protection to immunosuppressed people after contact with chicken pox.

Effectiveness and safety

In the laboratory the likely potency of vaccine may be assessed by a variety of methods such as calculating the number of live organisms in a dose, assay of antibody responses to the vaccine, inoculation of animals before exposure to the infection and measuring the degree of protection.

The effectiveness of a vaccine within a population can be calculated by the following equation:

$$\frac{\text{Attack rate in unvaccinated} - \text{attack rate in vaccinated}}{\text{Attack rate in unvaccinated}} \times 100\%$$

Assessment of safety may be made by injection of large doses of the vaccine into laboratory animals and observing for signs of toxicity. They need to be tested for absence of contamination. In the field, trials of a new vaccine will estimate safety prior to general use. Continuing monitoring of safety is provided in the UK by the mechanism of reporting reactions to the Committee on Safety of Medicines by the 'Yellow Card' system.

Uptake and herd immunity

It is not always necessary to immunise all individuals in order to protect the total population. In some situations, such as tetanus, all individuals need immunisation because of the ubiquitous nature of the organism. For other infections such as polio where infection spreads directly from one person to another and where the vaccine is highly effective, high levels of uptake in the community (probably >90%) will prevent epidemics. This provides protection for unimmunised people and eventually could lead to eradication of the organism. Immunising one group of people can protect another group; ensuring a high immunisation rate in older children against whooping cough, reduces the spread of infection and thereby protects very young children prior to completing their immunisations. The issue of vaccine uptake and herd immunity is important in the design of immunisation programmes.

Immunisation programmes

The decision to initiate an immunisation programme, the practical aspects of running such a programme and its final success depend on many factors.

Political. At national level it is politicians rather than doctors who decide on national programmes and campaigns. They are influenced by doctors but also by individual pressure groups and publicity. Politicians may also affect people's responses to immunisation programmes, either by support, by casting doubts about effectiveness or emphasising side-effects. Whether they are well or ill informed, what they say is reported in the press. Moral issues will also influence political discussion; introduction of a vaccine against HIV will probably be surrounded by controversy.

Economic. The budget available for health care is not unlimited; one group of priorities must be weighed against another. In the case of an immunisation programme the cost of prevention must be weighed against the cost of treatment. For instance, the falling rate of tuberculosis in the UK led to consideration of giving up routine immunisation of adolescents, because it might no longer be economically justified; some Health Authorities in the UK have already decided this and stopped. Against the cost of developing a vaccine programme must be weighed the hours lost by parents from work and consequent fall in productivity caused by the disease; factors such as distress and unhappiness are hard to measure. Common respiratory infections must be very expensive in these terms.

Medical. The medical task is to assess the trends in morbidity and mortality from the infection, and assess the possible influence of an immunisation programme. Once a programme is established, it is not easy to determine what would be the effects of its withdrawal. Where there are no recorded cases of polio in the country, the presence of a reservoir of infection abroad, combined with the severity of the disorder would seem to warrant continued whole population immunisation. Obviously the benefits of the immunisation must outweigh the risks for the individual as well as the community as a whole.

Public motivation. This may range from antipathy and fear when there has been adverse publicity, to apathy particularly when the dire consequences of the illness are not within the experience of the community, to panic when an outbreak occurs. All three reactions have been seen with pertussis immunisation over a period of time as short as 10 years. These changes in public attitude stress the need for health education and presentation of accurate, clear information to public figures and journalists.

Administration of immunisation programmes

I   Register of susceptible individuals
II   Explanation of benefits – appropriate literature
III   Obtain consent
IV   Call and recall system (manual or computer)
V   Immunisation clinic – appropriate clerical, medical, nursing staff
                        – arrangements for transport and storage of vaccines maintaining the cold chain
VI   Record of attendance and uptake of vaccine
VII   System for identifying and immunising non-attenders (opportunistic or home immunisation)
VIII Monitoring uptake

Recommended immunisation programme for UK (1992)

Age	Immunisation	
Neonatal	BCG	High-risk infants
2 months	Diphtheria Pertussis } DPT Tetanus Poliomyelitis Hib	1st dose primary course
3 months	DPT Polio Hib	2nd dose primary course
4 months	DPT Polio Hib	3rd dose primary course
12–18 months	Measles Mumps } MMR Rubella	
4–5 years	Diphtheria Tetanus Polio	Booster
10–14 years	Rubella	For those girls who have not already had it
	BCG	If Heaf negative
15–18 years	Tetanus Polio	Booster

Immunisation schedules

Schedules should not be rigidly interpreted. Primary courses can be commenced at any age after the first 2 months, though clearly the immunisation schedule is designed to protect against infectious disease as early as possible and at the ages of particular risk. The intervals between immunisations are the minimum required. If the intervals between immunisations in the primary course are longer than those indicated in the schedule, there is no need to restart the course but simply to carry on where the course was interrupted. This is most important with tetanus where the risk of reaction increases the greater the number of doses given.

Immunisation uptake

Factors affecting uptake can be divided into two broad categories, professional knowledge/attitudes, and administrative problems. Many studies on uptake rates have identified inappropriate advice received by parents of unimmunised children. This may be inaccurate or outdated advice on contraindications (e.g. asthma as a contraindication for measles vaccine). Inconsistent advice from different professionals is quoted by parents as a reason for avoiding immunisation. There have been many changes in the field of immunisation in recent years and this will continue with new vaccines becoming available and more information on vaccines currently in use. All those involved (administrative and clerical as well as medical and nursing staff) need to have regular updating of their knowledge.

Another consistent feature of studies is that the uptake rate recorded is inaccurate; children who are recorded as having no immunisations or partial immunisation are found to have been fully immunised. This may be because they have been immunised in another clinic, or have moved into the area following immunisation. Other problems arise when reliable recall systems are not in place and appointments are not sent. Children may have failed to attend appointments, but when they turn up to a clinic for some other reason the information on missed immunisations is not available so the opportunity is missed. Good information systems, either manual or on computer, should identify children due immunisations. This information can then be used to encourage attendance at appointments or to tag the records (perhaps of the whole family) in order to enable immunisations to be given opportunistically. Some groups may need a specially tailored system such as immunisations taken into the home.

Uptake of immunisations (%), England and Wales

Year of birth	Measles	Diphtheria	Pertussis	Tetanus	Polio
1970	34	80	79	81	79
1972	52	81	79	81	80
1974	53	80	77	80	79
1976	47	75	39	75	75
1978	53	81	41	81	81
1980	58	84	53	84	84
1982	63	84	65	84	84
1984	71	85	67	85	85
1986/87*	80	87	75	87	87
1987/88	84	89	78	89	89

Primary course completed by 2 years of age
*Recording changed from calendar to financial year

Target payments for family doctors achieving 90% (higher rate) and 70% (lower rate) were introduced in 1989, with success.

POLIO

There are three distinct strains of poliovirus – types 1, 2 and 3 – and there is very little antigenic overlap. Type 1 has been associated with most of the major epidemics and shows the greatest propensity to cause paralytic forms of the disease.

Vaccine. Oral poliovirus vaccine (OPV, Sabin vaccine) is a mixture of live attenuated strains of virus types 1, 2 and 3, grown in monkey kidney or human fetal diploid cell cultures. This vaccine is given orally on three separate occasions during which both local gut immunity and systemic immunity are established. This may not occur to all three strains on the first occasion so the dose needs to be repeated in order to ensure immunity to all three types. Inactivated poliovirus vaccine (IPV, Salk vaccine) is an inactivated vaccine containing all three strains given by injection. It provides satisfactory systemic immunity and will prevent polio illness; it does not provide local gut immunity so that the virus can still replicate in the gut and be transmitted to other people.

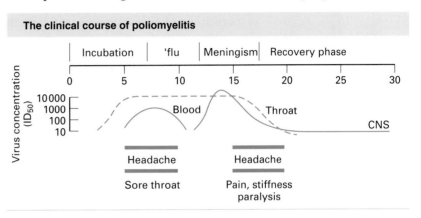

The clinical course of poliomyelitis

Effectiveness. Introduction of the two forms of vaccine has led to the elimination of indigenous polio in the UK and some other countries. It is hoped that it may be eliminated worldwide by the end of the century. With OPV the attenuated virus is excreted in the faeces and may spread to other members of the family and immunise them as well. However there is a slightly increased risk of reversion to a more virulent form in this situation, so it is preferable to immunise susceptible carers at the same time as the child. In the UK and the USA the benefits of herd immunity from OPV, the acceptability of an oral vaccine and the lower cost are thought to outweigh the rare complication of vaccine associated polio. Other countries such as Holland, which had an outbreak of polio in a group opposed to immunisation, use IPV.

Contraindications. Polio vaccine is contraindicated in pregnancy unless at very high risk of the disease. It is also contraindicated in those with immune deficiency; close contacts of those with immune deficiency should receive IPV because of the risk of transmission of the vaccine virus.

Reactions. Vaccine associated polio resulting from reversion to a more virulent form in the gut occurs in recipients of OPV in about one case per 4–5 million doses and in unvaccinated contacts in one case per 2–3 million doses given.

MEASLES

The maculopapular rash of measles appears first behind the ears and on the face, spreading downwards to form a confluent blotchy appearance.

Encephalitis affects 1 in 5000 children who have measles; 15% of these will die and 25% suffer cerebral damage. In developing countries in the presence of malnutrition, the severity and mortality of measles is much higher than in the UK. Uncomplicated measles requires only rest, fluids and an antipyretic. Prophylactic antibiotics are not indicated. Where secondary infection does occur this is likely to be a mixed bacterial infection and a broad spectrum antibiotic is required. The patient is infectious from a few days before, to 7 days after the onset of the rash.

Measles notifications

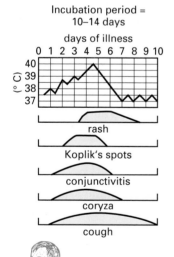

Number in 3 months

The vaccine is a freeze dried aqueous suspension of live attenuated measles virus grown on fibroblast tissue derived from chick embryos. It is given at 12–18 months of age with mumps and rubella. It can be given safely even if the child is thought to have had measles infection or during the incubation period. If the vaccine is given from 12–15 months of age, it is highly effective. Under the age of 1 year a significant number of children fail to seroconvert because of the presence of maternal antibodies to measles. A new vaccine (Edmonston-Zagreb) that is effective in the presence of maternal antibodies is being investigated in developing countries because of the high risk of measles illness under 1 year in these countries. In the USA, where high levels of measles immunisation have been achieved, they came close to eliminating indigenous measles in the 1980s. However small outbreaks are still occurring particularly among the very young, prior to immunisation, and in adolescents and young adults. The duration of immunity of the early vaccines has been questioned and the role of a 2 dose schedule is debated.

Contraindications. Live vaccines should not be given to children with any immune deficiency. Severe allergy (anaphylaxis) to eggs may be a contraindication because the vaccine is grown on chick embryo fibroblasts and there is a theoretical risk of cross reaction. However, immunisation can probably be safely carried out under controlled conditions. The vaccine may contain small amounts of various antibiotics

Measles

Incubation period =
10–14 days

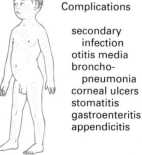

Complications

secondary
  infection
otitis media
broncho-
  pneumonia
corneal ulcers
stomatitis
gastroenteritis
appendicitis

(e.g. polymixin, neomycin) and should not be given to those known to be allergic to the particular antibiotic in the vaccine being used. If there is a history of febrile convulsions it is important to stress antipyretic measures.

Reactions. It is not uncommon for children to develop a fever, mild irritability and even a measles-like rash 5–10 days after the immunisation. There is a small increase in the risk of a convulsion during this time (1 per 1000). Because it is a live vaccine, any of the complications of measles illness can occur but much less frequently than with the illness.

Passive immunisation. Suppression of measles can be achieved by giving human normal immunoglobulin and may be indicated at certain times in exposed unimmunised children with chronic heart, lung or malignant disease.

MUMPS

The distinguishing feature of mumps is the enlargement of the salivary glands, usually the parotids. There may be a prodromal illness with fever, headache and malaise lasting 1–2 days. Aseptic meningitis occurs in about 1 in a 1000 cases though a mild form may be much commoner. Sensorineural deafness, usually unilateral, can occur and mumps is thought to be the commonest cause of this. Orchitis affects 20% of post-pubertal males but sterility following this is rare.

Vaccine. This is a live attenuated virus grown on chick embryo tissue culture. It is given combined with measles and rubella at 12–15 months.

Effectiveness. It is a highly effective vaccine. Since its introduction in the UK in 1988, there has been a noticeable fall in mumps illness.

Contraindications. As for measles.

Reactions. A mild mumps illness occurs in about 1 in 100 children about 3 weeks after immunisation. Aseptic meningitis may occur but is less frequent than in the mumps illness. It is usually mild and then recovery is complete.

RUBELLA

Rubella is a mild illness with a maculopapular rash, occipital lymphadenopathy and mild fever. Arthritis and thrombocytopaenia are occasional complications. Its importance lies in the effects on the fetus, which can be devastating. Diagnosis of congenital rubella relies on a combination of the clinical features, antibody levels and isolation of virus from the urine. High specific IgM titres indicate a recent infection,

Rubella notifications

Number of children aged 1 year with congenital rubella

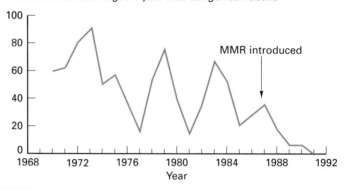

whereas IgG levels may be positive indefinitely. Virus may remain in the urine for up to a year.

Vaccine. This is a freeze dried suspension of live attenuated virus grown in tissue culture cells of human or rabbit origin. It is given in combination with measles and mumps vaccines at the age of 12–18 months. Until 1988 in the UK, rubella immunisation was only given to girls at the age of 11–13 years and to susceptible women in the child bearing years. This policy helped to reduce the incidence of congenital rubella, but there were still affected children born each year and terminations for possibly affected pregnancies. By 1987/88 the national immunisation rate for 14 year olds was 86% leaving a potential 14% susceptible girls with epidemics of rubella still occurring regularly. In 1988 the policy was changed to universal immunisation at 12–18 months, in order to try and get herd immunity and stop epidemics. Until these children reach 11 years, the programme to immunise older girls needs to continue. The vaccine is still offered to all sero-negative women of child bearing age.

Effectiveness. After the initial rise, antibody levels slowly decrease over the subsequent years though after 30 years there is still normally adequate immunity serologically. Reinfection is known to occur and though this does not normally affect the fetus, it may do so.

Contraindications. Rubella vaccine, as with all live virus vaccines, is contraindicated in pregnancy, though there have been no cases of congenital rubella caused by the current vaccines. Accidental immunisation during pregnancy would therefore not be a reason for termination of pregnancy. Other contraindications for live virus vaccines also apply. If children have arthritis, it would be wise to discuss immunisation timing because of the association of rubella illness with exacerbations of arthritis.

Reactions. Mild fever, rash and lymphadenopathy are sometimes seen. Arthritis and arthropathy are rare complications.

WHOOPING COUGH

Pertussis is caused by the bacterium, *Bordetella pertussis*, though milder infection may occur with *Bordetella parapertussis* or *Bordetella bronchiseptica*. A variety of viruses can also cause pertussis-like illnesses. The incubation period is 7–14 days, the catarrhal phase 7–14 days, the paroxysmal phase 4–6 weeks and recovery usually takes a further 2–6 weeks. Complications include bronchopneumonia, convulsions, apnoeic spells, and rarely now, bronchiectasis. The child remains infectious from 7 days after exposure to 21 days after the onset of the paroxysmal cough.

Erythromycin given in the catarrhal phase may attenuate the infection and it may be helpful if given as prophylaxis amongst infant contacts. Otherwise treatment depends on good nursing care, which may include oxygen, suction and tube feeding, plus the treatment of complications as they occur.

Prognosis is worst under 1 year of age. There was a case fatality rate of 0.9–2.6/1000 notifications in the 1977–9 epidemic, and large numbers required hospital admission. There may be an association between whooping cough and cot death as epidemiologically there are parallels.

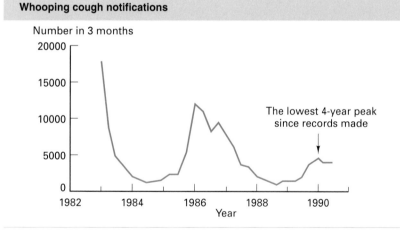

Vaccine. This is made from killed organisms of several serotypes of *Bordetella pertussis*. It is usually combined with diphtheria and tetanus vaccines in 3 doses in early infancy, but can be given at any age. It is particularly important that children with chronic illness or handicap are immunised since they will be at particular risk from whooping cough. Acellular vaccines have been developed which comprise parts of the organism that are thought to be the main antigens but excluding parts that are reactogenic. Vaccines with fewer side effects have been developed but at the expense of efficacy. There are now vaccines becoming available which seem to combine efficacy with low reactogenicity, but they are still undergoing trials.

Effectiveness. Protection rates of 85-90% are achieved, and if the illness does affect immunised children it is likely to be milder.

Reactions. Mild reactions are common. These may consist of local pain and swelling or a transient irritability, pyrexia and fretfulness. These are not contraindications to further doses. A few children have a more severe reaction with marked swelling and redness of the injection site or severe systemic upset. These children are likely to recover fully. Immunisation against pertussis became the subject of considerable controversy in the UK in the mid 1970s, following well publicised reports of neurological damage associated with reactions to pertussis vaccine. The frequency of such reactions and the incidence of pertussis illness and its complications were not known and varying figures were reported. The debate led to a considerable fall in the immunisation rate to about 31% in 1978 and as a consequence there was a bad epidemic of whooping cough in 1978–80. It became clear that pertussis was still a serious disease especially in infants. There were at least 30 deaths in England and Wales. At the same time the efficacy of the vaccine was clearly demonstrated. Attempts have been made to establish the risk of encephalopathy following pertussis vaccine, but there is no conclusive evidence of a link. On the other hand the risks from pertussis illness are well established. Immunisation rates have risen again in recent years with a resulting fall in the number of cases.

Contraindications. A severe reaction to a preceding dose is a contraindication to any vaccine. In the case of combined DPT vaccine there is a problem because the cause of the reaction could be any of the components. All three may be omitted, or pertussis alone may be omitted with the rationale that this is the most frequently associated with reactions. The definition of a severe reaction is set out in the Department of Health Guidelines which are regularly updated. There are other children with 'problem histories' such as an increased risk of fits or those thought at higher risk of having a neurological problem. In these children care must be taken to counsel the parents fully on the small risk of fits following the immunisation but also on the increased risk of severe problems of the illness. Most of these children can be safely immunised.

TUBERCULOSIS

Although tuberculosis has declined in incidence it remains an important disorder in the United Kingdom. Between 1987 and 1990 the incidence has remained static, with an increase in the number of notifications in families originating in the Indian sub-continent. In other countries there has been an increase in incidence attributed to the rise in HIV infected people who are particularly susceptible to reactivation of tuberculosis. There were 478 deaths from tuberculosis notified in the United Kingdom in 1988. In developing countries it is still an important cause of death. Transmission is by droplet spread from an individual with open TB. This may be an elderly relative or in the case of school children, an adult with undetected illness working in the school. Many infections are sub-clinical.

Presentation of tuberculosis. Unlike chicken pox or measles, the diagnosis of tuberculosis cannot be made simply and quickly on clinical grounds alone. The diagnosis requires a high level of clinical suspicion.

Asymptomatic subjects. Tuberculosis may be identified by tuberculin testing of contacts of known cases or by routine testing prior to BCG immunisation. It may also be identified in people having routine chest X-rays. If a contact has a negative tuberculin test it should be repeated after a further 6 weeks because the test may not become positive in the incubation period of the illness.

Sensitivity reactions. Where primary infection has been recent, children may present with a febrile illness, erythema nodosum or phlyctenular conjunctivitis.

Vague ill health. Children may present with primary tuberculosis with very ill-defined symptoms. There may be complaints of lethargy, tiredness and poor growth. Liver or spleen enlargement may be felt.

Pulmonary tuberculosis. This may present as (a) pleural effusion, the onset often being with acute breathlessness, pyrexia, pain and occasional cough; (b) caseation and cavitation; the child has a cough, is constitutionally ill and has a pyrexia. If the cavity connects with the main bronchi, the bacilli may be found in the sputum or gastric washings; (c) bronchial obstruction due to lymph node enlargement. This may cause either collapse or hyperinflation of part of the lung.

Miliary tuberculosis. This may be acute or slow in onset. The features are again non-specific with fever, weight loss and lethargy. The liver and spleen may be enlarged and choroidal tubercles may be seen as yellow dots along the retinal vessels.

Tuberculous meningitis. This is another feature of haematogenous spread and presents with a lymphocytic meningitis, low CSF sugar and bacilli visible on microscopy of the fluid.

Bone or joint involvement. This may present as synovitis or osteitis which may affect the spine, hip, knee, ankle, elbow, wrist, hands or feet.

Primary tonsillar infection with cervical lymphadenopathy. This is usually caused by the bovine type of tuberculosis.

Abdominal tuberculosis. This is a very rare presentation in the UK and is also caused by bovine infection. It presents with abdominal pain and the findings of a doughy mass in the abdomen. If the mesenteric lymph nodes rupture, tuberculous peritonitis will occur.

Diagnosis. The diagnosis is not always easy. The various forms of tuberculin testing to be described below probably provide for the easiest approach. Radiology is sensitive but non-specific, sputum microscopy is specific but very insensitive, and culture is slow.

Mantoux test. An intradermal injection of 10 units of PPD (purified protein derivative) in 0.1 ml is made on the flexor surface of the left forearm. If active tuberculosis is suspected a lower starting dose of 1 unit should be used. The date, time, position of injection and strength of solution are recorded and the site inspected 72 hours later. An area of induration of 5 mm or more is regarded as a positive reaction. This is not generally used for routine screening because of the difficulty of intradermal injections.

Heaf test. A Heaf gun with disposable single use heads is now recommended. If you are using a re-usable Heaf gun, it should be set to penetrate the skin at 2 mm, except for children under 2 years when it is set at 1 mm. The gun is sterilised by immersion in spirit and then flaming. The gun must be allowed to cool before use. Purified protein derivative equivalent to 100 000 units per ml is applied to the skin over the flexor surface of the left forearm. Sites containing superficial veins should be avoided. The result is read between 3 and 10 days later. Grade I and Grade II reactions may be due to avian tuberculosis or to previous BCG. All children with Grade III or IV reactions require X-ray and follow-up.

Reading the Heaf test

Negative: minute puncture scars; slight erythema may be present, no induration

Positive:

      Grade I : induration of at least 4 puncture points

      Grade II : coalescence forming a ring of induration

      Grade III: extensive induration 5 – 10 mm

      Grade IV: severe induration 10 mm possibly with central blistering

---

False negative results may be obtained from using materials that have deteriorated, if the material is injected too deeply, if the test is read too soon or too late, or if the test was performed near an inflamed site so that rapid removal of tuberculin occurred. False positive results may be obtained by a burn from the Heaf gun, local infection or a rupture of small blood vessels.

BCG. (Bacillus Calmette-Guerin) is a freeze dried live attenuated bovine strain of *Mycobacterium tuberculosis*. It is derived from the original bacillus grown by Calmette and Guerin in 1921. The vaccine is given by intradermal injection of 0.1 ml into the skin at the insertion of the deltoid. Most Health Authourities in the UK offer BCG to all tuberculin negative children at 10-14 years. It is also given to newborn

BCG

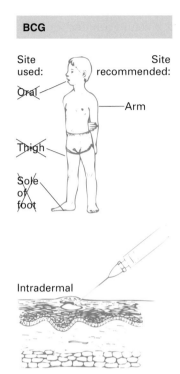

Site used: ~~Oral~~

Site recommended:

Arm

~~Thigh~~

~~Sole of foot~~

Intradermal

babies of high risk families (certain ethnic groups and families with a close rela-tive with recent tuberculosis) in a dose of 0.05 ml. Immunisation results in a small papule appearing 7–10 days later which enlarges over a few weeks and often ulcerates. Peeling occurs in 6–8 weeks with a residual scar forming. Mantoux conversion occurs within 3–4 weeks of immuni-sation though this is slower in babies. Abnormal reactions to BCG are often the result of faulty injection technique. If given subcutaneously there is much more likely to be abscess formation. Ulcers that are slow to heal are best treated with simple dressing and with tetracycline oint-ment if secondary infection has occurred. If an abscess develops or lymphadenopathy, this may need treatment with anti-tuberculous drugs and should be dealt with at a specialist clinic.

Effectiveness. Immunity seems long lasting with an 80% protective effect after 15 years. TB can occur after BCG immunisation but it effectively prevents the development of miliary TB or TB meningitis.

The decision to immunise against tuberculosis at birth depends upon the incidence of the disease. The World Health Organization recommended that where 5% of children aged 10–14 years have been infected, BCG should be given at birth. Where the rate is more than 2% but less than 5% it should be given on school entry and in places with less than 2% affected BCG should be given at 12–13 years. Where tuberculosis does occur in people who have already received BCG the diagnosis may be delayed.

Chemoprophylaxis. This may be given in several circumstances. If the mother of a newborn baby is infected with active pulmonary tuberculosis the baby may be given isoniazid by mouth and isoniazid resistant BCG. Secondary chemoprophylaxis is given to those with asymptomatic disease. This will include children with strong tuberculin reactions on routine testing, children who are contacts of patients with tuberculosis whose tuberculin test converts, and any tuberculin reactor under the age of 5 years. Chemoprophylaxis currently recommended is isoniazid for six months or isoniazid and rifampicin for three months. A local chest physician or Consultant in Communicable Diseases will normally co-ordinate this.

TETANUS

Tetanus is caused by a Gram positive anaerobic spore bearing organism, *Clostridium tetani,* found universally in the soil. The disease is caused by the neurotoxin produced by the organism. After an incubation period of 5–14 days there are progressive intermittent muscle spasms, often triggered by stimuli such as noise or touch. Tetanus is now rare in this country because of immunisation. When the disease occurs it still carries a high mortality.

Vaccine. This is a formol inactivated toxoid given in conjunction with an adjuvant by intramuscular or deep subcutaneous injection often combined with diphtheria and pertussis vaccines. After a primary course of three injections in infancy and the booster at school entry, immunisation is only required every 10 years. It may be that a further two boosters is sufficient for lifelong protection. If a wound occurs outside that 10 year period a single booster dose only is required. Too frequent reinforcing doses, as may occur in children who have frequent accidents, are unnecessary and can provoke severe hypersensitivity reactions. Human tetanus immunoglobulin may be given to unimmunised people suffering from major wounds with a high degree of contamination.

DIPHTHERIA

Diphtheria is caused by one of three strains of *Corynebacterium diphtheriae*. The infection may be caught from infected individuals or healthy carriers. The incubation period is 2–7 days after which the toxin causes destruction of the superficial epithelium of the respiratory tract producing obstruction. The toxin can also produce a myocarditis and lower motor neurone symptoms.

Vaccine. This is a formol inactivated toxoid adsorbed to an adjuvant. An adult form (more dilute) should be used for children over 10 years, because of the small possibility of the child already being immune to diphtheria and therefore having a severe reaction to the standard dose.

HAEMOPHILUS INFLUENZAE TYPE B (HIB)

There are number of different serotypes of *Haemophilus influenzae,* but it is the encapsulated type b organism that is the one that almost always causes invasive disease. This organism is one of the main causes of meningitis in young children. There is a high morbidity with 10 to 15% of children developing severe neurological sequelae such as profound deafness, cerebral palsy and epilepsy. The mortality rate is 3 to 4%. Hib is the predominant organism causing epiglottitis and can cause other invasive diseases.

Vaccine. A vaccine has been available for some years but was only effective in children over 2 years of age. Since the main serious effects of the illness occurred in children under this age it was not routinely used in the UK. Vaccines have now been developed which are effective in infants. The polysaccharide capsule of the organism is conjugated with a protein. The vaccine is only effective against type b infection. This vaccine was introduced in the UK in 1992 and is given at 2, 3 and 4 months, at the same time as DPT. Booster doses are not needed. It is a highly effective vaccine with low incidence of side effects.

HEPATITIS

Hepatitis A is the commonest cause of jaundice in older children and has an incubation period of 15–20 days or sometimes longer. Ourbreaks sometimes occur in schools or other situations where the level of hygiene is in question. In children the illness is normally mild. The period of infectivity is from 1–2 weeks before to 1 week after the onset of symptoms. Good hygiene remains the main method of control.

Vaccine. Passive immunisation may be considered for family and close contacts and for those travelling in high risk areas. A vaccine is now available which is recommended for those frequently travelling abroad or spending prolonged periods abroad.

Hepatitis B is transmitted largely by the parenteral route. This means that it is only likely to be acquired in special circumstances, i.e. contamination by blood, blood products or other body fluids. Once the virus is acquired it may cause a fulminating hepatitis, chronic hepatitis or be asymptomatic. Many people who acquire the virus become carriers, unaffected themselves but at risk of transmitting it to others. Children are most likely to become infected with hepatitis B virus by vertical transmission before or during birth from an infected mother. In the past, transfusion or injection of blood products was a source of infection, but many countries including the UK, now test blood products. Close contact with body fluids is another source of infection, as may happen in institutions for children with severe learning difficulties who may bite and scratch. In adolescence sexual intercourse and drug addicts sharing needles need to be considered.

Vaccine. There are two types of vaccine available. One is an inactivated virus obtained from human plasma, and the other is surface antigen produced by a recombinant DNA technique. Two doses are given six months apart. Serological testing should be carried out following this and if unsatisfactory immunity is demonstrated a further dose should be given. The vaccine is not offered routinely to all people in the UK, but is recommended in certain high risk groups, such as health workers, emergency workers, infants of infected mothers. All high risk mothers (certain ethnic groups, drug addicts) should be screened in pregnancy and if appropriate the infant can be immunised at birth.

OTHER VACCINES

Influenza vaccine is available and can provide 60–70% protection from the illness, but only for the following year. The nature of the vaccine is changed periodically to keep up with the change in the virus. It is recommended for certain high risk groups, particularly the elderly, but also children at risk with chronic heart or lung disorders and possibly neurological disorders.

Pneumococcal vaccine is of value in certain high risk children, particularly those with absence of the spleen. Children with sickle cell disease often have a non functioning spleen and may be at risk. It is only effective in children over 2 years of age.

Varicella/zoster vaccine has been developed but at present is not available in the UK.

TRAVEL ABROAD

The most important factors in preventing infection while travelling are those involved with good hygiene, care in what is eaten and drunk, and physical protection against bites. Routine immunisations should be up to date. Depending on the country to be visited, some additional immunisations may be recommended, e.g. typhoid, yellow fever, meningococcus C. Some countries require certificates of vaccination before allowing entry. Up to date advice on this and other recommendations can be obtained from the Department of Health leaflets (T2 and T3), from local travel clinics or from the London School of Hygiene and Tropical Medicine.

REFERENCES AND FURTHER READING

Immunisation against infectious disease 1992. HMSO, London
Rudd P, Nicoll A 1991. A manual on infections and immunisation. OUP, Oxford
Wood M J 1992 Infectious diseases. Commentary and selection of abstracts from
    The Lancet

Eating Well

It is difficult to over-emphasise the importance of early nutrition. New-born babies do little more that feed, sleep and grow. Parents know that an increase in weight indicates that their child is thriving. Doctors know that loss of weight is often the first sign of underlying illness. Good growth in the early months of life not only promotes early success, but may also have a major impact on adult size, well-being and longevity. Now in Western countries where food is plentiful and the food industry is able to prepare and present foods in many forms and to add whatever extras might be thought to be beneficial, the questions on what to feed infants and children is getting more challenging.

NATIONAL ADVICE

It is, and has been, the advice of all authorities, national and international, that breast feeding is the best way to feed healthy babies, but that is not to say that infants cannot be reared successfully without breast milk. Weaning is not recommended before 4 months of age, but healthy babies do not appear to come to any harm if they are given weaning foods earlier. Young children should be given an interesting varied diet, but some appear to thrive on 'junk foods' hurriedly swallowed. Clearly if we are to give advice it has to be based on a sound knowledge of nutrition and to be realistic within the lifestyle and culture of the child and his or her family. In the UK, we are fortunate in having regular national surveys. The ones quoted throughout this chapter are:

> DHSS Report 10 'A nutrition survey of pre-school children 1967–68'
> DHSS Report 32 'Present day practice in Infant Feeding',
> DHSS Report 36 'The Diets of British Schoolchildren'
> D of H Report 41, 'Dietary Reference Values for Food Energy and Nutrients for the United Kingdom.'

Another report on the study of the diets of preschool children is due. The last study over 14 years ago still contains some interesting information; for example in the report on school children, social class differences in height, obvious in 11 year olds, were already apparent by

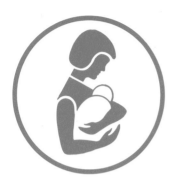

2 years of age. The government has also established a working group in 1991 to advise on weaning diets.

Government reports do not always make easy reading, they confine themselves in the main to reporting the facts. However the Department of Health (DoH) has produced some clear guidance in a number of pamphlets. In this chapter we have quoted from one of them, 'Feeding Today's Infants' (taken from DoH 1988). It is important that health professionals do not give contrary advice without very good reason. The Logo is taken from official reports produced by the HMSO. Not infrequently data are not available to answer specific questions of what is best, or what can be permitted, or whether the recent food fashion is potentially harmful or not. We then have no option but to express opinions based on general principles.

DIETARY REFERENCE VALUES (DRVs)

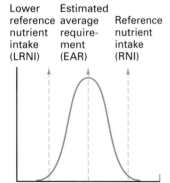

Frequency distribution of individual requirements

Lower reference nutrient intake (LRNI)   Estimated average requirement (EAR)   Reference nutrient intake (RNI)

|←2 SD→|←2 SD→|

In an attempt to answer the simple question, what is an adequate diet, the government took expert advice and then made recommendations. In 1969 the standards were called Recommended Daily Intakes (RDIs), and in 1979 Recommended Daily Amounts (RDAs). Both were misunderstood as being suggested requirements for nutrients, when in fact they were the amounts of nutrients thought to be required to prevent deficiency in the majority of the population. Hence, in excess of requirements for most. To avoid this misunderstanding new Dietary References Values (DRVs) have been published giving the average daily requirement (DoH 1991). They are based on what a population eats and are in line with WHO guidance. Assuming a normal distribution of intake, an estimate is made of 2 standard deviations above and below the mean. The level 2 SD above the mean is called the Reference Nutrient Intake (RNI); an intake at this level should be more than sufficient for the great majority. The RNI is equivalent to the previous RDI.

Terms relating to energy and nutrient intakes

RDI   – Recommended Daily Intakes of Nutrients for the United Kingdom, 1969.
RDA   – Recommended Daily Amounts of Food Energy and Nutrients for Groups of People in the United Kingdom, 1979.
DRV   – Dietary Reference Value. A term used to cover LRNI, EAR, RNI and safe intake (see below).
EAR   – Estimated Average Requirement of a group of people for energy* or protein or a vitamin or mineral. About half will usually need more than the EAR, and half less.
LRNI – Lower Reference Nutrient Intake for protein or a vitamin or mineral. An amount of the nutrient that is enough for only the few people in a group who have low needs (usually <3%).
RNI   – Reference Nutrient Intake for protein or a vitamin or mineral. An amount of the nutrient that is enough, or more than enough, for most (usually at least 97%) people in a group. If average intake of a group is at RNI, then the risk of deficiency in the group is very small.
Safe intake – A term to indicate intake or range of intakes of a nutrient for which there is not enough information to estimate RNI, EAR or LRNI. It is an amount that is enough for almost everyone but not so large as to cause undesirable effects.

As excess energy leads to obesity only an EAR has been set for each category.

For many nutrients there is insufficient data to establish the DRVs with any confidence. Nonetheless they provide the best guide that we have. It is important that we do not misuse them. The values should not be applied indiscrimately to individual children, particularly sick children. There is wide variation in need between children of similar age, weight, activity and feeding patterns due to differences in food absorption, utilisation and metabolic efficiency. For some nutrients, an intake below the LRNI may not lead to a deficiency state, and for others an intake above the RNI may cause no harm. In special situations it is helpful to read the evidence on which the values are based. Throughout this chapter will be examples of these values.

INFANT FEEDING

Breast feeding

All experts are agreed that breast feeding is the proper way to nourish an infant over the first months of life. Many books have been written on the benefits to the mother and the infant. At times the debate has been both heated and confused. The arguments in favour can relate to the mother, physically, emotionally and socially, and to the infant, physically, emotionally and socially. It follows that the balance and weight of the arguments will vary with cultures, economies and climates as well as the biological effects on mother and infant. The reasons why mothers choose to breast feed or not are instructive and particularly relevant if we wish to promote breast feeding.

It is helpful to view the breast feeding mother and infant as a dyad. In survival terms, it is the survival of this unit which was and is critical. There is an economy of supply as well as the need to satisfy, so simple statements like 'nature knows best', and 'breast milk is the ideal nutrient for babies' are not helpful to the debate for neither can be sustained.

Composition of mature human milk

Mean values for pooled samples of expressed milk (per 100 ml)

Energy (kcal)	70
Protein (g)	1.3
Lactose (g)	7
Fat (g)	4.2
Minerals	
Sodium (mg)	15
Potassium (mg)	60
Chloride (mg)	43
Calcium (mg)	35
Phosphorus (mg)	15
Magnesium (mg)	2.8
Iron (µg)	76

Mothers' reasons for planning to breast feed according to birth order (1990 Great Britain)

	%
Breast feeding is best for the baby	82
Breast feeding is more convenient	36
Breast feeding is natural	14
Breast feeding is cheaper	17
Closer bond between mother and baby	23
Mother's own experience	15
Breast feeding is best for mother	8
Cannot overfeed by breast	1
Influenced by medical personnel	2
Influenced by friends or relatives	1
No particular reason	1
Total*	3186

* Percentages do not add up to 100 as some mothers gave more than one reason

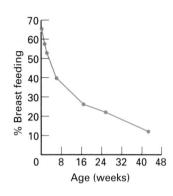

Nor are over-statements on the protective effects of breast feeding against the development of allergies or infections useful. Clearly if there is an effect it is not a major one in a Western Society.

So having put some of the unhelpful debating points to one side we can again state that all authorities agree that breast feeding is the appropriate way to nourish infants. Breast milk contains a range of nutrients which meet all the requirements of the great majority of infants. The sugar is lactose, which is released attached to protein. That is why it is difficult to produce a lactose free milk based on milk protein. The protein is 60 per cent whey and 40 per cent curd (casein). The whey protein is an interesting mixture of many different proteins including IgA, which is probably not digested, lactoferrin and lysosyme, which probably protect against infection, and lactalbumin. But it also contains traces of the protein from the mother's own diet, so hypersensitivity can develop to protein the mother has digested. The fats more directly reflect what the mother has eaten. If the mother is on a high essential fatty acid diet, then the milk fat will contain up to 10–15 per cent EFA. If the mother eats mainly carbohydrate or saturated fats then the milk fat will contain as little as 1–2 per cent EFA. 'Nature' produces both, and at the present we have no evidence that one or the other leads to benefit.

The debate becomes a little fraught when we consider Vit A & D and iron. European governments hold different views about the desirability of breast fed infants needing supplements of vitamins and iron! At the present in the UK it is recommended that all infants are given supplements of vitamins A, D and C from 6 months to 5 years.

Human milk has the advantage that it is ready to feed, sterile, at the correct temperature, has varying constituents and is convenient for the mother. But this last point, in a two income family, or with a single working mother, is its disadvantage, for it needs the mother to be in attendance! It is a target for the WHO and for many countries including the UK that a larger percentage of infants should be breast fed. The figures have not increased in the last 10 years.

In a major national initiative to improve the situation the following recommendations have been made.

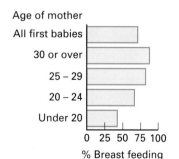

Age and breast feeding

Successful breast feeding is facilitated by:

- Putting the baby to the mother's breast very soon after birth
- Correct positioning at the breast
- Feeding on demand rather than at set times
- Not giving complementary feeds
- A positive and relaxed atmosphere
- Supportive and consistent advice

Samples of infant formula should not be given to mothers.

The reasons why mothers elect not to breast feed are many and need to be known by those who seek to 'improve' the situation. Likewise the reasons why mothers give up breast feeding are many and complex and simple remedies are unlikely to work here either. Advice on safety of drugs in breast feeding is given in the British National Formulary (1991 no. 2).

Reasons given by mothers for stopping breast feeding at different ages (1990 Great Britain)

Reasons for stopping	Under 1 week	2–6 weeks	4–9 months
Insufficient milk	35	60	30
Paintful breasts or nipples	30	14	2
Baby would not suck/rejected breast	25	8	22
Breast feeding took too long/tiring	6	13	6
Did not like breast feeding	10	3	0
Domestic reasons	3	6	2
Mother had inverted nipples	4	1	0
Baby was ill	7	6	2
Baby could not be fed by others	1	3	3
Embarrassment	1	2	0
Returning to work	1	2	15
Had breast fed as long as intended	1	1	42
Other reasons	3	1	7
Total	482	575	796

Percentages do not add up to 100 as some mothers gave more than one reason

Breast milk substitutes

Whilst we may wish, where it is possible, for an infant to be breast fed, we must also accept that every mother has a right to choose what she feels is best for her and her baby and support her in her decision.

Mother's reasons for planning to bottle feed according to birth order (1990 Great Britain)

Mother's reason	%
Other people can feed baby with bottle	39
Mother's own previous experience	26
Did not like the idea of breast feeding	21
Would be embarrassed to breast feed	7
You can see how much the baby has had	6
Medical reasons for not breast feeding	3
Expecting to return to work soon	5
Persuaded by other people	–
No particular reason	3
Other reasons	6
Total*	1852

Percentages do not add up to 100 as some mothers gave more than one reason

Feed volume and number by age

Age	Volume	No.
1–2 wk	50–70	7–8
2–6 wk	75–110	6–7
2 mths	110–180	5–6
3 mths	170–220	5
6 mths	220–240	4

These figures are a guide only. The needs vary from day to day and feed to feed

She will need advice on how to prepare and how to present feeds, and more to the point she will want to know how much she should offer. The commonly used requirement is 150 ml per kg body weight. This provides about 2.3 g protein and 100 kcal per kg when using infant formulae. However there is considerable variation from one baby to another. Bottle fed babies like breast fed babies should be fed on demand and allowed to find their own pattern. A rough guide is shown in

Composition of infant formulae

Per 100 ml	WB	CB
Energy (kcal)	66	66
Protein (g)	1.5	1.9
Casein (%)	40	80
Whey (%)	60	20
Fat (g)	3.6	3.4
Sat. fat (%)	41.1	41.1
Unsat. fat (%)	56.2	56.2
Carbohydrate (g)	7.3	7.3
Sodium (mg)	18	25
Potassium (mg)	65	100
Chloride (mg)	40	60
Calcium (mg)	54	85
Magnesium (mg)	5.0	7.0
Phosphorus (mg)	27	55
Iron (mg)	0.5	0.5

WB = whey-based,
CB = casein-based (Cow & Gate)

the table. A baby given too much may either vomit, have frequent bowel actions or become obese, or all three. On these matters the infant's 'appetite' is not to be wholly trusted. As with breast fed infants, they too may become obese.

The next question is, which artificial feed? There was a time when anything that succeeded was acceptable. Thirty years ago infants were reared on condensed milk offered on a spoon with water drinks! During the war 'National Dried Milk' was barely modified reconstituted cow's milk. Now it is required that infant feeds are as like human milk as possible.

Whilst the 'energy', water, protein, carbohydrate and fat, may in general be similar to human milk, the constituents themselves are very different, the protein is cow's milk protein, the fats are vegetable fats, and the carbohydrate may or may not be lactose or a mixture with lactose. There are five manufacturers in the UK which between them offer four main groups of products: whey based formulae, casein based formulae, soya based formulae and 'follow-on milks'. Here the question is which of the first two should a mother choose?

The 'whey based' formula has a whey/casein ratio similar to human milk, ie 60/40, but the proteins are still cow's milk whey and cow's milk casein. These are the 'highly modified' 'humanised' feeds. The 'casein based' formula has a whey/casein ratio of 20/80 which is as it is in cow's milk. The protein is less modified. It is generally recommended that infants are fed on whey based formula and that this is sufficient for any infant's needs. The casein based formulae are promoted on the basis that they are more satifying, thus it is implied that the infant will settle more quickly after the feed, sleep sounder, and perhaps grow sturdier. There is no evidence to support this view. Mothers choose a feed that they have heard 'works'. They also like to try a change. Thus some mothers start on WB and move to CB but others move the other way. No conclusions can be drawn from what mothers find effective. What is interesting is why mothers change, and what problems mothers have with feeding.

Reasons given by 1924 mothers for changing the infant formulae used (OPCS Survey 1985) (%)*

Reason	WB to WB	WB to CB	CB to WB	CB to CB	Other change
Still hungry/not satisfied	41	85	46	71	15
Kept being sick	32	11	30	18	28
Constipation	15	7	21	14	5
Allergy	1	1	3	3	33
Other reason	22	5	17	7	29
Total*	392	1301	245	374	115

percentages do not add up to 100 as some mothers gave more than one reason
WB = whey-based, CB = casein-based

Measuring milk powders according to manufacturer's instructions!

Target weight 14 g

	Mean	Range
Primigravida	16.4	14.7–21.3
Multigravida	17.4	12.4–26.0
Midwives	20.9	18.4–24.1
Nurses	17.1	15.6–20.1

They all tend to be too generous! (Source: Wilkinson et al 1973.)

There is little to choose between the different brands. How the industry markets breast milk substitutes is subject to an international code. These are particularly relevant to the developing countries but apply to all. In the UK the promotion is primarily directed at health visitors and parents. Each product vies at being most like human milk. As we know this to be a variable feast, this argument presents difficulties of interpretation. When it was discovered that taurine, an amino acid important in kittens for retina development, and used in man to manufacture bile salts, was abundant in human milk but not found in cow's milk, then taurine was added and used as a promotion feature. Likewise with carnitine, a simple protein used in the transfer of acetyl CoA across mitochondrial walls. There is no evidence in man that term babies suffer from the lack of either if fed on formula not containing them. The current 'interest' is in the addition of nucleotides. The race is on to manufacture human whey proteins like lactoferrin and to add them to infant formula. They may also be added under the general requirement that infant formula should be as like human milk as possible. The authorities will have to reassure themselves that they are safe.

Whilst the health professionals will be concerned about the contents, mothers are also influenced by the physical presentation (packet or tin, powder or granules) and the convenience and cost. The convenient ready to feed formulae are much more expensive. The others are made up, one scoop plus 1 fl oz (30 ml) water. This should not be varied without very good reason. Giving too concentrated feeds contributes to the dangerous hypernatraemia which develops in some infants when they fall ill with a fever or develop gastroenteritis.

WEANING

Weaning is the transition from an all milk liquid diet to a varied diet using solid foods. The term means 'to accustom to' and this suggests a slow process of adaptation and not milk today and solids tomorrow.

Weaning

- Very young babies do not need food other than milk. It is best to wait until the baby is at least 3 months old before introducing solids
- By 6 months, most babies will need to take an expanded diet
- By the age of 9 or 10 months, babies can be given a wide range of home-made and commercial food. A varied diet is most likely to provide all the nutrients needed for normal growth and health during infancy and childhood
- To avoid hypernatraemia, weaning foods should not contain excessive amounts of salt

Weaning does not need to start at the same age or weight in all infants. Very few infants require solid foods before 3 months but the majority should be offered a mixed diet not later than 6 months, yet over 60 per cent babies have had solid food before the minimum recommended age. The early introduction of solids is undesirable for a number of reasons.

Before the age of 3–4 months most infants do not develop the ability to bite or chew, nor are they eager to experiment with foods of different flavour, texture and consistency. The infant gut may be more vulnerable to infection and sensitisation and the use of energy dense foods could predispose to obesity.

On the other hand delay in introduction of solids is undesirable because infants may not achieve an adequate nutritional intake on milk alone after six months of age. The infant by this age has developed a biting/chewing reflex which should be encouraged. It is also about this age that the store of iron laid down in fetal life runs out. Weaning foods high in iron become important. Iron fortified cereals form the major source, but liver, red meat and green vegetables also supply good amounts.

In the survey (Martin & White 1988) mothers who gave their babies solid food by 6 weeks tended to use rusks and cereals. By the age of 4–5 months most were having solid food and of these 82 per cent were using commercial baby foods. It is sad that only a small minority used food prepared at home. Perhaps many thought the commercial babyfoods were better, or maybe they are just more convenient.

Weaning is the process of changing from breast/bottle to spoon, liquid to solid, smooth to texture, warm to a variety of temperatures and milk to a variety of tastes. In other words a process of adopting a new way of eating and it should be carried out in a slow, staged manner. The spoon can be offered first, smooth and plastic, without anything on it. Milk can be given from the spoon to show that food comes in ways other than breast or teat. Plain rice cereals mixed with milk to give a very sloppy texture is the next step then stewed and pureed fruit or vegetables avoiding added sugar and salt. Only one new food should be offered at a time enabling any dislikes or intolerance to be seen. If a food is rejected it should be tried again after a while.

The amount given should be very small starting at one feed and slowly building up. These initial stages should take a few weeks to introduce new tastes, texture and temperature and then the quantities offered slowly increased. The baby will start to cut down milk as the amount of solid food increases. At this stage small quantities of protein food, eg meat or fish should be included. Using commercial babyfoods does not allow this gradual process as each jar or packet is a pre-determined mixture of foods, all of exactly the same texture.

The aim of weaning is to have the child eating normal chopped family food by 9–12 months. These stages are given in more detail in the British Dietetic Association leaflet 'After milk – what's next', 1989.

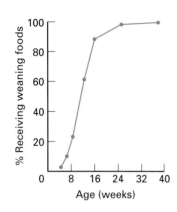

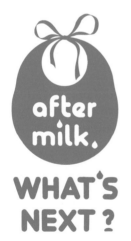

FOODS FOR INFANTS

Milk

The onset of weaning does not mean that breast milk or formula should stop. An extended period of mixed feeding is to be encouraged. There

Composition of cow's milks per 100 ml			
	W	S-S	S
Energy (kcal)	63	45	31
Protein (g)	3.1	3.2	3.2
Lactose (g)	4.5	4.5	4.6
Fat (g)	3.8	1.6	0.1
Vitamins			
A (µg)	53	24	1
Riboflavin (µg)	160	165	170
C (mg)	1.4	1.4	1.4
D (µg)	0.03	0.01	0
Minerals			
Sodium (mg)	53	54	55
Potassium (mg)	140	145	145
Calcium (mg)	110	115	115
Magnesium (mg)	10	10	10
Iron (µg)	49	50	51
Copper (µg)	10	10	10
Zinc (µg)	350	360	360

W = whole, S-S = semi-skimmed, S = skimmed
*Source: Ministry of Agriculture, Fisheries and Food

are advantages in continuing breast milk or infant formula throughout the first year (DHSS 1988).

Doorstep cow's milk has been recommended for infants from 6 months onwards and in a variety of forms – diluted, boiled, 'skimmed', with added sugar etc. Cow's milk is poor in iron and high in protein. That is why manufacturers have introduced 'follow-on milk'. These have been available for a number of years and are commonly used in Europe to bridge the gap between formulae and doorstep milk. They contain more iron and vitamin D and less protein than cow's milk but have no real advantage over continuing with breast milk or infant formula to 1 year.

Soya formulae have no milk in them at all. These were initially made available for use by the medical profession in the treatment of proven cow's milk intolerance. They cost half as much again as an infant formula and are now generally available. They are safe but have no obvious advantage over other formulae. They are often misused. There was concern recently that soya feeds had high aluminium levels. Bishop et al (1989), recommended caution in the use of soya milks in pre-term infants and infants in the first few weeks of life because they have immature renal function. The media extrapolated this to suggest that children fed on soya milk were likely to get Alzheimer's Disease, ignoring the fact that aluminium is very widespread amongst foods other than soya milk, particularly vegetables.

Goat's milk. Some mothers offer goat's milk to their children who appear not to tolerate cow's milk. It is also widely used in children with eczema. Neither goat's milk nor ewe's milk is a suitable feed for infants.

Pre-term formulae. It is unlikely that infants will be at home on the special energy dense preterm formulae as they are only available to hospitals in a ready to feed form. Preterm formulae are designed for the low birthweight infant during the first weeks of life when their requirements for protein, energy, sodium, iron, calcium, phosphorus and vitamin D are very high.

Infant drinks

A wide range of infant drinks, fruit and herbal varieties, are available for babies. Most breast and bottle fed babies in this country do not need extra fluid until solids are used, nevertheless they are popular. Recent concern over the effect of sugar on teeth has resulted in the requirement that no sugar is added. In fact the *actual* sugar level in some of them has remained high because of the use of concentrated fruit juices. Some contain as much as 9 per cent sugar which is equivalent to 5 teaspoons of sugar in a mug of coffee. Others have a much lower sugar content and all have lower acid levels than natural fruit juice. They are best used as flavourings and diluted as much as possible. If they are taken with meals, then the sugar and acid will be buffered by the other foods.

Vitamins

Clinical manifestation of vitamin deficiency is extremely rare in Europe. Many of the foods marketed for infants contain added vitamins and conventional household diets properly prepared also contain a variety of vitamins, apart from vitamin D. The main source of this vitamin is from the effect of sunlight on the skin.

Poor intake of vitamins may occur in children who have delayed weaning, bizarre eating patterns, food aversions and improperly treated food intolerances. Currently the Department of Health recommendation acts as a safety net by recommending the use of supplementary vitamins, 5 drops daily from 6 months up to 2 years and preferably 5 years.

Fluoride

When fluoride is added to water at levels of 1 ppm there is a decrease in incidence of dental caries by 50–60 per cent. Despite the evidence, some areas do not have a fluoridation programme. An approved daily supplement of 0.25 mg fluoride has been advised by the British Dental Association for children from 2 weeks to 16 years so in areas where water is not fluoridated it would be prudent to advise supplementation up to these levels taking into account any fluoride from other sources or dental treatments. Fluoride is available in drops or tablets.

Recommended supplements (mg/day)

Age (years)	<3.0 ppm	0.3–0.7 ppm
0–2	0.25	0
2–4	0.5	0.25
4–16	1.0	0.5

No supplement needed if water level >0.7 ppm.

FEEDING PROBLEMS IN INFANTS

Hypernatraemia

This is no longer the common problem it used to be due to the level of sodium in infant formulae, particularly the whey based formulae. In the days of National Dried Milk there were sodium levels nearly seven times higher than current milks.

Feeding problems experienced by mothers when babies were about 4 months old (stage 2) and 9 months old (stage 3) (1990 Great Britain)

	4 months			9 months		
	Breast	Bottle	All	Breast	Bottle	All
Baby hungry	20	15	16	5	2	3
Baby ill	15	24	21	25	34	33
Baby did not like milk	25	11	15	21	4	4
Baby vomiting	5	13	11	0	7	6
Baby got too much/too little wind	4	5	5	2	1	1
Baby constipated	3	4	3	2	1	1
Sore/cracked nipples	4	1	1	5	–	1
Baby could not latch on	1	0	1	0	0	0
Baby would not take solids	9	12	11	13	11	11
Baby would only take certain solids	3	5	5	22	21	21
Babies went off milk for a while	6	8	8	4	6	6
Other	23	15	17	30	4	22
Total*			903			626

Percentages do not add up to 100 as some mothers experienced more than one type of problem

Wind

Wind is air that has been swallowed. Some air is swallowed with feeding whether from breast or bottle, and babies swallow a lot of air when crying. Feeding too quickly or too slowly may be the cause of excessive wind, so may vigorously shaking the bottle just before feeding. It is not a serious problem but worries mothers and rarely may distress infants. The first step is to watch the baby having a feed.

Possetting

Regurgitation of small quantities of feed is quite common in infants. Again it is usually not a serious problem, however it is messy and smelly and families vary in how much they can tolerate. The problem may be due to overfeeding or incompetence of the sphincter at the end of the oesophagus. Reflux usually only occurs when the stomach is full so oesophagitis is uncommon. It usually resolves with age as the diet becomes more solid and less liquid and the child becomes more upright.

Various types of feed thickeners

	Description	Quantity rqd	Cooking	Comments
Gaviscon	Alginic acid Magnesium trisilicate Aluminium hydroxide Sodium bicarbonate	1 sachet per 4 oz (120 ml)	No	High sodium content Requires prescription
Instant Carobel	Galactomannas gelling agent (from carob bean seeds)	0.5–1% (scoop provided)	No	Mainly non-digestible May cause bulky stools Requires prescription
Nestargel	Hemicellulose gelling agent (from carob bean seeds)	0.5–1% (scoop provided)	Yes	Mainly non-digestible May cause bulky stools Requires prescription

Colic

Three-month or evening colic is the common term used to describe the harmless but distressing condition when infants, usually in the evening, cry for long periods of time, drawing up their legs as if in pain. The cause is unknown but various feeding practices have been incriminated. It is obviously uncomfortable for the baby and parents fearing something is wrong, need reassurance. Even then, it is distressing for them to see their helpless infant in pain. Many remedies have been tried but nothing appears to be effective. The condition is self limiting.

Constipation

The passage of hard stools causes straining and discomfort and needs correcting. The passage of a normal soft motion once a week is not uncommon and does not require intervention. Constipation is more common in formula fed than breast fed babies. Increasing the volume of fluid by offering cooled boiled water is often sufficient. If not, diluted fresh fruit juice or even prune juice may help.

Cow's milk intolerance

There are few symptoms that haven't been attributed to cow's milk intolerance. Estimates of incidence vary considerably. The promotion of soya feeds to avoid cow's milk intolerance is one reason why mothers make the diagnosis and begin treatment before they seek advice. True protein intolerance is rare.

When it is diagnosed a totally milk free diet is required. If the baby is breast feeding, this should be continued. If not, a nutritionally complete milk substitute is necessary. Two groups of product are available – soya formulae or hydrolysed protein formulae.

Soya formulae are available on prescription for proven milk intolerance. There are other soya 'milks' available in liquid and powder form which are diluted soya bean and not suitable for infant feeding. Hydrolysed protein formulae such as Pepti-Junior (Cow & Gate) and Pepdite (SHS) are sometimes used in preference to the soya formulae particularly where gastrointestinal symptoms are present and there is a significant risk of soya protein intolerance.

The remainder of the diet must also exclude milk so the advice of a dietitian should always be sought, as milk is widespread amongst manufactured foods, particularly the commercially prepared baby foods. Parents should be given an up-to-date list of suitable foods and items to look for on an ingredient label which indicate milk, eg hydrolysed whey, lactose, casein, etc.

Children tend to become more tolerant of cow's milk protein as they grow older. The time to introduce a 'challenge' will vary from child to child. Often it happens in error when a child gets hold of a chocolate or drink that contains milk. The introduction should be slow over a period of about a week.

Children who do not take a nutritionally adequate milk substitute in amounts of approximately 500 ml daily will require calcium supplementation until the diet is back to normal.

PRE-SCHOOL CHILD

Two reports appeared in the early 1980s on healthy eating, neither making specific recommendations for children. The Health Education Council (HEC 1983) published a discussion paper which became known as the NACNE report. It stressed the dangers of modifying children's diets on the basis of recommendations for adults. The DHSS Report on cardiovascular disease (DHSS 1984) specifically excluded children under 5 years of age.

Diet and cardiovascular disease

For adults, the COMA Report (DHSS 1984) on diet and cardiovascular disease made the following recommendations:

- No more than 35% of food energy should be derived from fat.
- No more than 15% of food energy should be from saturated fatty acids.
- Fibre-rich foods containing complex fibre-rich carbohydrates are preferred to simple sugars.
- Excessive intake of common salt should be avoided.

Notwithstanding, their guidelines are being extended to children within families without proper attention to their requirements for growth and nutrition. The changes recommended included decreased total fat and increased fibre both of which could have major effects on the diets of young children. The term 'muesli-belt malnutrition' has been coined to describe the problems of young children in families following healthy eating principles and who do not appreciate the different needs of the preschool child.

> **Recommendations for the pre-school child**
>
> - Full fat milk is preferred for children under 5 years. Semi-skimmed milk and dairy products, but not skimmed milk, may be progressively introduced from the age of 24 months, provided the overall diet is adequate.
> - The misuse of sugary foods should be avoided because they may lead to dental caries.
> - Fresh fruit and raw vegetables make good snacks.
> - The toddler's diet should not be over-salted, and it is wise not to add salt at the table.

Fat

Suckling infants obtain about 50 per cent of their food from fat, so a proposed change to 35 per cent (COMA) or 30 per cent (NACNE) would be very significant. Fat intakes as low as these can only be achieved by making major changes in the dietary habits of adults, whose energy need per unit body weight is only one third of that of a young child. No one would argue against the cautious limitation of high fat foods such as chips and crisps but this would in no way meet the targets set. Fat in milk forms an important part of the diet of many children. If the amount of milk is decreased the child loses a major source of calcium, riboflavin and protein. Changing to reduced fat milks would decrease fat but also energy. One pint of full cream milk replaced by one pint of skimmed milk leaves an energy deficit of 780 kJ. To make up the deficit from carbohydrate the child would need to eat an extra four small slices of bread every day.

Decreasing the fat content of food decreases the energy density so that more of the food needs to be eaten to give the same total energy. This is a problem for the young child who has a small capacity and energy requirements three times greater than adults. Fat is also the source of essential fatty acids and fat soluble vitamins in the diet. For these reasons skimmed milk should not be given to children under 5 and semi-skimmed milk should only be used from the age of 2 years providing that the energy deficit could be made up elsewhere. In other words, cow's milk for the under fives should be full cream.

Fibre

High fibre foods are more bulky and as such have a lower nutrient and energy density. It has been suggested that children on high fibre intakes may not be able to take in adequate energy. What exactly constitutes a high fibre intake is not known, as there are no recorded desirable intakes for this group. Increased fibre in the diet also increases associated components such as phytates which will affect absorption of important minerals. A moderate increase therefore seems sensible through use of wholemeal bread and wholegrain cereals which should be gradually added when weaning is established and an increase in amounts of fruit and vegetables.

What should a child eat?

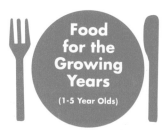

Individuals vary a great deal in their nutrient intake and requirements, so in the non-obese child appetite is a good indicator of when the child has had enough. There is no one food that must be eaten or must be avoided from a healthy diet, but a good mixed diet should be based on milk, lean meat, poultry, fish, eggs, cheese, fruit, vegetables, bread and cereals (preferably wholegrain). These foods have a good nutrient density and will provide the necessary protein, vitamins, minerals, fibre and energy.

Sugary foods and drinks should be avoided as they play a major role in dental caries and provide only energy. Fried foods and high fat foods such as chips, pastry, fatty meat products and crisps should be limited. It would be unrealistic to expect children to totally avoid these foods.

This age group is renowned for food fads and refusals. These should be seen as a natural part of child development and parents advised to ignore them. They should never 'give in' and replace a refused meal with a packet of crisps. This purely reinforces the wrong behaviour.

> **Three safeguards for dental health are important:**
>
> - Promotion of good general health and oral hygiene.
> - Adequate but not excessive exposure to fluoride by the use of fluoride-containing toothpaste and an intake of fluoride from the water supply or from supplementary drops.
> - Avoiding too many sugary foods, especially between meals, as these may lead to dental caries.

The child will eventually get hungry and eat if replacements are withheld. Milk is an important source of calcium, riboflavin and protein and children should normally be having one pint full cream milk, or its equivalent daily. For children who dislike milk drinks, milk can be given as puddings or equivalents ($^1/_3$ pint milk is equivalent to 1 pot yoghurt or 1 oz cheese).

Department of Health vitamin supplements should be continued unless there is no doubt about the adequacy of the child's diet.

COMMON PROBLEMS

Toddler diarrhoea

A small number of children pass frequent loose stools containing particles of undigested food three or more times each day. Whilst the diarrhoea may be profuse and unpleasant, the child continues to grow and gain weight adequately. The problem usually presents during the second half of the first year until early childhood.

Two dietary adjustments may help. If the child is on a low fat intake, which often occurs if milk has been reduced after weaning or if full cream milk has been replaced by semi-skimmed milk, adding fat to the diet may increase the transit time. Secondly, a decrease in fruit and vegetables may help particularly if taken in excess. Parents should be reassured that the problem is self-limiting and that their child is not ill. Toilet training, though difficult, may help.

Poor weight gain

Failure to thrive and failure to rear are both complex problems and they are considered at more length in other chapters. If there is a poor weight gain, the commonest 'final pathway' is that the child is not being offered, or is not eating enough food. Poor dietary habits may be the central problem. Some young children lose interest in food; children who continue to drink milk and squashes and only nibble snacks fail to gain weight. They are continually 'grazing' and never really get hungry. This can be a problem in Asian families where cow's milk is introduced early and weaning delayed.

The solution is simple in theory, but difficult to carry out. Parents need to be able to discuss the problem with someone who understands their fear that withholding the drinks and snacks and limiting milk might cause the child to starve. Reassurance that the child will eat when hungry is essential.

Nutritional surveys do not reveal major differences in energy intake between the wealthy and the poor. Nevertheless hidden poverty may result in poor weight gain. The nutritional problems of poverty cannot be solved by simply giving advice on cheap food. Cheap filling foods are not always 'healthy'.

Excessive weight gain

Obesity is an easier problem to prevent than solve. Overweight is relatively uncommon in young children and does not necessarily persist into adulthood. Where it does the parents are also likely to be obese. It is unusual for the obese child to come from a family with good eating habits and it is essential when treating the obese child that the whole family's way of eating is changed.

There needs to be a balance struck between the provision of foods with low energy density and high nutrient density otherwise growth may be affected. The major sources of energy should be avoided: fats as butter, margarine and oils and carbohydrate as sugar, confectionery, jams, sweetened drinks etc.

The fat content of milk should be reduced to either skimmed or semi-skimmed and kept to a maximum of 1 pint daily. Fruit and vegetables should be allowed freely and sensible use of cereals, bread, potatoes, pasta, etc. limited to mealtimes.

The child should be encouraged to 'grow into his height' or advised to lose small amounts depending on the degree of obesity and target weight. Sudden major weight losses are not helpful in the long run.

Food intolerance

This is a fashionable diagnosis ranging from intolerance to one food, eg strawberries, through to multiple intolerances of many nutritionally important foods.

There is no other way to make a diagnosis than to withhold the offending substance with relief of symptoms, followed by re-introduction and the return of symptoms. Most food 'intolerances' are not food 'allergies'.

Dietary exclusion should never be attempted without referral to a suitably experienced paediatric dietitian, unless the culprit is obvious and nutritionally unimportant, for example prawns causing a rash. The dietitian will advise an exclusion of the likely foods and design an appropriate nutritionally adequate diet around what is left. It is not uncommon for the diet to be more of a problem that the initial symptoms.

Advice for potentially allergic children from atopic families

- Breast feeding should be encouraged and care taken to avoid the early introduction of any other foods.
- A soya-based infant formula may be used instead of one based on cow's milk, but these formulae may also be allergenic.
- From 6 months, infant formula or follow-on milk, may be less allergenic than fresh cow's milk.
- It is wise to delay the introduction of fresh cow's milk, eggs, wheat, nuts and citrus fruits. These foods should first be given in small amounts.
- For infants with suspected food allergy: The suspected food may be withdrawn for a short trial period. Prolonged dietary change (for example cutting out all milk) requires expert advice.

Behaviour

Food intolerances and behaviour have been linked ever since the Feingold diet came to Britain from the USA. This was a diet avoiding some artificial colourings and preservatives, which claimed to improve the behaviour of overactive children. The validity of this has been questioned and trials do not support any link. Despite this the Hyperactive Children's Support Group (HACSG) has continued to recommend it widely and sometimes link it to other diets.

No doubt some children are affected by certain additives. Mothers describe children who have phases of erratic, uncontrollable behaviour following, for example, ingestion of coloured sweets. Avoiding that colour may help, but evidence is hard to find. Food additives must not be blamed for the erratic behaviour of children or for badly disciplined children. Avoiding such additives need not affect the nutritional value of the diet; it may improve it. This is not so when the more strict dietary regimens, recommended by some self help groups, are followed. These can lead to a diet inadequate for growth and development.

Food additives can be avoided by 1) Eating more fresh, natural food and 2) Looking at food labels when using processed food. To make labelling easier, additives used in the European Economic Community (EEC) have been given a number ('E' number). Those numbers with no 'E' prefix are awaiting EEC approval. Additives are grouped according to their function:

E100–200	Permitted colours e.g. E102 tartrazine
E200–321	Preservatives and antioxidants
E322 onwards	Various e.g. emulsifiers, stabilisers etc.

Most books on allergy, diet and behaviour etc give a list of 'harmful additives to avoid'. These are purely personal to the author and no such list will be given here.

OLDER CHILDREN AND ADOLESCENTS

Once the child starts school a number of changes take place which have an effect on diet. The child usually eats one meal in a different environment either as a school meal or packed lunch away from home.

Getting to school in the morning is often a rush and breakfast can be missed altogether or eaten on the move. Breakfast is still an important meal for young children with high requirements and small appetites and should not be missed. School meals should be an ideal time to introduce or reinforce healthy eating to a captive population, particularly the younger school child. Sadly, this is not usually the case. Since the 1980 Education Act there is no requirement of local authorities to provide any meal at all. Some still do so, but there is no longer any nutritional standard to aim for. Prior to 1980 a meal conforming to prescribed nutritional standards was provided for all who wanted it. ($^1/_3$ of child's RDA for energy and 40 per cent of RDA for protein.)

Estimated average energy requirements for children and adolescents

Age	MJ/day (kcal/day)	
	Boys	Girls
0–3 months	2.28 (545)	2.16 (515)
4–6 months	2.89 (690)	2.69 (645)
7–9 months	3.44 (825)	3.20 (765)
10–12 months	3.85 (920)	3.61 (865)
1–3 years	5.15 (1230)	4.86 (1165)
4–6 years	7.16 (1715)	6.46 (1545)
7–10 years	8.24 (1970)	7.28 (1740)
11–14 years	9.27 (2220)	7.92 (1845)
15–18 years	11.51 (2755)	8.83 (2110)

DRVs for iron (mg/day)

Age	LRNI	EAR	RNI
0–3 mth	0.9	1.3	1.7
4–6 mth	2.3	3.3	4.3
7–12 mth	4.2	6.0	7.8
1–3 yr	3.7	5.3	6.9
4–6 yr	3.3	4.7	6.1
7–10 yr	4.7	6.7	8.7
	Males		Females
11–18 yr	8.7		11.4

As a result of this change in policy the government agreed to review the dietary habits of school children (DHSS 1986,1989) and found that although they usually met recommended intakes for protein and energy, they were high in fat and sugar and as such unhealthy. This was particularly so in those children who skipped school lunch (over 10 per cent of older children) and ate out in local cafes. Here overall diets were poor, as the deficiencies in the lunchtime meal were not made up at other mealtimes.

Health promotion groups have been lobbying the Departments of Health and Education to re-introduce nutritional standards for school

DRVs for calcium (mg/day) for calcium (mg/day)			
Age	LRNI	EAR	RNI
0–12 mth	240	400	525
1–3 yr	200	275	350
4–6 yr	275	350	450
7–10 yr	325	425	550
	Males	Females	
11–14 yr	750	625	
15–18 yr	750	625	

meals to meet recommended intakes within current healthy eating guidelines. Some schools do attempt to provide healthy meals based on local feeding policies, so that parents can be satisfied that their child is getting a reasonable midday meal.

Trends in the way we eat tend to show up a lot in the older school child and adolescent, when peer pressure exerts a great effect. In general, eating has become less formal and eating out and take-aways have become more common. The tendency to miss out breakfasts becomes more common as children get older and along with freedom of choice at lunchtime could have disastrous consequences.

Adolescents often want to try out new ways of eating before becoming 'set in their ways' and it is not uncommon to see a phase of vegetarianism, particularly in girls. There is a tendency to miss out meat and fish and replace them with cheese and eggs or nothing at all. This leads to a very high fat intake when cheese and eggs are used or a poor protein intake without it and iron deficiency is also common. Advice on suitable meat alternatives should be offered. The Vegetarian Society is very helpful and produces useful leaflets.

School children are still growing at a varying rate so requirements will fluctuate. During the adolescent growth spurt, which occurs from 11–14 years in girls and 13–16 years in boys, the requirements for energy and nutrients are high. Appetite is usually increased and family food bills rocket. Although healthy eating is still very important, more energy dense foods are necessary to meet requirements. Fat and sugar intakes in excess of those recommended are necessary to meet these increased needs while keeping the cost of the diet within practical limits.

EATING FOR THE FUTURE

Teenagers are aware of the basic principles of healthy eating, but time is of the essence in this age group and convenience foods are generally not the most healthy. This is an important area which needs the cooperation of the food industry. School seems to be the main source of knowledge on nutrition and healthy eating. Teachers have an important role to play in promoting healthy eating within the context of health education both by example and within the curriculum.

Healthy eating guidelines of decreasing sugar and fat while increasing fibre, become more important after the adolescent growth spurt when requirements for nutrients for growth cease. A way of life becomes channelled, they may leave home for college or just for independence and take total responsibility, maybe for the first time, for their own way of eating.

Vitamin and minerals

There have been concerns expressed recently about the diets of school children, particularly with reference to vitamins and minerals, due to the increase of junk foods and decrease in family meals. Surveys have not shown significant deficits, but one study has suggested that the diets of some children are deficient and that supplementing them with vitamins and minerals may improve non-verbal performances. These findings were criticised because of study design and analysis, but still resulted in a huge increase in the sales of vitamin and mineral supplements as a result of the media attention. Another study, designed to meet the criticism of the first, was repeated by other investigators. No significant effect could be shown.

What is a sensible diet?

The basic principles of healthy eating apply to all members of the population even in patients on prescribed therapeutic regimens. Here the diet should only be modified as much as necessary to treat the condition. The remainder should conform to healthy eating guidelines.

Food is made up from the nutrients protein, fat, carbohydrate, vitamins, minerals, fluid and roughage, which in the correct proportions and quantities should give a healthy balanced diet. But people think in terms of food and not nutrients, so 'food groups' help people to understand how to eat well. Foods with similar nutritional properties are grouped together and suggested amounts from each group given. For example five groups may be used.

Meat group – meat, offal, poultry, fish, eggs, beans and pulses.
Main sources of protein in the diet. May also be high in fat so choose lower fat alternatives.
2 helpings, daily from this group.

Milk group – milk, cheese, yoghurt.
Another good source of protein. Major source of calcium. May also be high in fat so choose lower fat alternatives where appropriate (not under 5 years).
1 pint full cream milk daily for children and teenagers (semi-skimmed may be used over 5 years). Cheese and yoghurt may replace milk : 1 oz hard cheese (30 g) = $\frac{1}{3}$ pint milk (200 ml) = 1 pot yoghurt (150 g).

Fruit and vegetable group – all fruit and vegetables.
Provides vitamins, minerals and fibre. Main source of vitamin C which is not very stable so foods should be eaten fresh and cooked quickly in very little water. Potato falls into this group as a vegetable though is sometimes included with cereals as it is a 'filler food'. Although only an average source of vitamin C, the amount eaten in the British diet means they contribute a lot.
Mimimum of two helpings daily, but two each of fruit and vegetables is preferable. Eat to appetite.

Cereals group – items made from flour, bread, breakfast cereals, rice and pasta. Source of energy and fibre. Known as 'filler foods'. Better to use unprocessed, high fibre alternatives.
Eat to appetite, including some at each meal.

Fat group – margarine, butter, oils, lard and dripping.
Source of energy, essential fatty acids and fat soluble vitamins.
Use only in small quantities.

The type of fat, whether saturated, monounsaturated or polyunsaturated is also important. A high intake of fat, particularly saturated, is a risk factor in coronary heart disease. Current thinking suggests an overall reduction in fat with an increased proportion of monounsaturates (eg olive oil) and polyunsaturates (eg sunflower oil). Some omit the fat group and use a four food group classification because, although a small amount is necessary to give the essential fatty acids and vitamins A,D,E and K, these will be provided by foods in the meat and milk groups.

Terms relating to fat

- **Fat** – dietary fat – usually triglycerides, i.e. 3 fatty acid molecules joined to 1 molecule of glycerol.
- **Fatty acid** – A molecule of variable length consisting mainly of a carbon chain to which hydrogen atoms are attached.
- **Essential fatty acid (EFA)** – One which cannot be made in the body and which must be supplied by food.
- **Saturated fatty acid (SFA)** – One which contains the maximum possible number of hydrogen atoms.
- **Monounsaturated fatty acid** – One in which each molecule has 2 hydrogen atoms missing. As a result, the molecule is said to contain one double bond.
- **Polyunsaturated fatty acid (PUFA)** – A fatty acid in which each molecule has more than 2 hydrogen atoms missing. As a result, the molecule is said to contain, respectively, 2 or 3 or 4 double bonds.
- ***Cis*** **and** ***trans*** **isomers** – Terms which relate to the spatial arrangement of atoms in molecules such as monounsaturated or polyunsaturated fatty acids. Most fatty acids which occur naturally in foods are *cis*.
- **Cholesterol** – It may be ingested in foods such as egg yolk and offal, but most is made in the body. An essential component of every living cell wall, it is transported round the body in blood and may be converted to vitamin D.

Other foods not in either classification are also eaten, eg sugar, confectionery etc. These should only be minor items in the diet.

Leaflets explaining healthy eating in this way are available from the British Dietetic Association and the Milk Marketing Board. A more complex review of food groups is given by Francis (1986) using three overlapping circles. The top circle contains all the protein sources but laid out in a way that the other circles, one of which contains carbohydrate sources and the other fat sources, overlap so that for example, the area in the protein circle overlapping the fat circle contains foods which are high in protein but also fat. This gives 7 sections or groups and is more appropriate for teaching health professionals to help them use the four or five food groups for teaching the general population.

DIET IN DISEASE

Modifying the diet may be central to the treatment of some diseases and relevant to the management of most. It is important that all who have care of the child or advise the family, understand the principles involved. Diets are prescribed treatments and should not be altered without discussion with the prescriber. Here is a brief summary of some of the diets used by families for the benefit of their children.

Phenylketonuria (PKU)

A deficiency of the enzyme phenylalanine hydroxylase leads to a failure to convert the essential amino acid phenylalanine (phe) to tyrosine. Infants born with this disorder get into difficulty when milk feeding is established. A raised level of phenylalanine in the blood is detected on routine neonatal screening. If it is not, brain damage will occur.

The amount of phe in the diet is restricted to that required for normal growth and development. The aim is to maintain blood phe levels within an acceptable range (120–350 µmol/l). This is above the normal range, but has been chosen to avoid low levels, which will result in poor growth and development. In infants this means giving breast milk or formula to provide that amount of phe required to maintain acceptable levels and to supplement these feeds with a low phe infant formula (Analog XP, Minafen). Daily blood monitoring is essential until the levels are stable, then weekly for the first year or so when the requirements may fluctuate, and then it is gradually relaxed to fortnightly, then monthly.

Weaning starts at the normal age with fruit and vegetables which are low in protein and specially made low protein foods. As weaning progresses, phe requirements can be provided by foods other than milk, eg potato, cereals etc, using a system of '50 mg phe exchanges' where a given weight of food provides 50 mg phe and a daily allowance of phe is prescribed. As the baby takes more solid food the amount of low phe formula and therefore phe free protein will drop. This is replaced by a mixture of aminoacids (minus phe) which is a concentrated protein substitute (Aminogran, Maxamaid XP). High protein foods – meat, fish, cheese and eggs – are totally excluded from the diet and lower protein foods, eg potato and cereals, given in weighed 50 mg phe exchanges to provide the necessary phe.

Foods allowed freely include sugar, jams and other refined carbohydrate foods and fats such as butter and oils. A wide range of specially manufactured products are available (bread, flour, biscuits, pasta, milk substitute). These are mostly available on prescription, as are the expensive aminoacid mixtures and vitamin and mineral supplements essential in such an artificial diet.

Diet restriction continues to 10 years of age in most centres and later in many. There is currently debate over the issue of diet for life. One major problem, only presenting since screening and treatment, is that of maternal PKU. The babies of PKU women are at great risk of severe brain and other organ damage from high maternal phe levels. Strict low phe diet is essential pre-conception and throughout pregnancy.

A well established parents' support group exists which produces information for PKU families and health professionals.

Cystic fibrosis	This is a condition, unlike PKU, where diet is not the sole treatment, but it is essential for a good management. Nutritional problems are related to the malabsorption caused by inadequate pancreatic enzyme function, but poor appetite, inadequate food intake and increased requirements due to recurrent infection also play their part.

Dietary fat restriction used to be recommended because of problems with steatorrhoea, but the modern pancreatic enzyme preparations, Creon and Pancrease, are very effective in improving malabsorption, so fat intake should be normal to high in order to take advantage of its concentrated energy. Enzymes need to be taken with all foods except pure refined carbohydrates, the amount varying from one child to another and with the type of meal eaten. Fat soluble vitamins in larger than normal doses are usually prescribed.

Dietary supplements in the form of milk shakes, glucose polymers etc, are often necessary during periods of illness, but should not be continued afterwards when all attempts should be made to meet nutrient needs from a proper diet, so that supplements can be reserved for periods of poor appetite and when growth begins to tail off. Maintaining adequate growth and acceptable body weight is a major problem in cystic fibrosis, particularly in older children who have problems with body image. Oral dietary supplements are useful, but longterm use leads to poor compliance. Overnight tube feeding is an option allowing the child to eat normally through the day and feed overnight.

Nasogastric and gastrostomy feeding have been tried with varying degrees of success. Gastrostomy feeding may be preferable where frequent coughing causes displacement of the nasogastric tube leading to inability to overnight feed at the times the child most needs it.

Families receive support from the Cystic Fibrosis Research Trust set up to promote research, but also to help sufferers and their families.

Diabetes mellitus

Diabetes in children is invariably type I insulin dependent diabetes and treatment involves insulin injections and modified diet with the aim of normalising blood glucose. Dietary treatment aims to provide a balanced diet, incorporating healthy eating principles, which gives optimal growth and weight gain. Current healthy eating principles apply very well to the diabetic diet – low fat, low sugar, high fibre. Carbohydrate intake is not so much restricted as regulated. The child needs normal amounts of carbohydrate but in an unrefined form.

An accurate diet history is taken from each child and/or parents and used as a baseline for dietary prescription. The current aim is to provide 50 per cent of energy as carbohydrate, but in practice this is rarely possible in children without resorting to refined carbohydrates. A commonly used 'rule of thumb' for assessing carbohydrate requirements is that of 100 g plus 10 g for every year of life, ie a 5 year old would require 150 g. In practice this only gives about 40 per cent of energy requirements as carbohydrate, so should be used as a minimum and is only a rough guide. Individual dietary prescription according to current eating pattern, age, height and weight should be decided by the dietitian and a balance found between what is acceptable in theory and in practice.

RED – STOP
– foods high in refined carbohydrate

AMBER – STEADY
– carbohydrate exchanges

GREEN – GO
– foods free of carbohydrate

A system of carbohydrate exchanges (1 exchange containing 10 g carbohydrate) is used as a method of teaching parents and children the amount of carbohydrate in foods, along with a traffic light system for recognising which foods do or do not contain carbohydrate.

The dietary prescription is given in terms of daily carbohydrate allowance which is spread between meals and snacks and filled out with foods free from carbohydrate, for example 150 g carbohydrate or 15 exchanges spread according to previous eating pattern.

Breakfast	Mid-morning	Dinner	Mid-afternoon	Tea	Bed-time
30	10	40	10	40	20

This is used as a guide and approximately this amount of carbohydrate should be taken each day. Carbohydrate requirements will increase with age so diet should be reviewed regularly in relation to growth. An extra 10 g carbohydrate each birthday is a useful guide and reminder.

The British Diabetic Association exists to offer advice and support.

Children are strongly recommended to join. Diabetic camps are organised to take children out of the home situation for a holiday with other diabetics of similar age, run by doctors, dietitians, nurses and other interested volunteers.

Renal disease

There is no one diet for renal disease. A number of nutrients and electrolytes will be affected by renal disorders creating a wide spectrum of dietary manipulation.

Nephrotic syndrome, the most common renal disorder in childhood, does not usually result in chronic renal failure and is usually steroid sensitive. During a relapse there is huge proteinuria but this resolves with steroid treatment making high protein, low salt diets unnecessary. The main nutritional problem here is obesity due to steroids. Patients are usually warned of this problem and given preventative advice at the same time as being advised on healthy eating.

Diet in renal failure, acute or chronic is a subject worthy of its own book, but one factor common to most stages is anorexia and the resulting poor nutrition and poor growth. Maintenance of a good nutritional state is of importance along with dietary manipulation of protein, energy, sodium, potassium, calcium and phosphate according to blood biochemistry.

Dietary prescription may alter quite frequently and depending on the type of renal replacement, may go from one extreme to another, eg low protein with conservative management to high protein with peritoneal dialysis. Parents and children must be fully aware of the reasons behind these changes, if they are to be expected to follow them.

The British Kidney Patient Association exists to promote research and offer family support.

Short bowel syndrome

A variety of disorders in early life may result in a short bowel, but the end result is characterised by diarrhoea and reduced absorption of all nutrients. The problems encountered can be divided into those immediately post-operatively which relate to severe diarrhoea and providing adequate nutrition and the longer term effects on nutrition and growth.

By the time children reach the community they may be well on the way to, or even past their first birthday. Long term total parenteral nutrition followed by repeated attempts to introduce oral feeding can be a long slow process. Elemental diets of protein hydrolysate/ aminoacids, glucose polymers, long chain triglyceride/medium chain triglyceride are all tried in various combinations in an attempt to provide adequate nutrition by the oral route. The child will normally be discharged on a prescribed milk substitute with or without a limited range of solid food depending on age and tolerance. The diet, rather than being 'free from ...' is restricted to only those foods already tried individually and known to be tolerated. New foods should only be introduced following discussion with the dietitian.

Intercurrent infections nearly always result in severe diarrhoea and the child becomes easily dehydrated. These children are often fluid restricted as large quantities of fluid lead to watery stools and 'gut rush' with further malabsorption of nutrients. As the child grows the remaining gut seems to grow and adapt and more normal diet can be cautiously tried. Nutritional deficiencies often relate to the section of gut remaining, for example vitamin B_{12} injections are necessary in children who have no terminal ileum. Vitamin and mineral status should be monitored.

Nutrition parenterally (using other than the enteral route) was until recently only carried out in hospital. Though still uncommon, it is now seen in the community in children with short bowel syndrome, cancer, and other rarer disorders. The most important concern is the care of the intravenous line and parents will be taught strict aseptic technique and no untrained professional should go near this 'life line'.

Nutritional aspects should be closely monitored by the hospital. A bag of total nutrition must contain all nutrients currently known, in the amounts required by the individual, in a stable form. This is carried out by co-operation between paediatrician, paediatric dietitian and pharmacy. Regular review of growth parameters and micronutrient status should take place, as the responsibility for the child's total nutrition lies with the prescriber. The child may be eating, so the intravenous feed may be supplementary. It is likely that attempts will be being made to increase oral intake and decrease intravenous intake as appropriate.

Special feeds

Product	Protein source	Fat source	Carbohydrate (CH)	Indications	Per 100 ml feed			
					Protein (g)	Fat (g)	CH (g)	Energy (kcal)
Pepti-Junior	Hydrolysed whey	50% maize oil, 50% MCT	Glucose syrup Tr. lactose	Lactose intolerance Whole protein intolerance, Malabsorption syndromes, Steatorrhoea associated CF	2.0	3.7	7.2	66
Pregestimil	Casein hydrolysate L-Tyrosine L-Cystine L-Tryptophan	Corn oil MCT Oil Lethicin	Glucose syrup solids Modified tapioca Starch	Multiple malabsorption Short bowel syndrome Whole protein sensitivity	1.9	2.7	9.1	66
Neocate	Mixture of synthetic L-amino acids	Coconut fat Ground nut oil	Maltodextrin (Maize)	Multiple malabsorption Short bowel syndrome Whole protein sensitivity	2.0	3.5	8.1	70

Feeding in cerebral palsy

This is an area which is slowly coming to the forefront in terms of nutritional care. Children with cerebral palsy are commonly wasted and have had feeding problems all their lives. In fact, feeding is often described as the biggest heartache by the parents. Reflux is very common in cerebral palsy as are swallowing difficulties resulting in regurgitation and possible aspiration of foods. Chewing difficulties and postural problems all add to the problem.

Early intervention is essential with a multi-disciplinary approach including medical, nursing and social work staff, but particularly in relation to feeding. Physiotherapy, occupational therapy, speech therapy and dietetic expertise all work together to improve posture, positioning, feeding technique and nutritional value of diet. Supplementation is necessary where weight and height gain are dropping away from the centiles. The possibility of tube feeding via naso-gastric or gastrostomy tube should be considered in an individual. Problems such as reflux, likelihood of feed aspiration and fears of parents, need discussing, as do the ethical issues and financial implications. The suitability or otherwise should be fully discussed by all team members before any decision is made. Little work has yet been done on tube feeding in this country but studies in America are encouraging.

If supplementary tube feeding is used in a particular child it is just as important to maintain all input from other therapists with the aim of eventually getting the child to take an adequate intake without tube feeding.

Cancer

Wasting and malnutrition is a common side effect of many types of cancer. A lot of childhood cancers are treatable and the outcome of treatment is bound to be affected by the nutritional state of the child. There is frequently loss of appetite and vomiting, particularly with chemotherapy. Anti-emetics may help, but children often stop eating altogether. Dietary supplements are essential to improve intake but they are often rejected orally because of nausea and anorexia. Tube feeding by nasogastric or gastrostomy route can be used with great success. The diarrhoea caused by chemotherapy may respond better to an elemental diet which because of its unpalatability may be better given by tube. Intravenous feeding is sometimes used for short periods when gastrointestinal symptoms prevent use of the enteral route.

Monitoring of weight gain may not be a particularly good indicator in cancer due to the diminishing size of the tumour with treatment. Mid-arm circumference and skin fold thickness give a better indication of nutritional state.

ACBS

Diets can be prescribed. What is available on prescription is determined by the Advisory Committee on Borderline Substances. This committee approves certain indications for which some food preparations may be prescribed, ie they allow certain food items to be classed as drugs for use in specified conditions. For example, gluten free bread is prescribable for coeliac disease and dermatitis herpetiformis but not for eczema sensitive to wheat. Prescriptions for these items issued in accordance with the committee's approval and endorsed 'ACBS' will not normally be investigated. It is by this method that the expensive products used in for example PKU are prescribed for children free of charge until 16 years of age. After this time prescription charges must be paid so pre-payment certificates, which become economical when requiring more than fourteen separate items in a year, are a must for such dietetic conditions.

Religion and diet

Religion	Pork	Beef	Other meat	Non-scaly fish	Eggs	Milk	Canned foods
Buddhist	No	No	No	No	No	?	
Hare Krishna	No	No	No	No	No		No
Hindu*	No	No			?		
Jain	No	No	No		No		
Jewish*	No			No			
Muslim*	No						
Rastafarian	No	No	No	No	No	?	No
Seventh Day Adventist	No	No	No	No			
Sikh*		No					
Zen (Macrobiotic)	No	No	No	No	No	No	No

Dietary restrictions may be greater if foods are not prepared in acceptable way

REFERENCES AND FURTHER READING

Bishop N, McGraw M, Ward N 1989 Aluminium in infant formulae. Lancet i: 490

British Dietetic Association 1989 After milk – what's next. BDA, Birmingham

Department of Health 1991 Dietary reference values for food energy and nutrients for the United Kingdom. HMSO, London

Department of Health and Social Security 1974 Present day practice in infant feeding. HMSO, London

Department of Health and Social Security 1980 Artificial feeds for the young infant. HMSO, London

Department of Health and Social Security 1984 Report of the Committee on Medical Aspects of Food Policy. Diet and cardiovascular disease. HMSO, London

Department of Health and Social Security 1986 The diets of British school children: preliminary report. HMSO, London

Department of Health and Social Security 1988 Present day practice in infant feeding: 3rd report. HMSO, London

Department of Health and Social Security 1989 The diets of British school children. HMSO, London

Francis D E M 1986 Nutrition for children. Blackwell Scientific, Oxford

Health Education Council 1983 Proposals for nutritional guidelines for health education in Britain (NACNE). HMSO, London

Martin J 1978 Infant feeding 1975: attitudes and practice in England and Wales. Office of Population Censuses and Surveys. HMSO, London

Martin J, Monk J 1982 Infant feeding 1980. Office of Population Censuses and Surveys. HMSO, London

Martin J, White A 1988 Infant feeding 1985. OPCS, HMSO, London

Royal College of Midwives 1988 Successful breast feeding. RCM, London

Taitz L S, Wardley B L 1989 Handbook of child nutrition. Oxford University Press, Oxford

Wilkinson P W et al 1973 Inaccuracies in measurement of dried milk products. British Medical Journal 2: 15–18

12 Growth

Growth represents the summation of all the processes which convert fetus through childhood to adult. The study of growth is therefore at the heart of paediatrics and serial measurement must be a priority in child health programmes. Primary care staff need to be instructed in the careful measurement of the main growth parameters, length or height, weight and head circumference. An individual child's readings should be part of his or her health record, and the readings should be assessed in comparison with valid population standards in order to recognise significant variation from the normal range or deviation from acceptable growth rates. Poor growth may be the first sign of an environmental or health restraint. Organic disorders of sufficient severity to alter growth are usually conspicuous, for example asthma or cardiac disease, but others such as coeliac disease and chronic inflammatory bowel disease are sometimes more insidious. Growth measurement is an essential tool in monitoring the progress of children with already identified chronic disorders. At a population level, growth monitoring can be used as an index of the general health and nutrition of that population and may be useful in comparing the effects of changes in social and economic policies. Lastly most parents are interested in how their children are growing and are keen for them to be measured at intervals.

Normal patterns of growth   The familiar height growth curve can be broken down into three components; infantile, childhood and pubertal; hence the ICP model of growth. This model is useful in that it highlights the main control of each phase. Infancy is a continuation of rapid fetal growth and is primarily dependent on nutrition. The childhood phase commences around age 18 months and is regulated by growth hormone as well as other hormonal pathways. Puberty represents an acceleration due to sex hormones; the tempo of growth is altered but not the final adult height which would otherwise be reached by prolonged and gradually slowing childhood growth.

After birth the rate of growth decelerates quickly and during the first 18 months or so many healthy babies change their centile position for both length and weight (see 'genetic influences'). Through childhood the velocity of growth decelerates before the onset of the adolescent growth spurt. As a rule pubertal acceleration is an early component of female puberty but is delayed until the second half (testicular volume > 8 ml) of male puberty.

Individual variations in growth/centile charts. There is wide variation in growth and puberty parameters amongst children at any age. Prepubertal height follows a Normal or Gaussian distribution which means that the mean measurement at a given age is the same as the 50th centile.

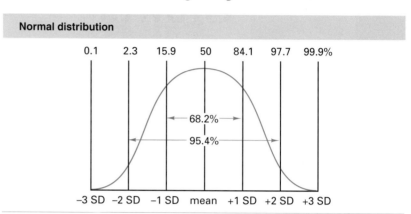

The 3rd and 97th centiles correspond to minus and plus 2 standard deviations respectively. These are the outermost centiles on height charts. However weight does not follow a normal distribution and therefore the outermost centiles (3rd and 97th) on a weight chart do not correspond to minus and plus 2 standard deviations. Centiles can be used whatever the shape of the curve and are a useful way of indicating variation.

By convention children whose measurements fall outside the 3rd or 97th centiles are considered to have possible pathology. On a screening basis this is fine but it must be borne in mind that most of these children will actually be healthy and that those with real pathology will have heights which are well beyond these centiles, e.g. about 50% of children with measurements of minus 3 standard deviations have a pathological cause for it.

Influences on growth

Genetic. It is recognised that there are variations in growth in different racial groups and that there is a secular trend within groups. Few countries have good population data and hence the wide usage of Tanner charts, though new charts based on contemporary UK data will soon be available. For example, it is well-known that Japanese children growing up in the USA in the 1950s were on average larger than their counterparts in Japan. However more recent data shows that Japanese in Japan, Hawaii and California no longer are so different in their heights, but they are still less tall than Hawaiians and Californians of European or African descent. Although there are differences in the absolute growth measurements between races, the ideal rate of growth does not vary that much between the different ethnic groups.

There are also familial trends in growth, in timing and in size and shape. These are most clearly seen in twin studies where monozygotic twins brought up in a similar environment resemble each other very closely in these measurements.

Some genes do not become active until after birth. This probably accounts for the poor correlation between parental heights and children's lengths in the first 12 to 18 months of life. Size at birth is more a reflection of uterine conditions than of genotype. During the first 18 months or so many healthy babies change their centile position for both length and weight, as their genetic programme for growth comes into play (Smith et al 1976). Another example of genetic influence can be seen in the age of menarche. There is considerably less difference between monozygotic twin sisters growing up in similar conditions, about 3 to 4 months, compared to that between dizygotic twins, about 10 months. Similarly there are high correlations in the ages at which the different stages of puberty are reached in monozygotic twins.

Nutrition. The effects of malnutrition on growth are well-known. 'Catch-up' growth is more likely to occur after a short period of acute starvation than after chronic malnutrition. A baby born with intrauterine growth retardation occurring in the later stages of pregnancy usually grows more rapidly than normal after birth and 'catches up' by the 2nd year of life. However a baby who has suffered chronic malnutrition in utero (usually symmetrically small in weight, length and head circumference) tends to remain small. During certain stages of growth, the child is more vulnerable to malnutrition than at others, i.e. the full growth potential may not be attained even after normal feeding is restored. Such times occur during early infancy and during the pubertal 'growth spurt'.

In affluent communities most children have more food than they actually need and overnutrition can also affect growth. Increased food intake during a period of rapid growth tends to speed up the rate of growth but the overall duration of the process is shortened (advanced bone age), i.e. most obese tall children have normal heights for bone age and do not become tall adults.

Emotional. Unhappy stressed children tend to grow less well. The effects may result from decreased appetite or disorganised meal patterns as well as from an effect on the hormonal control of growth. It is sometimes difficult to separate emotional factors from socioeconomic ones and there is often a relationship with nutritional and feeding difficulties. Removal from the stress, if possible, may have a dramatic effect on growth.

Endocrine. No single hormone on its own regulates growth but interaction between several hormones is necessary for growth to proceed.

Growth hormone (GH) is secreted by the anterior pituitary gland. Its release is mediated by the hypothalamus, an interplay between growth hormone releasing hormone (GHRH) and somatostatin, and can be stimulated by a variety of stimuli, physiological such as physical exercise, deep sleep, food and anxiety, and pharmacological such as clonidine

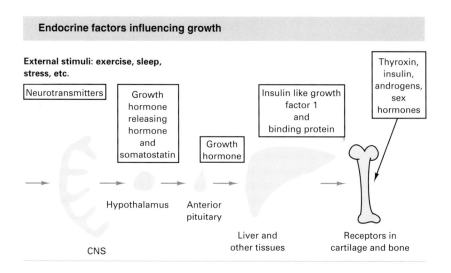

Endocrine factors influencing growth

and glucagon. For its effects on growth, GH works through intermediary growth factors, notably IGF-1 (insulin-like growth factor). IGF-1 acts as both a circulating hormone, its release from the liver being dependent on GH and nutrition, and as a local or paracrine factor after local secretion from a variety of cell types. IGF-1 regulates the proliferative zone of cartilage. GH secretion is episodic. Most of the time the blood level of GH is undetectable by conventional assays but 8 or 9 times a day the level rises sharply for 10 to 20 minutes. These peaks occur at irregular intervals but more often at night. The amount of GH secreted per 24 hours increases during puberty, and its production coincides with the peak of the growth spurt. After the end of the spurt the amount falls again to the young adult level. The increase in the secretion of GH at this time seems to be stimulated by the rise in the sex hormones.

The action of growth hormone is species-specific and prior to the development of methods such as recombinant DNA technology, GH had to be extracted from human pituitary glands, a process which limited the supply and also carried risks of developing 'slow virus' infection, e.g. Creutzfeldt-Jacob disease.

Thyroid hormone (thyroxine) acts synergistically with GH. It is necessary for normal growth from fetal life onwards and for normal function in both children and adults. It affects protein synthesis and is essential for the proper development of the brain. Thus a child born with thyroid hormone deficiency (incidence about 1 in 3000 births) will be mentally handicapped unless treated as soon as possible. Routine screening for TSH in newborn infants is now carried out to identify such infants.

In older children deficiency of thyroid hormones has a more noticeable effect on growth and on skeletal and dental maturity. When treated with thyroxine these children show catch-up growth and provided they are treated promptly they reach near-normal adult height.

The secretion of thyroxine by the thyroid gland is stimulated by thyroid stimulating hormone from the pituitary (TSH) which in turn is controlled by thyroid releasing hormone (TRH) from the hypothalamus.

Thyroxine itself regulates TRH secretion, in a classical feedback loop. TSH is produced in a pulsatile manner, about 6 peaks per 24 hours.

Cortisol has an anti-growth effect if it is present in excess. In this situation growth in height slows down, skeletal maturity is delayed and there is an increase in fat. Examples of this effect may be seen in children treated with high dose steroids for severe asthma, renal disease and rheumatoid arthritis.

Androgens produced primarily by the adrenal zona reticularis of the prepubertal child appear to have a role in skeletal maturation. They may be responsible for the modest growth acceleration seen normally between ages 6 to 8 years. Some children have a more conspicuous 'adrenarche' with a late childhood growth spurt and relatively early pubic hair growth (pubarche). This is usually an isolated and innocent event which does not lead to early true puberty ('gonadarche').

Testosterone is secreted by the Leydig cells of the testis. Luteinising hormone (LH, or Leydig-cell-stimulating hormone) from the pituitary controls its release. In the male fetus its level rises from about 11 postmenstrual weeks till birth. It causes differentiation of the external genitalia into the male type and may also have an effect on the brain, causing the hypothalamus to develop into the non-cyclical, male type. After birth, testosterone levels fall rapidly but rise again during the first 6 months before declining to very low levels throughout childhood. The pubertal increase follows the increasing amplitude of LH pulses and increasing testicular volume. During this period testosterone stimulates development of the secondary sexual characteristics and together with growth hormone, it causes the growth spurt of the skeleton. Testosterone stimulates secretion of growth hormone but in addition it has a direct effect on the growth of bones and muscles. It also accounts for the male growth pattern, characterised by a relatively greater spine length increase.

Oestrogen production by the ovaries is controlled by the pituitary. The levels of oestrogens are low throughout childhood until puberty when a large rise occurs. They are responsible for the development of the female secondary sexual characteristics and also for the growth spurt in adolescent girls since the increase in oestrogens stimulates increased release of growth hormone. Once menstruation begins, the level of oestradiol fluctuates with the phase of the cycle.

MEASURING GROWTH

How to measure?

Height and supine length. The principle is to measure the distance between flat surfaces applied to the top of the head and the soles of the feet.

Supine length is measured in children below the age of 2 years. It is also useful for older children who are unable to stand. Two observers are necessary. Length can be measured using a Harpenden infant measuring table with the child's head held in position at the fixed end by one observer and the movable footpiece brought up to the feet and heels by a second assistant who ensures the body, legs and feet are in a straight line.

Height is measured from the age of two years. There is a standard position for the head; namely the outer canthus of the eye should be on the same horizontal plane as the external auditory meatus. The child should not stand on tiptoe and the heels should touch against the wall/door.

Measuring height

MEASUREMENT OF HEIGHT

Head upright, looking forward
Back straight and against wall
Knees straight
Heels down

Looking down
Back curved
Knees bent
On tip-toes

Five points of correct technique
1   Child's hands by sides
2   Child looking forward
3   Your hand under child's chin with fingers on mastoid processes, exert gentle upward pressure
4   Your other hand on child's feet to keep back straight and to prevent heels rising
5   Keep Microtoise against wall

The 'gold standard' for height measurement is the stadiometer, calibrated against a 1 metre steel measure. However this is not a portable piece of equipment and in a community setting a microtoise (CMS Weighing Equipment Ltd) or a Raven minimetre (Castlemead) are more suitable. The latter can also be used to measure supine length, provided a fixed end can be obtained. In a growth clinic sitting height is also measured to obtain a measure of the child's proportions. The accuracy of the instrument should be checked against an object of known height/length and ideally the people who do the measuring should check on their technique at intervals. The standard deviation of measurement should be no more than 0.2 to 0.3 cm (*see also Errors*).

Weight is the most frequently recorded measure of growth in the first months of life. It is easily done but is potentially laden with errors. Accurate scales are essential of course. However weight is affected not just by the mass of the body tissues but also by changes in water balance and by factors such as a recent meal. Weight measurements are therefore of more use during periods of rapid growth, e.g. early infancy or following an illness, than at other times. Taken in conjunction with height (body mass indices) e.g. weight/height-for-age ratio as described by Cole et al (1981) it can be useful in the assessment of obesity (see *The fat child*).

Head circumference is usually measured at birth and at the six week check. If there is excessive moulding or oedema following birth this should be recorded and the measurement repeated after a few days. If there is any doubt about these measurements or if there is concern about the child's growth or development then further measurements are needed. The occipito-frontal circumference is the measurement usually taken. It is best to use a narrow metal tape measure rather than one made of paper or linen.

Puberty is recorded by the changes in pubic hair and in the external genitalia in boys, and in breast development in girls. The stages described by Tanner are in common use. The size of the testes is measured by volume and is assessed with an orchidometer.

Errors

In any measurement accuracy is essential if the observations are to be of any use. It must be emphasised that errors may be introduced by the instrument, the observer and by the subject (Wessex Growth Study). The instruments used should be correctly installed, properly and regularly calibrated and maintained. Although in the Wessex Growth Study Voss et al (1990) showed that a large proportion of the error in height measurement is contributed by the child, the people doing the measurements should be adequately trained in the methods of measurement, care of instruments and in the recording of the results. Each observer should obtain their own standard deviation of measurement, which should not be more than 0.2 to 0.3 cm.

When to measure?

The times at which children are measured vary from one district to another. In *Health for all children* (Hall 1991) it is suggested that height measurements should be made at around three years of age and between four and five years. Beyond the age of five years, the report suggests that height should be measured if there is doubt about the significance of past measurements or if previous records are incomplete or missing. There is debate about the value of continued height monitoring after school entry and more research is needed to clarify this issue. Since the childhood (growth hormone dependent) growth phase starts at around 18 months of age, there is a strong case for length to be measured at this age as well. In Nottingham at present, children are measured at about three years old, then in their first year at infant school (age 4–6), first (age 7–8) and fourth years (age 10–11) at junior school and in the second (age 12–13) and fourth years (age 14–15) at secondary school.

Recording measurements

Each measurement should be recorded in figures with the date and also plotted on the appropriate centile chart. It is important to calculate the child's age correctly. Ideally the measurements should be plotted with dots rather than open circles or crosses. The charts most frequently used for height and weight are those constructed from the data of Tanner & Whitehead. Growth charts are also available for children with Down's syndrome or Turner's syndrome (Castlemead). With the introduction of the national parent-held child health record, which incorporates the appropriate charts for height, weight and head circumference there should be no reason why each child's measurements should not be plotted.

By using centile charts it is possible to see whether the child's height, weight or head circumference is within the normal range for his/her age. When serial measurements are made and accurately plotted, it is easy to see on a chart whether growth is progressing at a satisfactory rate.

Interpretation

Most of the following discussion will centre on height measurements but also applies to the other measures. Should one or more of the child's measurements fall outside the normal range, proper interpretation and action depends on a number of factors.

Firstly, the child's state of health should be checked, looking for symptoms and signs of disease which may affect growth. A family history of growth problems e.g. short stature or delay in growth and puberty should be asked about.

Secondly, the parental heights should be obtained (by direct measurement if possible) and plotted with the necessary adjustment on the child's chart i.e. 12 cm is added on to the mother's height for a boy or subtracted from father's height for a girl. From these the midparental centile can be seen. If the child's height centile falls within ± 8 cm of the midparental centile, his/her height is compatible with that of the parents. A child whose height appears to be inappropriate for parental heights should be referred for further investigations.

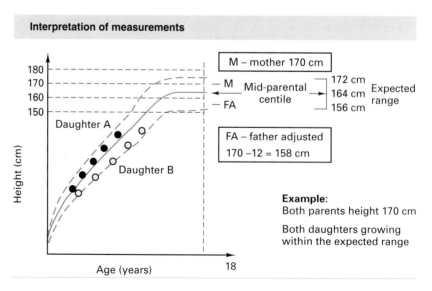

Interpretation of measurements

Lastly, the stage of puberty should be recorded and an assessment made as to whether it is appropriate with the other clinical findings. Even if the child's measurements are within the normal range, should these have crossed centile lines from previous measurements, he/she merits a more detailed assessment along the lines described above.

Referral criteria

Some indication of when children should be referred for further growth assessment and investigations has been given above. From the health visitor and school nurse point of view, all children who are below the 3rd centile or seem to be crossing centiles should be referred to the doctor. Those children who are below the 3rd centile but above −3 SD of the mean and who are well, should have their growth monitored regularly to check that they are growing parallel to the 3rd centile i.e. growth velocity is within normal range. The doctor should use the following guidelines to decide further action:

1. Any child whose height is −3 SD below the mean.
2. Any child whose growth is crossing the centiles, i.e. growth velocity decreasing or whose growth velocity is accelerating. As a general guide for children between the ages of 2 and 10 years, the 'Middlesex chart' shows the normal range of height velocity and indicates when further assessment is necessary. Another useful guide is that the pre-pubertal height velocity should at least be 5 cm/year.
3. Any child below the 3rd centile whose parents are tall.
4. Any child whose height is above the 97th centile without tall parents.

In a community paediatric setting, further action would involve carrying out basic investigations if feasible and/or referring to a growth specialist.

Basic investigations

The bone age measurement gives the skeletal maturity. Each bone begins as a primary ossification centre, enlarges and is shaped in a number of stages, acquires one or more epiphyses and finally reaches adult form when these epiphyses fuse with the main body of the bone. The sequence of events for each bone is the same with all individuals. Thus for a particular child comparison of the appearances of his/her bones with standards obtained from the those of normal children will allow the bone age to be obtained. Any delay or advance in skeletal maturity will be apparent.

Most commonly an x-ray is obtained of the left hand and wrist. However in children less than 18 months old, these bones are not very informative and the legs and feet are used. Assessment of skeletal maturity uses either the method of Greulich and Pyle or more precisely the bone-scoring method of Tanner and Whitehouse.

Depending on the clinical findings, it may be justified to carry out basic blood tests, looking for chronic bowel disease (ESR, anaemia, antigliadin antibodies), thyroid dysfunction, renal disease (creatinine), chromosomal abnormalities (e.g. Turner's syndrome). If it looks as though the child requires more complicated assessment and investigation, he/she must be referred for specialist advice.

Disorders of growth

A structured approach to history, examination and interpretation of growth charts allows the majority of growth disorders to be categorised without recourse to specialist investigation. The community paediatrician is well placed to advise the primary health care team on this assessment. Much of the medical management of children with growth disorders is supervised by specialists. However the community paediatrician needs to have some knowledge of such disorders to be able to liaise with the specialists and to provide advice and support to school, the family and the child whenever the need arises.

SHORT STATURE

Being small may be the first sign of pathology. It is also seen as a disadvantage in our society, more so with boys than girls, and can result in psychological problems and considerable unhappiness, particularly during the teenage years. Excessive smallness brings with it difficulties with coping with normal daily life and can be a serious handicap (Law 1987).

Classification of short stature	
Non GH deficient	GH deficient
Idiopathic (short normal)	Idiopathic
Delay	Organic i.e. known cause
Intrauterine growth retardation	• congenital e.g. septo-optic dysplasia,
Syndromes	empty sella syndrome
• Chromosomal e.g. Turner's, Down's	• pituitary/hypothalamic tumours e.g.
• other, e.g Noonan	craniopharyngioma
Diseases of other systems	• cranial irradiation
• malabsorption	• other acquired e.g. trauma, CNS
• renal, respiratory, cardiac	infection
Skeletal dysplasias e.g. hypochrondroplasia	
Other endocrine disorders	

Familial short stature/normal genetic shortness/idiopathic stature. Even if a child is on or below the 3rd centile in height, provided that he/she is within the normal limits for his/her parents and assuming that neither parent has had abnormal growth, then that child can be considered to be normal, and their growth usually follows a normal pattern. However in some children there is additional growth delay.

Constitutionally short

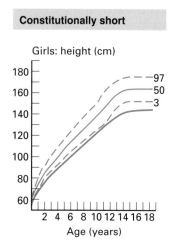

Girls: height (cm)

Constitutional delay in growth and puberty. This is a common cause of short stature especially in secondary school children. The delayed tempo of growth may already have been manifest as relative short stature in childhood, becoming more conspicuous in the early teens. Puberty is also delayed and is an essential feature for the diagnosis. There is usually a family history of delay, e.g. mother had a late menarche at about 15 or 16 years, father was on the small side during his school years and 'shot up' in height only after leaving school, a brother or sister or uncle or aunt showed delay. In these children there is nothing abnormal to find on examination. The bone age is delayed by about 2 years and matches the pubertal delay.

Explanation and reassurance may be all that is required. However

Delayed maturity

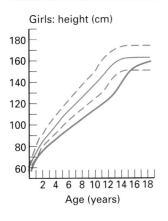

Girls: height (cm)

Age (years)

there are psychological pressures on such children, more so in boys, particularly at the time when their peers are becoming established in puberty and they themselves remain prepubertal and seem even smaller (Crowne et al 1990). There are a number of treatments which can be offered to accelerate growth and the appearance of secondary sexual characteristics. These treatments do not affect final adult height. Such treatments must be supervised by specialists. For boys, testosterone or a testosterone-like synthetic drug, e.g. oxandrolone may be used (Buyugebiz et al 1990). For girls, treatment is not so frequently requested. Low doses of oestrogens can be used to accelerate growth and stimulate breast development.

Intrauterine growth retardation. Small-for-gestational age (SGA) infants may result from maternal disease or malnutrition, from placental failure to supply adequate oxygen and other nutrients to the fetus, or from some fault in the fertilised ovum. Most of these infants show 'catch-up' growth and grow within normal centiles but often do not reach their full growth potential, i.e. seem small for their parents' centiles.

However some of these SGA infants do not follow this pattern and remain small and thin with characteristic facial features - a triangular face with large eyes and small lower jaw, prominent forehead, rather low set protruding ears. In addition there may be facial, limb or trunk asymmetry and clinodactyly. They are not mentally retarded. These features are seen in the Russell-Silver syndrome. In these children growth proceeds at a normal rate so they remain short. In some of them growth hormone supplementation accelerates growth but it has not yet been shown that it improves adult height.

Chromosome disorders

Some of the chromosome disorders are associated with short stature. Two well-known examples are Down's syndrome (trisomy 21) and Turner's syndrome.

Turner's syndrome affects approximately 1 in 5000 liveborn girls. In some of these children the karyotype is 46XO, the remainder being mosaics 46XX/46XO. It is probable that all surviving girls with Turner's syndrome are mosaics although this may not be revealed by conventional analysis. They may present at birth with puffy hands and feet but the diagnosis of the syndrome is often delayed. They are all very short, mean adult height being around 143 cm (4 ft 8 in), but those with tall parents tend to be taller. Although physical features of the syndrome include webbing of the neck, a broad chest with widely-spaced small nipples and lack of puberty and amenorrhoea due to the absence of functioning ovaries, many of these girls have less conspicuous features and escape diagnosis in spite of attending ENT and eye departments.

Few of these girls have growth hormone (GH) deficiency, but large scale national trials suggest that high dosage GH therapy does increase both growth rate and final adult height. Girls treated before age 10 years have a better response. In the UK, Turner's syndrome is an approved indication for HGH therapy but there are still unresolved concerns about the real benefits of this highly expensive treatment and the uncertainties about late side-effects.

Induction of puberty is effected with the female sex hormones, initially with oestrogens to stimulate breast and pubic hair development and later progesterone-like hormones are added cyclically to produce an artificial menstruation. These girls are infertile but with the development of assisted conception techniques some of them may in the future be able to become pregnant using donated oocytes.

Endocrine disorders

Growth hormone deficiency and thyroid hormone deficiency are the two main endocrine causes of short stature.

Growth hormone deficiency is a spectrum of congenital and acquired disorders of the hypothalamo-pituitary axis. Examples of the latter are destruction of the gland by tumour, e.g. craniopharyngioma, or by surgery or radiotherapy. In many cases however the cause of the deficiency is not known. It may be an isolated deficiency or occur with other endocrine abnormalities such as in panhypopituitarism.

Idiopathic growth hormone deficiency occurs in about 1 in 5000 births in the UK. It is more common in boys, and may occur in families. Affected children are short with infantile proportions and excessive subcutaneous fat. They have delayed bone age.

Classical or severe GH deficiency is readily identified and confirmed by showing that there is little or no rise in growth hormone level to a stimulation test, such as by clonidine or by hypoglycaemia induced with insulin. Insulin provocation is a potentially hazardous test with an increasingly limited place in modern paediatric endocrinology and its use should be restricted to experienced departments.

The modern view is that there is a continuous range of GH secretory capacity between absolute deficiency and the borderline normal responses seen in short normal children. This spectrum explains the many equivocal GH responses and emphasises that the decision for or against GH therapy has to be based on accurate growth data, and excluding other restraints, e.g. hypothyroidism.

Treatment is with human growth hormone (HGH), now produced by DNA recombinant technology. It is given by daily subcutaneous injection. There is usually a period of 'catch-up' growth following the start of treatment and then it settles down to a normal rate. Provided treatment has been started early enough (by age 6 years), the outcome is excellent. The longer the delay in starting treatment the more difficult it is to achieve the genetic potential.

Hypothyroidism in childhood is usually insidious, and short stature with markedly delayed bone age may be the first manifestation. It is important to establish whether the hypothyroidism is primary, e.g. autoimmune thyroiditis, or secondary, a component of panhypopituitarism. In primary hypothyroidism, thyroxine therapy results in some 'catch-up' growth but final height is often less than predicted from the

Growth hormone deficiency

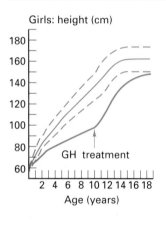

Girls: height (cm)

Age (years)

initial bone age delay. Part of this persisting height loss arises from disordered and abbreviated pubertal progress. Treatment needs to be lifelong for all the other actions of thyroxine.

Diseases of other systems

Malabsorption stunts growth. On a worldwide basis, chronic diarrhoeal illness is a common cause of poor growth. Other examples are coeliac disease and inflammatory bowel diseases such as Crohn's disease. Although these disorders usually present with bowel symptoms, poor growth may sometimes be the only sign and they should be considered in the differential diagnosis of short stature or pubertal delay.

Poor growth is a manifestation of chronic renal disease. It is also a major challenge both before and after renal transplantation and the impact of high dosage GH is being studied. Cardiac and respiratory diseases which cause a reduced amount of oxygen to reach the tissues may also result in small stature.

Iatrogenic causes. Fortunately current treatment options mean that few children with chronic disease are subjected to the growth suppression of high dosage corticosteroids. Inhaled steroids are valuable in the treatment of asthma but there is growing awareness that sustained high dosage can suppress the hypothalamic-pituitary GH and adrenal axes. Second-generation inhaled steroids with increased first-pass metabolism have reduced systemic and endocrine side-effects. Radiotherapy is part of many treatment protocols for malignant tumours. Irradiation of the spine may directly reduce spinal growth and hence final height. Cranial irradiation may cause growth hormone deficiency. Insulin hypoglycaemia and other provocation tests may produce a normal GH response, but profiles of spontaneous secretion show blunted and disorganised pulsatility i.e. neurosecretory dysfunction. Surgical removal of tumours in the region of the hypothalamus and pituitary may result in damage or destruction and cause growth hormone and other endocrine deficiencies. Particularly threatening to final height is partial GH deficiency combined with inappropriate early puberty e.g. girls who have been treated for acute lymphoblastic leukaemia. Careful monitoring of the growth of such children and endocrine investigation when indicated is therefore an essential part of their management.

Psychological disorders

Children with eating disorders, not necessarily low calorie intake, often grow slowly. Children suffering from psychosocial deprivation will demonstrate increased growth when placed in a happier environment. It has also been shown that emotionally deprived children have a reduced growth hormone response to a stimulation test which is reversible when the child has been removed from the depriving situation. The diagnosis and management of such growth disordered children is often very difficult but is one of the areas in which community paediatricians not uncommonly become involved.

Bone and cartilage disorders

Affected children are small and are not in proportion i.e. they have short limbs or trunk or both. There are many disorders which produce this appearance, almost all of them rare and many of them inherited. The most well-known of these, but not the most frequent, is achondroplasia. Although most of these conditions are conspicuous, in some e.g. hypochondroplasia which is a relatively common variety, the disproportion is relatively mild, becoming more obvious in puberty. At present there are trials of high dosage GH underway but the results are uncertain. There is also the option of surgical treatment to lengthen the limbs, a technique carried out in a small number of specialist centres.

TALL STATURE

Parents and children who seek advice because of tallness are far fewer than those who are concerned about small stature. Part of the reason for this is probably because being tall is seen as an advantage in our society. However excessive tallness can be as much of a handicap as being small. A 5 year old who is as tall as an 8 year old is expected to behave as the older child, and may be labelled as clumsy or aggressive because of his/her large size in relation to peers. In teenage years particularly, being very tall may cause additional problems with forming relationships with peers and emotional difficulties may develop.

Classification of tall stature		
Not dysmorphic		**Dysmorphic**
Normal velocity	Increased velocity	
Familial	Hypothalamic/pituitary disease	Marfan syndrome
Obesity	Hyperthyroidism	Klinefelter syndrome
Growth advance	Adrenal disease	Cerebral gigantism (Sotos
	Gonadal disease	syndrome)

Familial

Sometimes parents who are themselves very tall become concerned that their tall daughter may grow up as a very tall adult, maybe exceeding parental heights. Particularly if they themselves had a difficult time coping with their tall stature they will seek advice for their children. In this situation it is helpful to have a prediction of final adult height. The TW2 formula for this includes chronological and bone ages, present height and, if known, the recent growth rate. If the predicted final height is excessive, treatment may be indicated and must be supervised by specialists. Essentially treatment does not affect growth which has already occurred and can only affect growth to come. For girls treatment is usually with oestrogens started at about 11 years old, and for boys testosterone can be used. Testosterone usually causes an initial increase in height velocity. In extreme cases, surgical intervention may be discussed.

Obesity

Fat children who are tall usually show moderate pubertal and bone age advance. Their height velocity is in the normal range and they do not necessarily become tall adults.

Growth advance

These children are tall for their chronological age and have a normal rate of growth but because of bone age advance they reach their final adult height sooner and do not become tall adults.

Endocrine disorders. Tall children who show an increased height velocity should be investigated for endocrine pathology.

Adrenal disease. Oversecretion of androgens is often associated with the appearance of some of the signs of puberty in either sex, i.e. skin changes, pubic hair and increase in size of the phallus and an increased growth velocity. Testicular palpation and ovarian ultrasound show the gonads to be prepubertal. Unless all the signs of puberty are consistent, adrenal disease must be considered. The usual causes of androgen excess are congenital adrenal hyperplasia and tumours.

Hyperthyroidism and hypothalamic/pituitary disorders resulting in excessive secretion of growth hormone are other causes of increased growth in childhood.

Precocious puberty. Early puberty is difficult to define exactly but according to convention, signs appearing before 8 years in girls and 9 years in boys should give cause for concern. It is more common in girls than in boys.

Causes of early puberty	
Physiological	Pathological
• Familial	• Intracranial tumours e.g. of hypothalamus, pineal area
• Tall obese girls	• Extracranial tumours e.g. of adrenal glands, gonads
• Isolated adrenarche	• Others such as hypothyroidism, mental retardation,
• Isolated thelarche	cranial radiotherapy, drugs

Early puberty particularly if associated with an increased growth velocity, or with signs which are not consonant, i.e. out of step with the expected sequence of pubertal events, requires further investigation. A careful history and full physical examination, with particular attention to assessment of growth and pubertal stages, the optic fundi and visual fields, are essential. Causes of precocious puberty include intracranial tumours, especially of hypothalamus, third ventricle, and pineal area, extracranial tumours such as of gonads, adrenal glands (as mentioned above) and of other organs which produce ectopic gonadotrophin e.g. hepatoblastoma.

Isolated early breast development (thelarche) is relatively common. As long as there are no other signs of puberty and growth velocity is normal, there is no need for further investigation. It is likely that premature thelarche is the response of an extremely oestrogen-sensitive gland to a transient activation of FSH release and ovarian follicle formation. Central or gonadotrophin dependent precocious puberty is usually without overt intracranial pathology in girls but it is frequently indicative of substantial problems, for example a brain tumour, in boys.

Familial or constitutional advance of growth and puberty accounts for relatively tall children with a rapid tempo of growth in late childhood.

Nutritionally obese children are commonly of above average height and enter puberty early.

Premature adrenarche describes a group with early pubic and body hair growth, often with increased sebaceous activity and body odour. They have only modest height acceleration and bone age advance before progressing into an otherwise normal puberty.

Dysmorphic syndromes

Syndromes associated with tall stature are rare. Three will be mentioned briefly.

Marfan's syndrome comprises excessively long limbs, arachnodactyly being a particular feature. Ocular abnormalities include lens subluxation, myopia and retinal detachment. Cardiac abnormalities in childhood are of the valve type but in later life become aneurysmal. There are variants and the diagnosis is a clinical one.

Klinefelter's syndrome is a chromosomal disorder (47 XXY) with the features of tall stature, long legs, small testes and often mild learning difficulties. Affected individuals often do not present in childhood and come to medical attention later because of hypogonadism and late puberty or with infertility.

Sotos syndrome (cerebral gigantism) usually presents in early childhood with tall stature, large hands and feet, delayed development and clumsiness. There is usually bone age advance so these children do not usually become tall adults.

THE FAT /OVERWEIGHT CHILD

It is not at all uncommon for community paediatricians to see children who are overweight. They may be identified by routine school nurse's or health visitor's measurements, by parental or teacher concern, or by the child him/herself. There may be difficulties with peer relationships, reluctance to take part in games, and unhappiness related to teasing.

Definitions of obesity are usually based on measurements such as skinfold thickness or body mass indices calculated from weight and height. None of these is entirely satisfactory. Standard positions on the triceps and subscapular areas are the usual places where skinfold thickness measurements are taken, using Holtain skinfold calipers. However these measurements are not easily reproducible. Body mass indices are various ratios of weight and height e.g. weight/height, weight/height^2 for age which are indirect measures of obesity. Since body fatness does not change with age as height does, there will be times when these indices could be misleading. These indices should therefore be used with caution (Fung et al 1990).

Uncommonly there is a pathological cause for the obesity. Useful clues are associated short stature and/or mental retardation. However obesity is seldom the presenting feature in these disorders, e.g. dysmorphic syndromes such as Down's or Prader-Willi syndromes, endocrine disorders such as GH deficiency, hypothyroidism. In these disorders, being overweight can be an additional handicap and part of the management should include weight reduction/control.

'Simple obesity' is the result of mismatch between calorie intake and energy expenditure. These children are tall for their age and for their parents. However there are complex factors involved, including social and psychological ones, and the management of such children is not simple. On an individual level the child and family must be motivated to lose or control weight. Lack of motivation is a frequent cause of treatment failure. General dietary advice, encouragement of regular exercise and enthusiastic support by family and friends and professionals involved with the child such as teachers, school nurse and doctor, GP, and dietitian, are essential on an individual basis.

On a wider scale, education and national policies regarding nutrition and health have their part to play (*Health of the Nation*). Garrow (1991) has suggested that one of the strategies to reduce the proportion of obese people in the population would be to develop a policy in primary schools to identify school entrants who are above the 90th centile for weight for height and to provide facilities for the children to increase normally in height but slightly less than normal in weight between the ages of 5 and 12 years. Whether such a policy can be implemented remains to be seen.

FAILURE TO THRIVE

Children, particularly infants, who are gaining weight slowly are often seen in community paediatric clinics. As described above, some healthy babies will change their centile positions for weight and length during the first few months of life. Others will be found to have an organic cause for their slow growth, a number of these have been mentioned above. Others will have 'non-organic failure to thrive'. It is a vast subject and this section will only discuss the controversy surrounding definition.

What is 'failure to thrive'? It is a term used to describe those children who are not gaining weight. However it can and does mean different things to different people. For instance, it could mean that a child is gaining weight steadily but below the 3rd centile or it might mean that the child's weight has crossed centiles.

The definition of 'failure to thrive' has recently been aired in the literature (Anon Lancet 1990, Edwards et al 1990 and ensuing correspondence). Edwards et al in Newcastle have summarised the various meanings of the term and suggest that since failure to thrive implies failure to achieve a normal rate of growth, the definition should include deviation for a defined period from the child's expected growth trajectory. They propose that children are failing to thrive if weight deviates two or more major centiles (3rd, 10th, 25th, 50th, 75th, 90th and 97th centiles) below the maximum weight centile achieved between 4 and 8 weeks of age for a period of a month or more. In their study they compared the birth weights and weight at 4 to 8 weeks with the weight at 9 and at 12 months for each of a group of children in Devon and in Newcastle. They found that there was closer agreement between the weight at 4 to 8 weeks and that at 12 months than between birth weight and weight at either 9 or 12 months. They used this definition to select a group of children without an organic cause for their slow weight gain whom they measured in the 2nd year of life. Each of these children was also matched with a control child. Compared with the control group, the children who had failed to thrive were lighter, shorter and had smaller head circumferences.

Although the definition is still being debated, all the workers agree that measurements of weight and height should be correctly plotted on centile charts so that poor weight gain can be observed and acted upon as soon as possible.

REFERENCES AND FURTHER READING

Anon 1990 Failure to thrive revisited. Lancet 336: 662–3
Brook C G D 1982 Growth assessment in childhood and adolescence. Blackwells, Oxford
Buyugebiz A, Hindmarsh P C, Brook C G D 1990 Treatment of constitutional delay in growth and puberty with oxandrolone compared with growth hormone. Archives of Disease in Childhood 65: 448–9
Cole T J, Donnet M L, Stanfield T P 1981 Weight-for-height indices to assess nutritional status – a new index on a slide rule. American Journal of Clinical Nutrition 34: 1935–43
Crowne E C, Shalet S M, Wallace W H B, Emminson D M, Price D A 1990 Final height in boys with untreated constitutional delay in growth and puberty. Archives of Disease in Childhood 65: 1109–12
Edwards A G K, Halse P C, Parkin J M, Waterston A J R 1990 Recognising failure to thrive in early childhood. Archives of Disease in Childhood 65: 1263–5
Fung K P, Lee J, Lau S P, Chow O K W, Wong T W, Davis D P 1990 Properties and clinical implications of body mass indices. Archives of Disease in Childhood 65: 516–9
Garrow J 1991 Importance of obesity. British Medical Journal 303: 704-6
Government White Paper 1991 The health of the nation. HMSO, London
Gregory J W 1991 Health of the nation (letter). British Medical Journal 303: 1059
Hall D M B (ed) 1991 Health for all children – A programme for child health surveillance, 2nd edn. Oxford University Press, Oxford
Law C M 1987 The disability of short stature. Archives of Disease in Childhood 62: 855–9
Smith D W et al 1976 Shifting linear growth during infancy: illustration of genetic factors in growth from fetal life through infancy. Journal of Pediatrics 89: 225-30
Tanner J M 1989 Foetus into man – physical growth from conception to maturity, 2nd edn. Castlemead Publications, Tunbridge Wells
Voss L D, Bailey B J R, Cumming K, Wilkin T J, Betts P R 1990 The reliability of height measurement (Wessex Growth Study). Archives of Disease in Childhood 65: 1340–4

13 Intellectual Development

This section is concerned with milestones as they are currently used in child health practice with respect to gross motor and fine motor skills, cognitive and social development. Development of speech, vision and hearing are described in the appropriate chapters. The ability to assess the development of a child cannot be obtained from written accounts alone and indeed a written account is only a very minor part of such training. Although charts, such as the Denver Developmental Screening Chart, acknowledge the enormous range of normal that exists, it is impossible within a single scale to record all the individual variations in the quality of response obtained. Obtaining rapport with the child and recognising for example the shy, nervous or withdrawn child who is not performing to his real level of ability, are important skills which only come with practice and experience. In a way, what is needed is observation of the subtleties and fine detail of behaviour rather than testing for the crude gross milestones of development which are used in screening. If we are particularly concerned about a child, more detailed and graphic descriptions are certainly required in order to highlight areas of difficulty where particular help may be provided. Those using the standardised tests of developmental progress such as the Stanford Binet intelligence scale, the Wechsler intelligence scale for children, the Bailey scales of infant development and the Griffiths scales must ask themselves the reason for doing so. Is it to provide a clinical description of the child, his abilities and his difficulties which would aid diagnosis and management, or is it to provide a comparison of an individual child with his peer group?

Assessment of development depends upon accurate observation and interpretation of those observations in the light of our knowledge about 'normal' development. It must not be forgotten that parents are the ultimate authority on the development of their own child, supplemented in the school age child by teachers' observations. Formal developmental screening is no longer part of our child health surveillance programme, with the realisation that parental observation and anxiety will lead to earlier diagnoses than screening tests.

Descriptions of normal development, linked to a child's ability to perform particular tasks at a particular age relate only to the performance of the 'average' child. For all milestones there is a very wide range of normal. The developmental charts illustrated in this chapter show

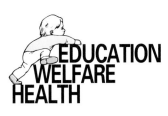

EDUCATION
WELFARE
HEALTH

Age range of ability

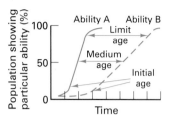

both the average and the range and are used to record a description of a child's progress, but should not used as a pass/fail test. Allowance must also be made for prematurity in interpretation of developmental information. The initial age is the age at which the first few most advanced children display the skill; the median age is the age at which 50% of children display the skill; the limit age is the age at which nearly all children have acquired the skill. Failure to acquire a range of skills by the limit age signals the need for more detailed assessment. The development of individual children does not occur at a constant rate so that single observations of development, particularly in very young children, have little predictive value. Serial observations are much more valuable and will highlight children who 'fade' in their developmental progress compared to their peers and those who shine brighter and brighter with time.

ASSESSMENT OF REFLEXES

Reflexes in the newborn are a useful way of studying motor development. Exaggeration of reflexes, diminished reflexes, asymmetry of reflexes, persistence of primitive reflexes or delay in the acquisition of secondary reflexes form a useful body of knowledge in the study of developmental progress.

Moro reflex

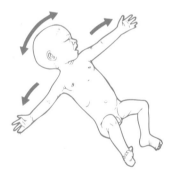

Moro reflex. This is elicited in the supine position, with the head supported by one hand a little off the table. The head is then suddenly released, causing first abduction and extension of the arms with opening of the hands, followed by adduction of the arms and crying. This reflex is present very consistently at birth and disappears around 5 months. Persistence after 6 months of age must be considered abnormal. Because this reflex can be elicited so easily in its classical form, any variation from this should be considered with suspicion. An asymmetrical Moro reflex may be due to a fractured limb as well as to neurological causes.

Galant's reflex. With the baby held in ventral suspension, sharp stimulation with the fingernails of the skin down each side of the back results in flexion of the spine to the stimulated side. The Galant's response is present in very preterm babies and its persistent absence in the newborn may well indicate a poor prognosis. Asymmetry is also important, as in the Moro reflex.

Stepping reflex

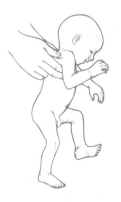

The stepping reflex. With the baby held vertically, contact of the soles of the feet on to a table causes reflex stepping movements of the legs. Persistence of the stepping reflex beyond the age of 6 months may indicate cerebral palsy.

Grasp reflex

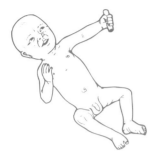

The palmar grasp reflex. Insertion of an object or the examiner's finger into the palm of the hand or on to the sole of the foot, produces reflex flexion of the fingers or toes. This produces a strong grasp with the palm and secondary contraction of the arm muscles sufficient to raise the baby from the supine position when traction is exerted by the examiner's finger. This reflex needs to be lost before voluntary grasping can occur. Abnormal persistence may indicate cerebral damage as may absence or asymmetry in the newborn period.

The asymmetrical tonic neck reflex (ATNR). Turning of the head to one side leads to extension of the arm and leg on that side and flexion on the opposite side. This has been likened in boys to the position required to use a bow and arrow or in girls to the posture required to brush the hair holding a mirror in one hand and a brush in the other. In early life it may be useful in directing the hand towards objects in the visual field. However, it may prevent rolling over or the hands being brought to the face. Abnormal persistence of the ATNR, particularly in an exaggerated form is very frequently found in infants with cerebral palsy.

Balance reactions. These are necessary in order for the child to develop ability in the sitting position. The response consists of extension of the arm to prevent falling when the child's body is displaced to either side in the sitting position. Similar saving reactions occur in the standing position.

The parachute reaction. The child is held in a ventral position and is rapidly lowered head first towards the table. The arms extend in order to 'save' the child. Failure to appear is frequently seen in children with neurological abnormalities.

POSTURE AND GROSS MOTOR

The rate of development within an individual child varies depending upon his state of health, the degree of stimulation that he receives and such events as the arrival of a new baby, admission to hospital or a change of house. Allowance also needs to be made for prematurity. For this reason data related to a child's development cannot be taken in isolation from the environment in which he is living. Furthermore the child's personality and temperament may distort his response to the test procedure.

Children follow different patterns of events leading to walking including crawling, creeping and bottom shuffling. Those who bottom shuffle are usually late to walk because it is more difficult to get to the upright posture from the sitting position than from the crawling position. When assessing children who are slow to stand and walk it is obviously important to enquire about other methods of locomotion.

Children who bottom shuffle tend to dislike lying in the prone position and thus do not develop crawling. Some children go straight from sitting to walking without an intervening stage. Negro babies are generally more advanced in early motor development than other babies.

Six weeks

At the age of 6 weeks when lying prone, the baby is just able to raise his chin momentarily. When he is pulled to sit from the supine position the child still shows head lag but is able to show some ability to raise his head, particularly in the half-way position of this manoeuvre. When lying in the supine position the baby still adopts a pattern of flexion at the elbows, knees and hips. A pattern of extension at this age, may be an indication of spasticity. Held in ventral suspension he can hold his head in line with the rest of the body. A large discrepancy in the performance of the baby in the prone and supine position with superior performance when prone, may indicate a developmental abnormality such as cerebral palsy. However, some babies such as those who are bottom shufflers, greatly prefer one posture to another. Others are not given the opportunity to develop their motor skills in a wide variety of postures.

Three months

By the age of 3 months there are some most impressive changes in the child's motor abilities. In the prone position, the child is able to lift the head and upper chest clear and is able to sustain this posture supported by the forearms. When pulled to sitting there is only minimal head lag. In ventral suspension the head is now above the level of the body. When held sitting, the back is straight and the head only occasionally drops forward. When held standing the child sags at the knees.

Six months

At 6 months of age, in the prone position, the baby can lift his head and chest clear, supporting his weight on extended arms and can roll over. Rolling is a very complex motor activity involving coordination of right and left sides, arms, legs, head and trunk. If the child is able to execute such a complicated manoeuvre it is most unlikely that any motor deficit exists. In the supine position he is able to lift his head from the pillow and in this posture grasp his foot. When pulled to sit the head is erect and the back is straight. He is able to sit against a wall requiring no lateral support. When held standing the baby is able to bear weight on his feet.

Nine months

By the age of 9 months most children will be able to sit unsupported for 10–15 minutes. This posture will be stable and the baby is able to maintain balance as he reaches out to grasp nearby objects. By this age the child can also stand holding on and may attempt to take steps if supported. In the prone position some may be crawling and most should be making some attempt at this manoeuvre.

ONE YEAR

At the age of 1 year the child can sit well and for an indefinite period of time. He can rise independantly from the lying position to the sitting position and from the sitting position is able to crawl effectively on all fours. Some children get along by either hauling using the arms alone, or creeping on the hands and feet, or by bottom shuffling: some miss out these stages altogether. The child is now able to get up and down from the standing position and is able to walk around the furniture, a manoeuvre known as cruising. He may be able to stand alone for a few seconds.

Fifteen months

At 15 months the child can get to the standing position without the aid of nearby objects. He is able to walk unsteadily on a wide base but frequently falls due to minor obstructions. Additional hazards to safety occur as the child learns to crawl upstairs but is unable to get down. He is also able to kneel with or without support.

Eighteen months

By 18 months of age walking skills are well developed and falls are seldom though there is obviously wide individual variation. He is now sufficiently stable to stoop and pick up an object from the floor without overbalancing. He can run for short distances and can push or pull toys around the floor. Carrying a large object does not result in falling over. He is able to sit down without help in a small chair. Getting upstairs can now be accomplished in an upright posture with the hand held and downward progression may occur by creeping backwards or by proceeding downwards step by step on the buttocks.

TWO YEARS

By 2 years of age the child can go up and down stairs holding on in the upright position. This is done step by step and does not follow the adult pattern of alternating feet on each step. Running is now more skilled and the child is able to change course to avoid obstacles. He may play in a squatting position from which he can easily rise to his feet. Climbing on and off furniture is performed with ease but often not with the approval of his parents. He is beginning to be able to both throw and kick balls without falling over in the attempt.

By the age of $2\frac{1}{2}$ the child can walk upstairs without holding on but cannot yet do this downstairs. He has now developed the ability to jump with both feet together and to stand on tiptoe following a demonstration of this.

THREE YEARS

At the age of 3 the child can walk upstairs with alternating feet but still has to use two feet on each step for descending. He can walk as well as stand on tiptoe and can also stand momentarily on one foot, a skill which many adults cannot demonstrate. The child can now pedal a tricycle as opposed to the previous manoeuvre of pushing it along with his feet on the ground. Increasing agility enables the child to climb nursery apparatus and to jump down one step. Others may attempt more than this but are not likely to succeed.

FOUR YEARS

By the age of 4 years the child can walk both up and down stairs using alternating feet. He can stand on one foot for 3–5 seconds and can also hop on one foot, though there is wide variation depending upon the opportunities and encouragement to develop these skills.

FIVE YEARS

By the age of 5 years the child is able to skip on alternate feet and to run lightly on his toes. His wide repertoire of motor skills will be illustrated by climbing, sliding, swinging, etc. There is increased skill in kicking, throwing and catching balls. He is able in 90% of cases to walk heel to toe. By the age of 5 the child has developed a basic repertoire of gross motor skills. Following this there are improvements related to greater strength, greater precision, greater speed and length of performance.

FINE MOTOR SKILLS

Development of fine motor skills depends on normal vision and appropriate opportunities for learning. Deprivation of either will result in delay of acquisition of such skills.

Six weeks

At 6 weeks the palmar grasp reflex operates but there are no voluntary fine motor movements.

Three months

At 3 months of age there is intense hand regard, in which the child stares continually at his own hand. This intense observation leads in the next few months to the development of voluntary use of the hand which is visually directed. At 3 months the child may reach out and hit objects such as pram beads.

Six months

By 6 months of age the child is able to pick up voluntarily any object such as a cube using a palmar grasp. Both the cube and his hand need to be within the same field of vision. At first this is only done with the greatest of difficulty and the cube is soon dropped. Lacking memory, the child does not look for the dropped object but seems to carry on unperturbed. Although voluntary grasp is established at this age, voluntary release is not seen for several months. At 6 months the child also begins to be able to transfer objects from one hand to another. However the child is not yet able to use this as part of a problem solving exercise. So, if the child is offered a second cube, he is likely either to ignore this cube or to drop the first one and use the same hand to retrieve the second object. Once the child has learned the ability to grasp objects he soon learns to be able to bring them to his mouth, and to add these sensations to his other means of exploring and understanding objects.

Nine months

At 9 months of age the child has developed a mature grip between thumb and index finger and can also use his index finger to approach and poke at small objects. Toys that are dropped are now sought for. The child has a wide range of manipulative skills, objects can be shaken, bashed, pulled, pushed or held.

ONE YEAR

By 1 year of age the practice of fine motor skills has enabled the child to pick up small objects such as crumbs. The child is able to use his fine motor skills to feed himself with a biscuit or hold his own bottle. He has developed the phenomenon of casting, in which toys are deliberately dropped and watched as they fall to the ground. Given two objects he may bring them together in the midline and match them or imitate a simple action such as banging two bricks together. If offered a third object, most children seem unable to transfer in order to grasp the third object but may become quite upset by this apparent dilemma and drop both of the original objects.

Fifteen months

At 15 months of age the index finger has developed as an organ for pointing to objects that he wants. Children are reported to be able to build a tower of two cubes though there is a wide variation between these abilities from various reports. This may well be highly dependent on the child's previous experience of bricks and his opportunity to practise. It cannot be assumed as perhaps some developmental tests do, that most children grow up surrounded by one inch cubes.

Eighteen months

By 18 months of age the average tower builder has progressed to a somewhat precarious edifice of three bricks. If given a crayon this will be used for spontaneous scribble usually in a preferred hand. The index finger may be used to point at objects in the book and the child can usually turn the pages two or three at a time, inflicting a variable degree of damage.

TWO YEARS

At 2 years of age the average tower builder is up to a tower of six cubes, again bearing in mind the wide variation in accomplishment in this task. Although performance with crayon and paper is still largely scribble this may begin to assume a circular form and the child might also be able to draw dots and imitate a vertical line. Page turning one at a time is now achieved though it must be remembered that many children do not have books and cannot therefore develop the skill. Between 18 months and 2 years most children are able to complete simple jigsaws involving fitting a circle, square, and triangle – initially by trial and error and only later by matching. Gains of skills and their level of development depend upon the availability of such toys as posting boxes, etc. Children may more readily demonstrate their fine motor skills in terms of manipulation of toys from activity centres up to small miniature toys, peg boards, jigsaws, dressing dolls, etc than in more standardised tasks which do not hold the same degree of interest.

At $2\frac{1}{2}$ years of age the child is able to build a seven block tower. He is also able to construct a 'train' from three blocks placed horizontally in a row and one block placed on top for a chimney. With a pencil he is able to imitate a circle and a horizontal line if this is demonstrated. Only at the next stage are they able to copy the completed symbol without a previous demonstration.

THREE YEARS

By 3 years of age the child's tower has grown to nine bricks and using three bricks the child can copy a bridge design. He can draw a circle from a copy and can now draw a cross if this is first demonstrated. The child is, at this stage, beginning to produce recognisable pictures and will produce the first crude picture of a person plus a variety of assorted parts. The Goodenough draw a man test is a useful and reliable way of assessing development of children between ages 3 and 10. The child is asked to draw a man. He is left undisturbed and given as much time as he wants. The final drawing is scored using 51 criteria which record the degree of complexity and the anatomical details shown. The child is given a basal age of 3 years and is accorded an extra 3 months for each of the features recorded in his picture.

FOUR YEARS

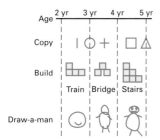

By the age of 4 years we have now reached the limits of tower building, bearing in mind the number of one-inch cubes the paediatrician can carry in his bag at any one time. The tower is now 10 or more cubes high. From about $4\frac{1}{2}$ the child is able to construct stairs with the one-inch cubes after an initial demonstration. He can now copy a cross without a previous demonstration and can also draw a square if the technique is shown first. The drawing of a man will now have a head and legs and the picture may or may not have a separate trunk. Most children will also be able to draw a very simple representation of a house. The child of 4 should be able to name the four primary colours in the one-inch bricks and is certainly able to match them. Some children may have been able to do this since the age of 3. A four year old can generally do buttons up, a useful practical skill which enables him to dress himself. However, absence of the skill probably indicates that the mother dresses the child because it is quicker.

FIVE YEARS

The 5 year old can draw a square and a triangle from a copy. (He will need to be 7 to be able to copy a diamond and 9 to be able to copy a parallelogram.) He can also draw a house with door, windows, a roof and a chimney. Using one inch cubes he can copy the step design without demonstration and also construct a 'gate'. Ideas of shape and copying ability have improved to the extent that the child can now learn to recognise and copy letters from the alphabet.

SOCIAL DEVELOPMENT AND PLAY

Although appropriate toys for each age group are inserted into the text it must be recognised that to a large extent, the toys without the parent are useless. Also the importance of play such as peep-bo, round and round the garden, and nursery rhymes which do not require any toys are a very important aspect of stimulation.

Six weeks

At 6 weeks of age the child smiles in response to a friendly human face. The child is visually very alert and will fixate and stare at the mother's face for long periods. As well as crying he develops a whole range of sounds; coos, glugs, grunts and laughter, which indicate mood. An awake baby in a carrycot only receives the stimulation that is brought to him. This may be obtained from mobiles suspended above the cot, by carrying him around or by the use of a bouncing cradle in which the baby reclines.

Three months

At 3 months of age the child begins to react with excitement to familiar and pleasant situations such as feeding and bathing. Similar responses occur when he is played with. From 3 months the child may attempt to hit toys suspended on a string across the pram. Although the child can do very little with toys, things to listen to, such as a musical box and things to look at, such as mobiles, are very useful.

Six months

At 6 months of age the child can successfully grasp suitable toys and transfer them to the mouth. He is capable of grasping a rattle and shaking it and may apply this strategy to many other objects. He is also able to play with his feet and take these to the mouth too. The child is now able to play with a wider range of toys of many different shapes and colours; they appear to enjoy those they can grasp or which make a noise like rattles and bells.

Nine months

At the age of 9 months the development of memory means that the child becomes much more wary of strangers and sensitive to separation from his mother. It also means that lost toys are looked for and he can play games such as peep-bo. He can feed himself with a biscuit, and attempts to hold his own cup or bottle. He may also try to grab the spoon. He can now handle toys which require a wider range of manipulative skills to make them work.

ONE YEAR

At 1 year of age children who have been given the opportunity are able to drink from a cup. However, many parents feed their children as this is tidier, so that they do not develop the skill until somewhat later. The same applies to spoon feeding which children can manage with help at this age but not all get the opportunity. At 12 months children understand how to cooperate in dressing, recognising that shoes go on feet and arms go in the sleeves. However, although many children do begin to cooperate with dressing at this stage, others who seem to dislike being dressed, develop the ability of doing the reverse of what is being required. The same can apply to nappy changing which can be a nightmare with a mobile uncooperative child. The child is now able to imitate gestures such as clapping hands and waving bye-bye. Some are able to produce this spontaneously in appropriate situations and others on demand. The child is also able to grasp quickly and imitate other actions such as ringing a bell or banging two bricks together. In play the child will often concentrate for long periods of time, putting objects in and out of boxes or quietly emptying mother's cupboards. Simple cooperative play is developing and the child will give a toy to the parent on request. Toys such as stacking beakers and pop-up men can be useful, though the child's skills are more directed towards taking apart than putting together. Rag books are also useful.

Fifteen months

At 15 months the curiosity and exploratory behaviour becomes more intense aided by the improved mobility and manipulative skills developed over this time. The child grasps anything within reach and cannot distinguish safe from dangerous objects. He will begin to be frequently told 'no' and reacts adversely if removed from unsuitable situations.

Eighteen months

The child of 18 months should be able to manage a cup without too much spillage and to be pretty adept at using a spoon independently. He may be able to take off shoes and socks, often in inappropriate circumstances. Negativism and the need for constant supervision are usually more marked than at 15 months. Domestic mimicry is seen in terms of the child copying mother sweeping. The beginnings of symbolic play are also seen, for example putting dolly to sleep or giving mother 'a cup of tea' in a toy cup. The child has progressed from toys that one pushes to trucks or cars, or fitting pieces into other types of shape fitting toys. Sand and water are most appreciated and the child will begin to be able to use drawing and painting materials in a chaotic uncoordinated and sometimes undesirable manner.

TWO YEARS

The 2 year old may be slightly less of a danger to himself than the child of 18 months. Greater awareness and knowledge and improved motor abilities may reduce some hazards but increase others. Negativism continues to be prominent and temper tantrums a common feature. The 2 year old should be pretty competent in eating and drinking. The 2 year old is also ready though frequently not willing to be toilet trained, however with greater or lesser difficulty, most children will become dry during the day around this age. The child's play shows further development in domestic mimicry. He begins to want to join in and 'help' with adult activities. Simple make believe play is also developing. Children of 2 years are unable to share their belongings and play along side one another rather than with one another. Useful toys are replicas of adult materials such as tools, cups and saucers, toy cars, simple wooden trains and, of course, picture books and being told stories.

The $2\frac{1}{2}$ year old is usually pretty reliable with using the toilet during the day. However many need help in that they are unable to pull down their pants or replace them. Make believe play is becoming increasingly elaborate with the child frequently talking to himself in play. Tray jigsaws may be very popular. Stories and picture books remain very popular. Scribbling with crayons and painting may just be beginning to emerge with some recognised form or pattern.

THREE YEARS

The three year old should at last be fairly independent with toileting and accomplish all the subsidiary functions such as pulling pants up and down and washing hands. He is also able to play together with other children and understands concepts such as sharing or taking turns. Many 3 year olds, and quite a number of younger children too, are

Gross motor development

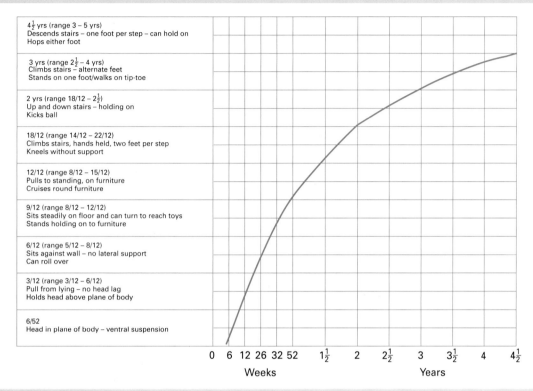

$4\frac{1}{2}$ yrs (range 3 – 5 yrs)
Descends stairs – one foot per step – can hold on
Hops either foot

3 yrs (range $2\frac{1}{2}$ – 4 yrs)
Climbs stairs – alternate feet
Stands on one foot/walks on tip-toe

2 yrs (range 18/12 – $2\frac{1}{2}$)
Up and down stairs – holding on
Kicks ball

18/12 (range 14/12 – 22/12)
Climbs stairs, hands held, two feet per step
Kneels without support

12/12 (range 8/12 – 15/12)
Pulls to standing, on furniture
Cruises round furniture

9/12 (range 8/12 – 12/12)
Sits steadily on floor and can turn to reach toys
Stands holding on to furniture

6/12 (range 5/12 – 8/12)
Sits against wall – no lateral support
Can roll over

3/12 (range 3/12 – 6/12)
Pull from lying – no head lag
Holds head above plane of body

6/52
Head in plane of body – ventral suspension

0 6 12 26 32 52 $1\frac{1}{2}$ 2 $2\frac{1}{2}$ 3 $3\frac{1}{2}$ 4 $4\frac{1}{2}$

Weeks   Years

Fine motor development

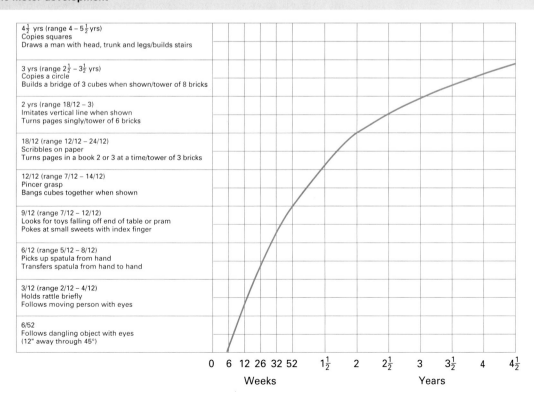

$4\frac{1}{2}$ yrs (range 4 – $5\frac{1}{2}$ yrs)
Copies squares
Draws a man with head, trunk and legs/builds stairs

3 yrs (range $2\frac{1}{2}$ – $3\frac{1}{2}$ yrs)
Copies a circle
Builds a bridge of 3 cubes when shown/tower of 8 bricks

2 yrs (range 18/12 – 3)
Imitates vertical line when shown
Turns pages singly/tower of 6 bricks

18/12 (range 12/12 – 24/12)
Scribbles on paper
Turns pages in a book 2 or 3 at a time/tower of 3 bricks

12/12 (range 7/12 – 14/12)
Pincer grasp
Bangs cubes together when shown

9/12 (range 7/12 – 12/12)
Looks for toys falling off end of table or pram
Pokes at small sweets with index finger

6/12 (range 5/12 – 8/12)
Picks up spatula from hand
Transfers spatula from hand to hand

3/12 (range 2/12 – 4/12)
Holds rattle briefly
Follows moving person with eyes

6/52
Follows dangling object with eyes
(12" away through 45°)

0 6 12 26 32 52 $1\frac{1}{2}$ 2 $2\frac{1}{2}$ 3 $3\frac{1}{2}$ 4 $4\frac{1}{2}$

Weeks   Years

Social development

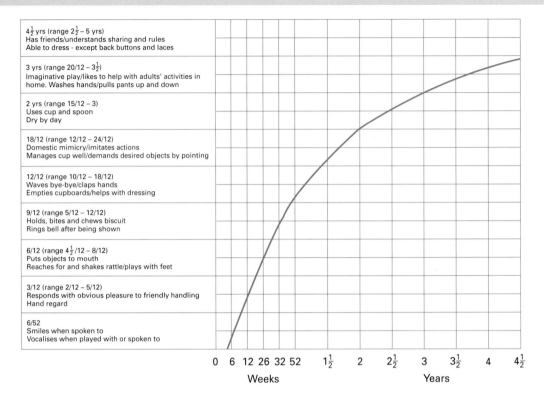

4½ yrs (range 2½ – 5 yrs)
Has friends/understands sharing and rules
Able to dress - except back buttons and laces

3 yrs (range 20/12 – 3½)
Imaginative play/likes to help with adults' activities in
home. Washes hands/pulls pants up and down

2 yrs (range 15/12 – 3)
Uses cup and spoon
Dry by day

18/12 (range 12/12 – 24/12)
Domestic mimicry/imitates actions
Manages cup well/demands desired objects by pointing

12/12 (range 10/12 – 18/12)
Waves bye-bye/claps hands
Empties cupboards/helps with dressing

9/12 (range 5/12 – 12/12)
Holds, bites and chews biscuit
Rings bell after being shown

6/12 (range 4½/12 – 8/12)
Puts objects to mouth
Reaches for and shakes rattle/plays with feet

3/12 (range 2/12 – 5/12)
Responds with obvious pleasure to friendly handling
Hand regard

6/52
Smiles when spoken to
Vocalises when played with or spoken to

0   6 12 26 32 52   1½   2   2½   3   3½   4   4½
Weeks   Years

confident enough to separate from their parents at nursery school or play group. Recognisable drawings of a human body or a house begin to be made. The 3 year old can begin to make real constructions out of bricks or construction toys of various types and can make sensible layouts using things like miniature animals, people, etc. The 3 year old is able to remember nursery rhymes and also stories. He is constantly asking questions about things that he sees.

FOUR YEARS

The 4 year old continues to ask questions though they are now of the 'why' or 'how' variety rather than the 'what' or 'who'. He can dress and undress except for difficult buttons and laces though the result may often be back to front or inside out. Imagination is shown strongly in play with such items as dressing up. He needs other children to play with and the idea of 'friends' becomes a well established need.

FIVE YEARS

The 5 year old is able to play games with increasingly complicated sets of rules. A wider time perspective occurs in play. Particular themes either in play or within school can be carried on over a prolonged period in time. A 5 year old can, but not always, be protective and responsible towards his younger brothers and sisters. The 5 year old can play and build constructively and copy or produce increasingly complicated designs. He has the ability to tell the time, recognise letters and numbers, beginning the process of learning to read.

EMOTIONAL DEVELOPMENT

There are many profiles of childhood describing behaviour at different ages. Theories based on these observations give us a means of understanding the process of learning, the development of reasoning and of emotional responses. Such theories have contributed towards educational progress and in our understanding abnormal or difficult behaviour. They provide a view of the child's world as the child perceives it, as opposed to our description of what the child does. The theories are not only clinically useful but also provide a fascinating insight into the world of a developing child. They are not mutually exclusive for each examines different aspects of child development and each makes its separate contribution towards our understanding.

GESELL

Arnold Gesell at Yale University, first made detailed observations of normal child development which he classified into gross and fine motor, adaptive, language and personal/social.

On the basis of these observations, he drew three conclusions:
- that there is a defined sequence of development
- that development proceeds in a cephalo-caudal progression
- that development proceeds from gross undifferentiated skills to precise and refined ones.

The important implication of these findings for management in cases of developmental delay is that the child should be helped to acquire skills according to the sequence. Thus, it is inappropriate to teach a child to walk when he is yet unable to sit. Gesell thought that development reflected maturation of the central nervous system, rather than the results of learning. This theory was supported by observations that motor skills developed in a normal way in infants who were swaddled, however the quality of their performance was not studied.

Gesell also observed that it was not possible to induce the earlier development of particular skills by specific training and practice. He concluded from this again that central nervous system maturation was the dominant factor rather than training. It would be wrong to draw the conclusion from these relatively limited observations that nothing need be done or can be done for the young handicapped child on the argument that progress awaits brain maturation. This approach is too simplistic and although it must be accepted that damaged or delayed maturation will cause delay in development, it cannot be accepted that appropriate therapy and stimulation are not required. Some aspects of development are certainly dependent upon external stimulation; thus, the development of visual function depends on appropriate stimulation of the retina. Deprivation of this stimulation by opacities or gross uncorrected refractive errors results in the failure of development of visual function if these ophthalmic problems are corrected late. Similarly, cutting off the whiskers of mice results in defective development of the parts of the brain which control these sensitive organs. Others have developed the idea of critical periods for the acquisition of particular skills which suggests that optimum learning occurs only if the required stimulation is obtained at a particular time in development.

In spite of these criticisms, Gesell has contributed an enormous amount towards our understanding of normal development, particularly motor development, and its clinical application to developmental diagnosis.

LEARNING THEORY

Learning theory and behaviour modification practice has wide application in many areas including the management of mentally handicapped children. Learning theory is based upon the assumption that, with the exception of reflex responses, all behaviour is learned. It therefore stresses the role of experience in the environment rather than that of cerebral maturation. Certain responses are learned following specific stimuli and appropriate responses are reinforced. This has led to the therapeutic tool of behaviour modification whereby new responses may be learned and reinforcement withdrawn from inappropriate responses.

The theory on which behaviourism is based rests largely on animal experiments starting with Pavlov's classical experiments conditioning dogs to salivate when a bell was rung, through to the later experiments of Skinner and of Watson. The extreme point of view that all behaviour results from external learning cannot be accepted, but taken in conjunction with the other theories explaining child development, behaviour theory has an important application to our understanding of certain aspects of normal development and certain abnormalities in behaviour. For example, children probably acquire their gender identification by means of the type of stimulation they receive. Thus boys are encouraged to model themselves on their father's behaviour and are given trains and guns to play with whilst little girls are encouraged to model themselves on maternal behaviour and are given dolls and pushchairs to play with.

Animal experiments have shown that there are critical times for acquiring certain types of behaviour, for instance monkeys reared entirely away from their own mothers do not exhibit normal maternal behaviour and are aggressive and not protective towards their offspring. This animal model parallels that of early childhood deprivation and the failure of those individuals to bond or take care of their children.

Behaviour theory has been very useful in that it has identified how certain types of normal social behaviour are developed. Some understanding of the genesis of disturbed behaviour is gained and why within some families they recur. However, all external influences act upon some substrate. It is clear that babies have particular personalities right from birth, and that these personalities are to some extent independent of external factors.

ERIKSON

Eric Erikson's psychoanalytical theory covers the whole of human life from birth to old age. He describes each stage in terms of conflicts between two opposing forces. These conflicts arouse anxiety. Failure to resolve the particular conflicts of each stage in development results in maladaptive behaviours which continue into adult life.

Phase I. Infancy (the first year of life)

- acquiring a sense of basic trust
- whilst overcoming a sense of basic mistrust
- realisation of hope

In this phase, the child is entirely dependent. His satisfactions are in being fed and in the process of bonding to his parents. Absence of these results in anxiety. It is easy to see how important it is for the child to acquire, early on, a sense of confidence in the world around him. If he fails to do this and the world is seen as a hostile, unpredictable place, then he is likely to be a 'difficult baby' and to have feeding and sleeping problems. As adults, those severely deprived in this early stage are likely to be emotionally detached and aggressive, being unable to form deep and lasting relationships with others.

Phase II. Early childhood (1–3 years)

- acquiring a sense of autonomy (own will)
- whilst combating a sense of doubt and shame
- a realisation of will

In this stage the child acquires confidence in his own ability as opposed to self doubt. He realises his own will and has the ability for independent action. He is, however, required to conform to certain behaviours and may feel guilty if he does not. Children of this age develop negativism, temper tantrums and toilet training difficulties. He needs to learn to balance his own wishes against those of others. If he is unable to realise the strength of his will then as an adult he may be lacking in confidence and initiative. On the other hand if he does not develop any form of censorship mechanism then he might have difficulty accepting the demands made by society.

Phase III. Nursery school age (3–5 years)

- acquiring a sense of initiation
- overcoming a sense of guilt
- realisation of purpose

From the self confidence acquired in Phase II, a child goes on to initiate social behaviour which goes beyond himself into group situations. He must learn to share attention, affection and materials. In this phase conscience formation occurs and the child internalises previously external standards of behaviour. He may feel anxious that his separate autonomous behaviour is not always in accord with that of the group and guilt may result from this or from the fear of being found out.

With the greater sense of initiative the child begins to assume responsibility for himself as well. The child obtains his primary identification as male or female. Sexual curiosity and erotic feelings may arise and the Oedipus complex of attachment to the parent of the opposite sex is often seen. The child develops ideas of the future and can postpone satisfactions or pleasures till a later time.

Success in overcoming the conflicts of this stage results in a confident, outgoing person who is able to generalise his confidence into the group situation. Failure to do so at this stage may result in nightmares, fears of the dark, animals, or physical injury.

Phase IV. Primary school age (latency) (5–11 years)

- acquiring a sense of industry
- whilst fending off a sense of inferiority
- realisation of competence

In this age group children acquire the drive to achieve whilst attempting to overcome a feeling of failure. This drive and competitive spirit applies in intellectual activities, physical activities and in social relationships. Success at these results in increasing self-esteem (and esteem from others) whereas failure or a sense of failure, can result in difficulties in learning and impaired relationships. Those involved with school health will be very familiar with the child who finds himself isolated outside the competitive and energetic world of this age group.

Phase V. Adolescence

- acquiring a sense of identity
- whilst overcoming a sense of identity diffusion
- a realisation of fidelity

This description is perhaps best illustrated by Gauguin's picture *'Ou venons nous ou sommes nous ou allons nous'* – 'where have we come from, where are we, where are we going to?' The child needs to acquire a firm sense of who he is, what he wants from life and where he is going. Failure to do this is described by Erickson as role diffusion.

In this stage the child acquires a time perspective and is able to work towards distant goals such as examinations. There is anticipation of particular achievements in the future. The role of leadership is further developed in this age group and for the first time idealogical identification is seen in terms of political attitudes. Sexual identity develops further.

At this age the child should have acquired sufficient self-certainty in preparation for an independent life and decision making. The drive towards decision making is combated by a sense of doubt and uncertainty. Role experimentation in terms of jobs, ideology, and allegiances may cause added conflicts with parents as the adolescent seeks to acquire his own individual identity. Understanding adolescent problems is understanding the balance between acquiring the self certainty and anxiety about the ability to do so.

Phase VI

- acquiring a sense of intimacy
- avoiding a sense of isolation
- a realisation of love

This is the phase of courtship and marriage.

Phase VII

- acquiring a sense of generativity
- avoiding a sense of self absorption
- a realisation of care

This is Erickson's description of parenthood and the ability of parents to put the demands of their own child beyond that of their own.

Phase VIII

- acquiring a sense of integrity
- avoiding a sense of despair
- a realisation of wisdom

This is maturity!

PIAGET

Jean Piaget, a Swiss Zoologist, based his explanations of child development upon precise observations, particularly of his own children. His observations on cognitive development have been widely incorporated into teaching schemes in primary education.

The sensori-motor stage. 0–2 years. In this stage the child acquires a permanent image of himself and of the practical world about him. He learns to understand his separateness (dualism) from his mother.

1. Reflex action. 0–1 month. At this time Piaget describes all reactions as being simply reflex. For example, the child sucks in response to any object put into his mouth and he cannot distinguish between his own finger and the nipple.

2. Primary circular reactions. 1–4 months. By this time the child has formed motor habits which Piaget calls schema. Having developed these motor habits they can be wilfully repeated for their own sake, e.g. wilfully sucking the thumb.

3. Secondary circular reactions. 4–9 months. Now actions are produced not for the pleasure of their doing, but for the results they produce in the external world. Intentional acts are carried out. The child tries out all his various schemata on a new object until he finds one which produces the most satisfying results. Coordination of vision and movement develop although the child only grasps an object if the hand and the object are seen simultaneously.

4. Coordination of schemata. 9–11 months. In this stage the child pursues a particular end rather than trying out all his various motor habits to look for a satisfying result. Therefore if the result is obtaining a particular object that he desires he might use his previous experience, such as tugging at the blanket on which the object is placed, to bring the object sufficiently near for it to be grasped.

Piaget describes memory developing at this time – the child realises that objects that have disappeared have not gone and that he should look to see where they have dropped or where they might reappear. A child will discover a block which has been hidden under a cup. He is able to imitate gesture and understand situational clues, for example preparations for a meal. With memory comes distress at separation from the parents. The child becomes much more discriminating in terms of adults and will not go willingly to a stranger. Children remember the Child Health Clinic and immunising injections. Anticipatory crying occurs in the expectation of receiving a further injection.

5. Tertiary circular reactions. 11–18 months. At this age, the infant seeks new results by active experimentation. Thus if he is dropping objects from a pram he may vary the position of dropping the objects to observe the variation in effect that can be obtained.

6. Invention of new means through mental combinations. 18–24 months. In this stage, the child may be seen to solve problems not by physical experimentation but through mentally working out the solution and then applying this knowledge. Thus if a chain is in a small box, which does not admit the child's fingers, his first action may be to invert the box so that the chain is expelled rather than make unfruitful attempts to get his fingers into it to grasp it. These observations of Piaget can be readily repeated. They are a most worthwhile and rewarding part of a developmental assessment.

7. Infantile realism. 3–7 years. By 3 years of age, the child sees himself as the centre of the universe. He cannot conceive that others can have a different viewpoint (egocentrism). Animism describes the child's belief that everything is alive and has thoughts, feelings and wishes, just as he does. Dreams exist and thoughts and wishes are just as powerful as real events. In his pre-causal logic, nothing happens by chance. There is always a cause and causes are motivational. For example, balloons go up into the air because they want to. The child's beliefs are based not on what he perceives but on an internal model of the world which may bear little relationship to what his senses tell him. For instance the child is insensible to the contradiction that babies come from a baby shop even though he has never seen one. In the authoritarian morality of this age, the child believes that the punishment arises out of the crime. Bad events are explained as a punishment for something that he has done. It is easy for the child to feel responsible for events that have taken place, particularly in view of his egocentric stand-point.

It is during this period of infantile realism that the child may suffer excessive anxiety if he feels that his bad thoughts and wishes may actually have come true or that having such thoughts may result in some punishment following automatically. The pre-causal child will see teaching about heaven or hell or stories of Father Christmas coming down the chimney as very concrete and real. Rules are rigid and unalterable. Thus the child in the back seat is happy to point out the red light the parents have just crossed or the double yellow line at the kerbside!

Although there is a rapid expansion of language ability, Piaget observed that children mainly talk to themselves and that their 'conversations' are really a collective monologue.

8. Concrete operations. 8–11 years. At the time of his move to junior school the child acquires the ability to think logically. He realises that words, thoughts and rules are separate from concrete objects and activities. He is able to learn to compare and to contrast, and to understand the relationship of parts to the whole, to be able to group objects in time and space, and to understand the principles of conservation of mass, weight and volume.

9. Formal operation. From age 12 years. From 12 years of age the child acquires the ability for abstract thinking. This involves a systematic approach to problems and the ability to understand hypotheses. There is a progressive ability to acquire an understanding of concepts of space, time, causation, number, definition, order, shape, size, motion, speed, force and energy. It is only within the secondary school that such concepts can be properly understood and taught within the syllabus.

DEVELOPMENTAL ASSESSMENT SCORES

A detailed description of an individual child's development recorded with accuracy in the notes will meet most clinical needs. This may be summarised in terms of 'levels' for fine motor, gross motor, language and social skills. For research, for example in looking at the effects of various interventions upon development, this description needs to be expressed as a measurement so that the range and performance of groups of children can be compared. Skill is required to perform these tests so that they yield reproducible results. They measure what the child is able to do on that day and are influenced by the mood of the child and familiarity with the tasks involved.

There are now many different developmental tests and scales, some very general and others measuring individual skills such as language, motor abilities, visual perception or emotional maturity. They may be used as a measurement of ability, or as a diagnostic tool for children with learning difficulties. Only three of the many scales are described here.

The Griffiths Scales. These are frequently used by paediatricians as a research tool. Users need to attend courses of instruction. Two scales cover the age range from birth to eight years. The scales are divided into A locomotor, B personal-social, C hearing and speech, D eye and hand co-ordination , E performance and F practical reasoning for older children. Results are initially scored as a Mental age (MA), in months for each of the areas A to F . These are converted to a sub-quotient using the formula MA ÷ CA x 100. The general quotient is obtained from the average of the six sub quotients.

Denver Developmental Screening Test. This graphical method of representation of development is often used in clinical practice. It is particularly useful because the boxes for each item show the 25th, 50th, 75th and 90th centiles for children attaining these abilities. The original scale was developed in the USA, but a UK modification, the Cardiff modification (Bryant et al 1974), is available.

Wechsler Intelligence Scale for Children (WISC), Wechsler Preschool and Primary Scale of Intelligence (WPPSI). These scales have been widely used in the past within the education services. They cover the age range 4 to 17 years. There are separate verbal and non verbal sections. They are used very little now for educational assessment as a measurement of 'intelligence' or attainment does not help with the practical task of identifying areas of difficulty that can lead on to practical advice on remediation.

REFERENCE AND FURTHER READING

Bayley N 1965 Comparisons of mental and motor test scores fof ages 1–15 months by sex, birth, order and race, geographical location and education of parents. Child Development 36: 379

Bryant G M, Davies K J, Newcombe R G 1974, The Denver developmental screening test: achievement of test items in the first year of life by Denver and Cardiff infants. Developmental Medicine and Child Neurology 16: 475

Buckler J M H 1979 A reference manual of growth and development. Blackwell Scientific, Oxford

Egan D, Illingworth R S, McKeith R 1971 Developmental screening 0–5. Clinics in Developmental Medicine No. 30. Spastics International Medical Publications and Heinemann, London

Erikson E H 1967 Childhood and society. Penguin Books, Harmondsworth

Frankenberg W K, Dodds J B 1968, The Denver developmental screening test. University of Colorado Press, Denver

Gessell A 1948 Studies in child development. Harper and Row, London

Gessell A 1966 The first five years of life. Metheun, London

Griffiths R 1967 The abilities of babies. University of London Press, London

Griffiths R 1970 The abilities of young children, Young and Son, Chard

Holt K S 1977 Developmental paediatrics. Butterworths, London

Holt K S 1991 Child development, diagnosis and assessment. Butterworth-Heinemann, Oxford

Illingworth R S 1979 The normal child, 10E. Churchill Livingstone, Edinburgh

Maier H L 1969 Three theories of child development. Harper and Row, London

Piaget J 1929 The child's conception of the world. Routledge and Kegan Paul, London

Piaget J, Inhelder D 1969 The psychology of the child. Routledge and Kegan Paul, London

Robson P 1970 Shuffling, scooting and sliding; some observations on 30 otherwise normal children. Developmental Medicine and Child Neurology 12: 608

Sheridan M 1973 Children's developmental progress. National Foundation for Educational Research

Terman L M, Merril M A 1961 Stanford Binet Intelligence Scale. LM Harrap, London

Wechsler D 1974 Manual for the Wechsler intelligence scale for children. Psychological Corporation, New York

14 Emotional Development and Disorder

Child psychiatric disorders are one of the most frequent reasons for child consultations to paediatricians and general practitioners. Between 20 and 30 per cent of all child health consultations involve a psychiatric disorder. A sound understanding of the causes and treatment of these common problems is therefore important for anyone dealing with children. This relatively high rate of psychiatric disturbance in children may seem surprising but similar rates are also to be found in adults who consult health practitioners and there is no reason to believe that children are somehow immune from mental disorder. Children who have a psychiatric disorder are often seen as difficult rather than disturbed. But the distinction between 'normal' and pathological behaviour is important because reassurance is appropriate in the first case and dangerous in the latter.

Behaviour, mood and cognition are the three main aspects of mental functioning and a disturbance in one is usually associate, with an abnormality in the others and may be classified as a psychiatric disorder if the change in behaviour, emotions or thought processes is so prolonged or so severe that it interferes with everyday life and becomes a handicap for the child or those who care for the child. The definition of a psychiatric disorder must also take into account the child's stage of development and the socio-cultural context in which the behaviour occurs. For example, lying on the floor, kicking and screaming in a temper for 2 minutes several times a day would not be unusual in a two year, but would be considered abnormal in most ten year olds – unless the child was developmentally delayed or if everyone else around the child behaved in the same way.

Definition of psychiatric disorder

- a change in the child's usual behaviour, emotion or thoughts
- persistent – for at least 2 weeks
- severe enough to interfere with the child's everyday life
- a handicap to the child and/or the carers
- taking account of the child's stage of development
- taking account of the socio-cultural context

Occasionally, a child's mental state may be so bizarre or extreme that it only has to occur once to be regarded as abnormal. For example, deliberate self injury or hallucinations are not part of normal experience and one event is enough to indicate mental dysfunction. Using the above definition of psychiatric disorder the overall prevalence rate is 10 per cent for child psychiatric disorder in the general population, which is much the same as in adults. This rate is influenced by a number of factors which are outlined in the table.

Summary of the main aetiological factors that increase the risk of child psychiatric disorder

Child factors	Family factors	Outside factors
Boys: more likely to develop behaviour problems when younger	Marital difficulties: separation and divorce	Bullying
Girls: more likely to develop emotional problems when older	Death of parent or close relative, or even loss of a favourite pet	School ethos and organisation
Physical illness: especially epilepsy	Poor discipline: inconsistent, hostile or weak	Socio-cultural factors
Difficult temperament	Abuse: physical, emotional, sexual and/or neglect	Peer group pressure
Developmental delay	Hostile rejection	Social policy
Communcation problems, e.g. deafness/language disorder	Poverty: poor housing unemployment, poor facilities	
Poor self image, low self esteem	Large family size – four or more children	
Mental handicap	Mother: psychiatric illness Father: criminal activity	

Assessment and aetiology

The assessment of child psychiatric disorders is a complex process in which the observations of others play a major part. Thus it is important to gain information about the child from as many sources as possible. Even so, a child's disturbance is often situation specific and there may be reports of difficult behaviour in one setting only. Psychiatric disorders that are only manifest in one situation do not necessarily mean that the cause of the problem must also be there: a child may be difficult at home due to academic failure at school; a child who has been abused within the family may present major problems at school but not at home.

The temptation to identify a single cause for any psychiatric disorder should be resisted. The aetiology is likely to be due to multiple factors, each interacting with the others in such a way that the whole is greater than the sum of the separate factors. The different contributing factors act together as part of a pathogenic process. Thus a child with mild physical handicap may induce overprotectiveness in the mother – resulting in immature, demanding behaviour at home. This in turn leads to a relative withdrawal of the father that only serves to make the mother/child interaction more powerful.

The assessment process will take account of a number of different factors, each interacting with the others in such a way as to generate the problem. It is helpful to start by considering the contribution that the child makes to the development of the disorder and then to go on to review the role of the family and finally the influence of school and the outside world.

THE CHILD

Labelling the child as the problem is often regarded as unacceptable and unfair because they are given responsibility for the problems that more correctly belong to the parents or to the family as a whole. But 'labelling' is often more of an issue for professionals than it is for parents and to identify the child rather than the parent, as the problem, will usually lead to a more positive and caring attitude on the parent's part.

Temperament

Obvious differences in temperament between one child and another exist from birth, if not before. At this early stage, temperament is defined in relatively simple descriptive terms, but there is a strong tendency for these characteristics to persist. Some children have a stable temperament from the start. They are relatively easy to bring up and are mostly predictable in their reactions. Others seem to be difficult from the start and require extra care and attention. The 'difficult child syndrome' consists of strong negative emotions, unpredictable behaviour and difficulty adapting to new situations.

The difficult child syndrome

- Intense emotions – *unhappy*, mainly negative reactions
- Slow to adapt to change – *unsettled* by any change in routine
- Variable physiological responses – *unpredictable* feeding, sleeping, etc.

Children who persistently show strong signs of adverse temperament from birth onwards are likely to prove especially difficult to bring up. However there is a tendency to improve spontaneously and by 5 years old, at least half of the children will no longer show the full syndrome. Those that have persistent problems will require 'super parenting'.

The requirements for parenting difficult children

- more structure and routine in everyday life
- more limit setting and clear boundaries for behaviour
- more intensive training of appropriate behaviour
- more love and affection

Gender and age

There are clear gender effects that influence the prevalence of psychiatric disorders and these differences give some clues about the aetiology of psychiatric disorders. Gender seems to have a limited effect on the rate of disorder in toddlers, but by school age there is a noticeable increase in the frequency of all types of psychiatric disorders in boys where they outnumber girls by almost 2:1. Any developmental disorder, such as enuresis, language disorder and clumsiness is associated with an even higher ratio of males to females. In adolescence the ratio gradually reverses with increasing age to the normal adult ratio where females outnumber males in the prevalence of most types of psychiatric disorder.

The gender effects are influenced by the diagnostic category as well as by age. All forms of behaviour problem are more common in boys throughout childhood. Emotional disorders on the other hand occur with equal frequency in younger boys and girls and then become more prevalent in girls during adolescence. It seems that the most likely explanation for the age/gender differences is that younger boys are developmentally more immature and constitutionally vulnerable than girls. This is most probably due to the reduced chromosomal material in the Y chromosome that allows unbalanced genetic influences to take effect. In adolescence, however, the sex hormone changes probably play a dominant role making females emotionally more vulnerable and boys more likely to react aggressively. Knowledge of these age and gender influences may not effect the way in which emotional and behavioural disorders are managed, but many parents find it helpful to have their child's problems put in a framework that makes them more understandable.

Intelligence

A child's ability to solve problems and to use abstract concepts are important aspects of general intellectual ability that influence the development of psychiatric disorder. There is an inverse relationship between intellectual ability and psychiatric disorder that holds true right through the full range of intelligence. Psychiatric disorder is five times more frequent in children with an IQ less than 50. At this severely limited level of ability, the normal gender differences are not seen. There are many possible reasons for the increased prevalence of psychiatric disorder in mentally handicapped individuals.

> **The chief factors that increase the risk of psychiatric disorder in children with severe learning difficulties**
>
> - Isolation from 'normal' society
> - Poor adaptability to new situations
> - Limited problem solving ability
> - Organic brain dysfunction
> - Low self esteem
> - Poor communication skills
> - Low expectations of parents and others

Physical state

Children who are tired, hungry, too hot or too cold are more likely to show signs of emotional stress or difficult behaviour. For example, tempers occur more frequently in the evening and before meals. Of course, this does not constitute a psychiatric disorder unless it is a persistent and handicapping problem. On the other hand, it can be helpful to know that there are high risk times for problem behaviour so that preventative action can be taken.

Physically ill children are also more likely to develop emotional and behavioural problems, but the effect is not as much as one might expect. This may be due to an emotionally strengthening and maturing effect of illness. In this case the child may actually gain skills and competence as a result of having to cope with being ill. Even children with life threatening conditions such as leukaemia and other malignant disease seem to cope remarkably well. What does seem to have an adverse effect is the number and intrusiveness of any investigations. Repeated invasive tests that the child is unable to influence in any way are most likely to result in psychiatric disorder. But even then the majority of children manage without having significant problems.

In addition to the child's reaction to the illness, the parent's own feelings will have an effect on the child. Overprotectiveness and overindulgence are common responses to illness in a loved one. It is likely that conditions affecting a vital organ such as the lungs, the brain or the heart produce strongest protective reactions in parents.

Emotional state

It may seem self evident the a child's emotional state can alter the threshold for behavioural and emotional problems. However, it is frequently overlooked and in any case the relationship is often a complex one. For example, a jealous child may become defiant and attention seeking. This may lead to a negative, punitive parental response which in turn could eventually result in the child's depressive withdrawal or apparently unprovoked aggressive behaviour by the child, all due to an original jealous emotional state.

The concept of emotional arousal is useful in explaining how stress can have a cumulative effect. A child starting at a new school can be expected to have an increased level of arousal. This will be raised even further if the child has previously experienced problems at school or if there are other current stress factors. Eventually, when the level of emotional arousal has reached a high level, a relatively small amount of additional stress such as being mildly reprimanded, may trigger a major emotional outburst. Unless it is understood that the outburst has occurred in the context of high emotional arousal due to the accumulation of multiple stress factors, it will be difficult to work out why it happened and what can be done to prevent another episode.

Children with immature emotions are more likely to present with emotional and behaviour disorders. Emotional immaturity can occur as a result of a number of different factors.

Factors that cause emotional immaturity

- developmental delay
- exposure to a severe emotional stress
- repeated experience of emotional stress
- inconsistent parenting
- lack of affection or frank rejection
- lack of training in stress management

Emotional maturity can be promoted by graduated and carefully supervised exposure to stressful situations that are within the competence of the child to cope with. At the same time the child is taught a variety of strategies that can be used to help manage the stress, but the details of these approaches are beyond the scope of this chapter.

Ways of coping with emotional stress

- talking with others about the stress
- conflict resolution (or avoidance if resolution impossible)
- graduated exposure to stress
- cognitive coping techniques
- relaxation

Self esteem

The sense of having a separate identity develops slowly during childhood. A clear sense of being a separate person has usually developed by two and a half years of age, but it is not until around 7–8 years old that most children develop self concept and have an understanding of what kind of person they are. Before this age a child might describe themselves as bad after doing something wrong, but the feeling of being bad will not continue for long. By 7–8 years old it is possible for a child to feel permanently bad and to have a low self esteem as a result.

Children who have experienced repeated failure, rejection and other negative experiences will eventually develop a low self esteem and poor self image. This makes children vulnerable to behavioural disorders. Children with low self esteem often behave badly deliberately in order to have it confirmed that they really are bad. This results in a paradoxical feeling of pleasure.

Low self esteem is therefore a powerful motivating factor for bad behaviour and emotional distress as well as a strong force that actually maintains the problems. It is also an important reason why the usual methods for treating behaviour disorders are often ineffective in children with a poor self image. Looked at the other way round, high self esteem is a protective factor against emotional and behavioural problems and good self image increases children's resilience to stress.

Communication problems

Anything that interferes with clear communication can easily lead to frustration and the development of difficult behaviour. All forms of speech and language disorder may cause problems as can deafness. Unclear or inconsistent communications from parents and other adults have just the same effect.

PSYCHIATRIC DISORDER AND THE FAMILY

Families come in all shapes and sizes, but there are distinct advantages of the traditional family with two natural or 'birth' parents. On the other hand a dysfunctional two parent family may cause considerably more problems for children than a stable and caring alternative family arrangement such as the single parent. All families, however they are constituted, have a number of basic tasks to carry out.

> **The basic tasks for the family**
>
> - Giving continuity of care throughout childhood
> - Providing food and protection from danger
> - Training children to be socially competent
> - Helping children adapt to life crises
> - Meeting the changing needs of children during development
> - Ensuring children have positive self-esteem
> - Encouraging children to reach their full potential
> - Promoting the child's physical and emotional health

Family breakdown

The institution of The Family has undergone dramatic changes in recent years. Rates of divorce and separation are reaching epidemic proportions with one in five children in the UK experiencing the break-up of their family at some stage during their childhood. In the USA, up to 40 per cent of children can expect to be separated from a parent before they reach adulthood. A high rate of psychiatric disturbance is associated with parental separation and divorce and in the year following parental separation, the rate of psychiatric disorder is as high as 80 per cent. Nevertheless, it is clear that many of the problems were already present several years earlier, reflecting the dysfunction of the family prior to the eventual breakdown. Emotional and behavioural problems are particularly frequent in children who have been exposed to persistent quarrelling and ill feeling between parents and where children have been used as pawns in the marital conflict. The effect of family breakdown is generally greater in boys than in girls, but in older teenagers, it is the girls who are more likely to show overt emotional distress. The increased vulnerability of boys to the effects of family breakdown are seen most noticeably in an increase in aggressive and anti-social reactions on the one hand, or withdrawal and anxious behaviour on the other. Both reactions are often associated with academic under- achievement in boys, but not in girls.

Overt parental conflict constitutes the most damaging aspect of the fraught relationships that are associated with family breakdown. Covert tension between parents seem to have much less of an adverse effect on children. There is evidence that some of the detrimental impact of marital breakdown on children is delayed as a 'sleeper' effect that only emerges many years later on in life. This is probably more likely to occur in women and to affect the parent-child relationship in the next generation. Most children who have experienced the separation of their parents continue to feel a deep sense of loss, even into adult life, and children who come from a broken home have a higher than expected frequency of marital failure themselves in adult life. Unfortunately, fathers often start to disengage from the family well before the divorce and within a few years of the divorce, more than 50 per cent of children have little or no contact with their father.

Forming attachments

The process of forming a bond of attachment and affection between parent and child develops for the parents from the moment that pregnancy is confirmed and reaches a peak in the first few days after birth. However, the child's attachment to the parent only becomes noticeable at around 6 months old when separation anxiety is seen for the first time. The child–parent bond then continues to strengthen over the next few years and should be securely established by the time the child starts at school.

Immediately after birth some 10 per cent of mothers have no feeling of affection for their baby, but within a fortnight this has reduced to less than 1 per cent. A very small number of mothers fail to form an attachment to their child with serious implications for the future development of childhood psychiatric disorder.

Attachment problems are more likely to occur if there has been reduced parent-child contact in the first few weeks after birth or if the mother has experienced a failure of attachment to her own parents. In spite of problems in the mother–child relationship it is possible for fathers to compensate for the adverse effects of this on the child. It is also important for parents to know that it is not necessary to have affectionate and loving feelings for their child all the time and that it is possible to do a reasonable job of parenting without them.

Bereaved children show a very similar range of emotional and behavioural disturbance to children who have experienced loss of a parent by separation or divorce. Nevertheless, the rate of psychiatric disorder following death is significantly less than following divorce. In fact young children may show surprisingly little reaction to the death of their parent provided that they receive continuity of good quality care. It is not until 7–8 years of age that children develop the concepts of time and of the uniqueness of the individual necessary to comprehend death.

Boys appear to be more vulnerable to the death of a parent, particularly to the death of a father. The long-term consequences for children who have experienced the death of a parent have been hotly debated. There is some evidence that there is an increased risk for developing depression in adult life, but it is unclear whether this is directly due to the loss or the result of the many changes in family function and fortune that follow the bereavement.

Family size and structure

Children who come from families with four or more children have an increased risk for conduct disorder and other anti-social behaviour. There is also an increased risk of reading difficulties and decreased verbal ability in children from large families. The effect of sibship position is less than one might imagine. Eldest and only children may be academically more successful and youngest and only children are slightly more likely to experience separation anxiety. The age gap between siblings also has little effect, although there is some evidence that academic achievement and social adjustment is better if the age gap between siblings is more than four years. A very close gap between the first born and the next child can be associated with a higher rate of anxiety and moodiness in boys.

Single parent families

Approximately 1.5 million children in Great Britain are being brought up in a one-parent family. Of these families about 20 per cent are headed by a lone parent who has never been married, 10 per cent of one-parent families arise through the death of a parent and another 10 per cent of lone parents are fathers. Although many children live for a while in a one-parent family, more than 50 per cent of lone parents have either re-married or are co-habiting within three years of the family breakdown.

Most one-parent families live in deprived inner-city areas and 60 per cent of them are dependent on local authority housing, compared with 20 per cent for two-parent families. More than 50 per cent of one-parent families are living in poverty. Therefore financial and social adversity have a major influence on children brought up in one-parent families.

> **Some of the adversities faced by children brought up in single families**
>
> - Financial hardship
> - Social adversity
> - Difficulty in maintaining continuity of care
> - Over-involved relationships more likely to develop
> - Less likely to have back-up for parent who is sick or tired
> - Less opportunity for parents to have time for themselves
> - Full responsibility for the family is born by one person
> - Lack of modelling of normal male/female relationships

In spite of all the difficulties that single parents face, many are highly successful in the child care that they provide – against all the odds. But children brought up in single parent families will continue to be at risk unless there are major social changes to provide more adequate support, and ways can be found for children to maintain satisfactory contact with their absent parents. The trend of dysfunctional parenting and broken relationships is likely to continue until training and help with relationships for children is given a higher priority by society.

Parental illness

There is a strong link between parental mental illness and psychiatric disturbance in their children. This is mostly due to adverse social factors and disturbed family relationships that are so frequently associated with illness. The degree of involvement of the child in the parental illness is the key factor in determining how disturbed a child may be. Thus, a child whose parent has schizophrenia may be less disturbed than one whose parent is suffering from obsessional neurosis or personality disorder involving the child in the parent's psychopathology.

It seems likely that parents with psychotic disorders are readily understood to be ill and children are therefore able to distance themselves from the illness.

Maternal depression has been shown to have a particularly adverse effect on children. There is some evidence that disturbed emotions and behaviour in children continues even after the mother has recovered from the depression. This suggests that the disturbed parent/child interaction that occurs during the period of depression sets up a chain of disturbances that easily become self-perpetuating. Although the depression probably has a direct effect on parenting ability, there is also evidence that the often associated social and marital difficulties also play a significant part. The move towards care in the community for parents who are either physically or psychiatrically ill has led to a much greater exposure of children to the social adversity and emotional stress of illness. A child's temperament seems to be a key factor in determining the nature of their response to a sick parent. Children with intense emotional responses, generally negative mood and poor adaptability, have been found to react badly to stressful situations at home.

Social adversity

Social factors alone are rather weak determinants of childhood psychiatric disorder. They generally seem to act by making children more vulnerable to health and educational problems. The concept of a cycle of disadvantage is the most helpful way of understanding the way social adversity operates. For example, families who live in rented accommodation are frequently found to have a higher rate of delinquency in their children. The important factor here is unlikely to be the rented accommodation itself, but rather the process that leads to families using rented accommodation. The children of teenage mothers are another example. Many are brought up in adverse socio-economic circumstances, but the most important factor that determines the outcome for these deprived children is the amount of personal and educational support that the mothers receive, rather than the level of social adversity.

There is good evidence that unfavourable social influences tend to occur together and affect children from an early age – even in utero. In spite of this, many children from socially deprived backgrounds can be successful, provided they receive consistent affection and predictable child care. There is little doubt that ethnic origin and family culture make a significant contribution to children's everyday life. It is less clear what role these influences play in the aetiology of child psychiatric disorder, but there is some evidence to suggest that as children grow older, socio-cultural factors become more significant. It might be expected that children from mixed race marriages would have a higher rate of psychiatric disorder, but there is little evidence to support this view once socio-economic factors are controlled for.

The birth of a child

The arrival of the first-born child leads to a radical realignment of relationships. The single 'diadic' relationship between the couple increases to three 'diadic' relationships and for the first time a 'triadic' relationship. It is the three person relationship that provides the fertile ground where jealously can develop. A well established bond between the parents is therefore necessary in order to maintain the family unit through this period of change and potential crisis. The birth of a second child leads to a further dramatic increase in the number of possible relationships within the family. The first-born typically becomes more naughty and confrontational and has to initiate more of the interactions with the mother. It is in this context that a previously satisfactory relationship between a mother and child can become strained, sowing the seeds for a long-standing behaviour problem. Once again, the key factors in determining whether or not the child will develop a psychiatric disorder are the child's temperament, the mother's state of health and the stability and security of the parents' relationship with each other.

Adopted and foster families

Children who are fostered have a higher rate of psychiatric disorder, but in the majority of cases this disturbance was present before the fostering took place. The breakdown of a fostering placement is associated with a particularly high rate of emotional and behavioural disturbance. Adopted children have a slightly increased rate of psychiatric disorder that becomes more noticeable during adolescence when young people are trying to come to terms with their origins in order to look to their future. There is also evidence from twin studies showing that genetic influences can have a powerful effect on behaviour which may only partially be compensated for by the environment within an adopted family.

Concerns have recently been raised about 'out of country' and 'mixed race' adoptions and anxiety is voiced about the adoption of children by homosexual adults. It seems reasonable to conclude that in each of these situations, an additional adversity is present. However, none of these conditions precludes the possibility that a child will receive a high standard of care. What evidence there is suggests that children brought up in these unusual families do not have a particularly high rate of emotional or behavioural problems.

CHILDREN'S EMOTIONAL DEVELOPMENT WITHIN THE FAMILY

It is difficult to be sure exactly what a new born baby is feeling and later on children still find it hard to put feelings into words. But describing and communicating feelings is a difficult task for most adults as well. Crying is one of the main ways that babies have for communication and most babies soon discover that crying quickly brings them full adult attention. The strong feelings that parents experience when they hear their baby cry is helpful because it is a signal that the child wants attention. Thus the ability to manipulate parents develops early on in life. In fact, manipulating people by using emotional pressure is a very primitive way of getting what you want and even very young children soon learn how to do it. It is important to recognise it for what it is and to help children to develop more acceptable ways of making their needs known.

There are both positive (enjoyable) and negative (unpleasant) emotions. Each positive emotion has its mirror image – a negative aspect of the same emotion. So for example, it is possible to cry with happiness. Love can easily turn to hate and it is not unusual to experience remarkably strong feelings of anger towards those who we also love the most. There are, of course, other more complicated emotions such as jealousy and humour, but they are not 'pure' emotions and are made up of several different feelings. Thus jealousy includes both anxiety and anger.

Pleasant and unpleasant emotions and their mirror images

Positive emotions	Negative emotions
Calm and relaxation	Fear and anxiety
Love and affection	Hate and anger
Happiness and excitement	Sadness and depression

Positive emotions

The first 'smile' may be seen soon after birth, but these are not the real thing since they often occur when the child is completely relaxed or even asleep. By 2 weeks old it may be possible to elicit a smile by any form of gentle stimulation, although the smile often occurs as much as 8 seconds after the event. At about 6 weeks babies are smiling in direct response to sounds (especially the mother's voice) and to smiling faces. Even eyes on their own can produce smiling and the reaction time gradually becomes less as time goes by. By 8 weeks the child's smiling becomes an essential part of developing social relationships.

Laughter is usually seen for the first time around 4 months of age as a reaction to strong stimulation by touch, sound or movement. By 9 months laughter becomes more responsive to social situations such as hiding games or behaving in a very different way from usual. However, at this stage the same behaviour may easily result in either laughter or in tears. Older children gradually develop a sense of humour and by 6–9 years most children have found their own unique brand of humour. At this stage children go through a stage of loving jokes that almost no one finds funny.

Fear and anxiety

Even very young babies show some signs of fear, but it is in a very uncomplicated form and is seen in the startle response to a loud noise or any sudden and unexpected change. It is not until about 6–8 months old that babies show the first clear evidence that they are experiencing a definite emotion. At about 6 months old the first signs of anxiety appear in the form of anxiety towards strangers and fear of separation. Anxiety is therefore the first emotion to develop in a specific way so that it is absolutely clear what the child is feeling. Anxiety is associated with a

The relationship between age and the physical symptoms of anxiety and emotional distress

Age	Symptom
2–6 years	Generalised aches and pains
5–8 years	Limb pains
6–12 years	Abdominal pains
7 years onwards	Headache

high level of physiological arousal and a wide range of psychophysiological reactions. Young children complain a lot about the physical symptoms of anxiety. Then as they grow older, their complaints become more specific and easier to relate to their worries. The table gives an idea about how children's symptoms of anxiety change with age. Children's fears tend to change as they grow older. At first the worries are to do with real dangers and specific objects, but later on in adolescence the anxiety becomes more to do with the imagination and ideas.

The change of anxieties and fears with age

Birth onwards	Loud noise
6 months to 3 years	Strangers
9 months onwards	Heights
2–4 years	Animals
4–6 years	Darkness, storms, imaginary monsters
6–12 years	Mysterious happenings
12–18 years	Social embarrassment, academic failure, death and war

Anger

The first sign of obvious anger that is clearly directed against a specific person, develops between eighteen months and two years of age. Before that time children scream and yell in what seems an angry way, but it is more likely to be aimed at the situation rather than the person. To be angry in a way that targets another person, it is necessary to be aware of oneself as separate from other people and from the rest of the outside world. This stage is not reached until between 2–3 years of age when children start to use 'I' when talking about themselves.

At first, anger is shown in a physical way by pushing, hitting, kicking and rolling on the floor, but by the time children are 4–6 years old, the anger is expressed more often in words. At the same time the outbursts of anger become shorter and are replaced with sulking instead. As children grow older they continue to react to frustration with anger and sulking which last much the same total length of time as a toddler's tempers. At all ages, anger is always associated with feelings of anxiety and the psychophysiological reactions of anger are similar to those of anxiety.

Sadness and depression

Although children can become sad and miserable in a reasonably clear way at an early age, this is not the same as being depressed. Depression is different from sadness because it has two additional essential components that are not necessarily part of feeling miserable

1. Feeling of worthlessness (self-concept required)
2. Feeling of hopelessness (concept of time necessary)

Children who feel depressed come to believe that they are useless failures and that there is little hope that things will get better in the future. In order to feel a failure and to have a sense of worthlessness, it is necessary to have a concept of what sort of person you are (self-concept). This develops at about 7–8 years of age. A sense of hopelessness requires a concept of time which develops around the same age of 7–8 years.

This means that it would be very unusual for a child less than 8 years old to become 'depressed' in the strict sense of the word. Younger children can certainly be sad and tearful, but that is not the same as the specific emotion of depression which has a very different significance. Depression is always accompanied by the psychophysiology of anxiety. It is also associated with the behaviour of anger such as irritability and withdrawal of affection.

Grief

Grief is the normal emotional reaction to loss. The most obvious form of grief is seen in the bereavement reaction to the death of a close friend or relative, but the same reactions also occur in children after the loss of a pet or if a friend moves away to another area. Surprisingly strong grief reactions may also be felt when an older brother or sister leaves home.

Very young children show little or no sign of grief provided that their everyday life is not unsettled and they are being well looked after. Before 7–8 years old, children have little real understanding of death and what it means. However, they quickly pick up how other people are feeling and react to that. Nevertheless, reactions to loss are clearly apparent in children over the age of about 6 months and the level of distress that is caused by loss and separation increases to a peak at around 3–4 years.

There are three phases for the response to separation:

1. PROTEST – crying, screaming and actively searching for the absent parent
2. WITHDRAWAL – becoming detached and quiet, showing few emotions
3. DESPAIR – resignation, misery and listlessness

As children grow older these 3 phases of emotional reactions to separation develop into the bereavement reaction which also has 3 stages:

1. SHOCK AND DISBELIEF (lasts up to 2 weeks)
2. OVERWHELMING EMOTIONS (lasts up to 6 weeks)
3. READJUSTMENT (lasts up to 1 year)

Grief is not the same thing as depression because self esteem is normally preserved and there are no feelings of worthlessness, but in other respects the symptoms and signs are much the same. Grief contains large amounts of anger, guilt and anxiety. Bereaved children show grief in different ways depending on their stage of development. Before 7–8 years of age children may show very little response to a personal loss, provided that their basic needs for care and affection are being met. Young children tend to take their cue from adults and to a large extent they mirror the emotions and behaviour of those around them. Older children can experience the full range of grief and in adolescence the experience of loss can result in the most acute feelings of any age.

Slow emotional development

Some children seem to take much longer to develop mature emotions.

The major causes of emotional immaturity

- generally slow development
- temperamental characteristic
- lack of training in emotional control
- lack of emotional security

Delay in emotional development is characterised by selfishness, rapid mood swings, and poor impulse control. Of course any child will react with immature emotions when under stress, but children with slow emotional development will behave in this way all the time, even in the absence of stress.

Ways of promoting emotional maturity

Fortunately, the emotions of most children develop naturally along the normal lines without parents having to think much about it. No child will be able to mature properly without a feeling of emotional security which requires the following type of care:

Emotional security requires

- a loving and affectionate atmosphere
- predictability of care and relationships
- consistent discipline and limit setting
- age appropriate expectations

If a child is emotionally immature, it is important not to take any of these requirements for granted. None of them is easy to achieve and immature children need them even more than mature children do and it would be pointless to attempt to promote emotional development if one or more of these needs is unmet. Assuming that everything has been done to provide for a child's emotional security, then the following approaches assist emotional maturation.

Ways of promoting emotional maturation

- setting a clear standard and model for emotional expression
- planning a graduated increase in responsibility
- avoiding any response to emotionally immature behaviour
- praising any mature expression of emotions
- training emotional control

REFERENCE AND FURTHER READING

Barker P 1986 Basic child psychiatry, 5th edn. Blackwell Scientific, Oxford
Bentovim A, Elton A, Hildebrand J, Tranter M, Vizard E (eds) 1988 Child sexual abuse within the family. Wright, Bristol
Garralda M E, Bailey D 1986 Psychological deviance in children attending general practice. Psychological Medicine 16: 423–9
Goodyer I M et al 1987 The impact of recent undesirable life events on psychiatric disorders in childhood and adolescence. British Journal of Psychiatry 151: 179–84
Graham P 1987 Child psychiatry: A developmental approach. Oxford University Press, Oxford
Herbert M 1987 Conduct disorders of childhood and adolescence, 2nd edn. John Wiley, Chichester
Hersov L, Berg I 1980 Out of school: modern perspectives in truancy and school refusal. Wiley, Chichester
Hill P 1989 Adolescent psychiatry. Churchill Livingstone, Edinburgh
Nicol A R (ed) 1985 Longitudinal studies in child psychiatry: practical lessons from research experience. Wiley, Chichester
Richman N, Landsdown R 1988 Problems of preschool children. John Wiley, Chichester
Rutter M 1983 Development neuropsychiatry. Guilford Press, New York
Rutter M 1985 Family and school influences on cognitive development. Journal of Child Psychology and Psychiatry 26: 683-704
Rutter M 1989 Isle of Wight revisited: 25 years of epidemiological research in child psychiatry. Journal of the American Academy of Adolescent Psychiatry 28: 633-53
Rutter M, Hersov L 1985 Child psychiatry: Modern approaches. Blackwell Scientific, Oxford
Rutter M, Tizard J, Whitmore K, 1970 Education, health and behavior. Krieber, New York
Rutter M et al 1985 Depression in young people: developmental and clinical perspectives. Guilford Press, New York
Taylor E A 1986 The overactive child. J B Lippincott, Philadelphia
Tonge B, Burrows G, Werry J, 1990 Handbook of studies on child psychiatry. Elsevier, Oxford

Poor Homes and Families

The term 'community paediatrics' implies an awareness of the importance of 'place' in the presentation and management of sick children, but in that sense, all paediatrics should be community paediatrics and hopefully in the future the adjective 'community' will not be necessary. The same might be argued for 'social paediatrics'. However here it is used in a limited sense for the care of children whose health is compromised by social disadvantage. The title of the chapter is deliberately ambiguous. The phrase 'inequalities in health' is used to describe differences that result from a poor environment, poor nutrition and poor access to health care. 'Neglect' is used to describe the standard of care a child receives and covers such areas as failure to provide adequate food, or to protect from danger, or provide adequate stimulation. The term 'deprivation' is often used to describe both inequalities and neglect for they often go together and are difficult to separate from one another. According to the National Child Development Study (NCDS), 4% of families in the UK suffer 'deprivation' on the basis of low income, poor housing and single parent or large families.

Social class

Social class for epidemiological purposes is derived from the Registrar General's classification of occupation. In child health it relates to the occupation of the parent, usually the father.

Social class I : professional, higher administrative
Social class II: administrative, managerial
Social class III: clerical and skilled manual (IIIn non-manual and IIIm manual)
Social class IV: semi-skilled
Social class V: unskilled

It is, to some extent, an artificial classification of a continuum of social positions. Nevertheless it does allow helpful comparisons to be made. There are considerable differences in child morbidity and mortality rates between the different classes. There are further examples given in the others chapters. Theories on the reasons for these social class differences based on political, social and behavioural concepts abound. As health professionals faced by a child who is ill we have to ask ourselves, has the child got a disease (biological), can the parents provide care (material) and do the parents, and the child if old enough,

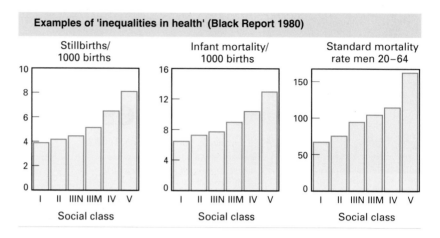

Examples of 'inequalities in health' (Black Report 1980)

know what to do and are they willing to do it (behavioural). The interplay between the biological, material and behavioural are complex.

In a recent study in Nottingham day nurseries mothers were asked to describe which factors they believed were healthy for their child and which were not.

Responses of a group of day nursery mothers

Things that are 'good' for my child	Things that are 'bad' for my child
Routine	Smacking
Discipline	Polish and dust
Insurance	Dangerous animals
Savings	Junk food
Dental checks	Worms
Love	Metal things on doors
Encouragement	Bleaches
Stability	Tight shoes
Comfort	Not having enough exercise
Protection (safety from strangers)	Windows (lack of catches)

Source: Blair M (unpublished data)

When the group was asked to explore some of the difficulties in adopting the first column it became clear how many restraints there are – poor parking space, unsafe play areas, inadequate cooking and storage facilities, difficulty in overcrowded accommodation and problems with violent and unstable personal relationships. 20 per cent of them described their children as having either sleep or feeding difficulties which were sufficiently worrying to seek help from a health professional. Many of these mothers were describing conditions of considerable deprivation and hardship.

In a local study comparing children who were admitted to hospital with a diagnosis of failure to thrive (weight less than 3rd centile) with a control group, three factors were found to occur more frequently in the mothers of cases; the mother perceived herself as having disturbed mood and used the word 'depressed' to describe her feelings, she came from a lower social class and her infant was more frequently of low birthweight.

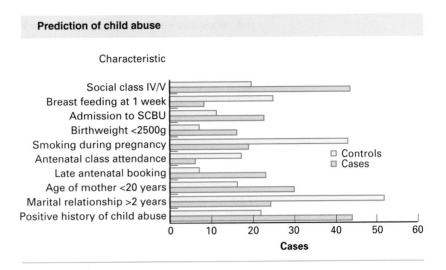

Prediction of child abuse

Characteristic

Another example of the complex interaction of biological, material and behavioural elements is shown by a study in Cardiff which used objective birth data to predict child abuse (Murphy 1981). The graph below summarises the main differences between cases and controls.

Deprivation

Deprivation is a relative lack of material and/or psychological support. In an attempt to direct resources according to need, measures of deprivation have been developed.

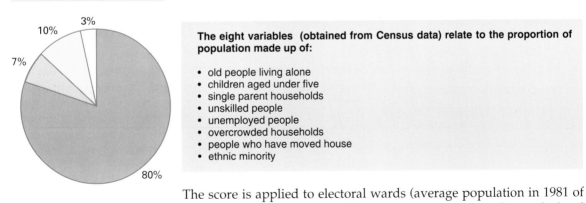

Children (0–18 years) and families (England and Wales 1982)

- Living with both parents
- Living with lone mother
- Living with mother and step father
- Living with neither natural parent

The Jarman index is derived from eight variables, each weighted according to how much GPs in a national study believed that it increased their workload.

The eight variables (obtained from Census data) relate to the proportion of population made up of:

- old people living alone
- children aged under five
- single parent households
- unskilled people
- unemployed people
- overcrowded households
- people who have moved house
- ethnic minority

The score is applied to electoral wards (average population in 1981 of approximately 5 000) and the GP receives payment according to the level of the score to reflect the workload implications (Jarman 1983). There has been criticism of this score: because of the size of the wards, there may be considerable pockets of deprivation within predominantly affluent areas and vice-versa, and the scores are derived from census data which can become quickly out of date in a highly mobile population. Another criticism is that it is based on GP workloads and the list does not *necessarily* reflect the health *needs* of the population served.

The Social Index was developed for use in the Child Health and Education Cohort Study and was designed to be more in tune with the home environment of the child than occupational class alone. It has been used to identify disadvantaged groups experiencing difficulties in health service use (Osborn & Morris 1979). By recognising these difficulties, resources can be targeted specifically at the most disadvantaged, for example, provision of a mobile immunisation service or an interpreter service.

The Inverse Care law. The availability of good medical care tends to vary inversely with the need for it in the population served. The 'Inverse Care Law' holds that market forces lead to this situation where the higher income groups are more able to obtain and use services. They receive more specialist attention; occupy more of the beds in better equipped and staffed hospitals; receive more elective surgery; have better maternal care, and are more likely to get psychiatric help and psychotherapy than low-income groups – particularly the unskilled (Tudor Hart 1971).

The impact of poverty on child health is seen in two main areas	
Physical	Behavioural
Infant mortality	Educational attainment
Childhood deaths	Truancy
Childhood morbidity	Teenage conceptions
Child development (height, weight and nutrition)	Pocket money
Racial disadvantage	Child labour
Homelessness and housing conditions	TV viewing
Clothing	Smoking
Child protection and child abuse	Drinking
	Drugs
	Juvenile crime

Data on the effects of poverty on the 'outcomes' listed above is available with varying degrees of completeness and accuracy. The challenge of paediatrics in the future is in developing methods of recording the health status and determinants for children at disadvantage and developing effective interventions to promote positive outcomes. Community Paediatricians are in a very good position to act as advocates for change.

Neglect

This is usually defined as the consequences of care rather than the process. In the 1989 Children Act, it is defined as:

*'the persistent or severe neglect of a child (for example, by exposure to any kind of danger, including cold or starvation), which **results** in **serious** impairment of the child's health or development, including non organic failure to thrive.'*

This definition relates to the question of whether or not a child should be placed upon the 'at risk' register. Neglect which has not yet led to a serious impairment may not be registered. It is the hallmark of community paediatrics that we wish to prevent these events from occurring. A child *may* be left to play alone in a street and *might* wander into the road and *might* be injured by a vehicle and this injury *may* be minor, serious or fatal. How do we decide what is neglect and who is neglectful?

Under the 1989 Children Act, a court may make a care or supervision order if it is satisfied that:

(a) *the child concerned is suffering or likely to suffer significant harm; and*
(b) *that the harm, or likelihood of harm, is attributable to :*

(i)   *the care given to the child, or likely to be given to him if the order were not made, not being what it would be reasonable to expect a parent to give to him; or*
(ii) *the child's being beyond parental control.*

The difficulty for the paediatrician, whose advice may be sought, is in the definitions of 'significant' and 'reasonable'.

Simple remedies which depend on one type of intervention such as providing more resources whether as aid, benefits, charity, punishment for wilful failure to provide care, education, or support and counselling are less likely to be successful than a broad approach. Inequalities and disadvantage are also likely to extend over many years and over successive generations of the same families. Programmes for intervention therefore need to be long term and sustained if there are to be benefits.

Prediction of neglect

Factors that may predict neglect antenatally, at the six week or subsequent checks are listed in the accompanying tables. These 'indicators' may be used to identify families who require more intensive support. A

Indicators

Antenatally	At six week check
• Not living with father of baby	• DNA
• History of 'in care' as a child	• Completed after three months of age
• Received special education for MLD or behavioural problems	• A combination of the following
• School attendance problems	– failure to thrive
• Moved house more than once during pregnancy	– widespread ammoniacal dermatitis that has
• Booked late or not booked	not been treated
• Poor attendance at antenatal clinic	– described as naughty
• Was abused as a child	– dislikes beign handled
• Smoking in pregnancy with no intention to cut down	– 'disinterested handling'
• Poor management of personal finances	– rough or impatient handling
• Has had social worker or probation officer	– dirty clothing
• History of violence	– mother noticed not to speak to child during check
• Age 21 or under	– mother noticed not to have direct eye contact
• Older children abused or neglected	with child
• Tattoos	– untreated or unrecognised infection
• Psychiatric history, mental illness, drug or alcohol abuse	– excessive crying or apathetic
	– difficult feeder
	– has not written in PHR
	– has ears pierced?

single indicator has little significance, but the presence of multiple factors should serve to highlight the extra needs of these families. Although a combination of risk factors may have both a specificity and sensitivity greater than 80% (Browne et al 1988), they cannot be used as a screening test as far too many false positives would be found. Browne estimates that such a process applied to a population of 10 000 births would identify 33/40 abusers, but also identify over 1000 false positives. The indicators can however be used to guide our professional judgements. The family characteristics of families that neglect and both neglect and abuse their children are quite different. The features described by Crittenden (1988) are very familiar to community paediatricians who work in deprived areas. There are, of course, protective factors that prevent neglect taking place even where there are multiple risk factors. These may relate to positive experiences in childhood, better education, family, community or professional supports.

INDIVIDUAL FACTORS AFFECTING THE WELL-BEING OF CHILDREN

The factors we shall discuss are those that influence the outcome for individual children. Some are capable of being changed by personal practice, others require action by local authorities or government but some such as genetic factors are not currently amenable to change. Graham (1988) lists the basic needs which if not met will impair health as: an adequate diet; adequate housing; adequate income; a stable, continuous source of affection and care, together with protection from physical, emotional and sexual abuse; cognitive stimulation and adequate education; safe environment; and access to preventive and curative health care.

Genetics

Studies of families of both gifted children and those with learning difficulties, show strong intergenerational continuities (Rutter & Madge 1976). In the Isle of Wight study, 37% of the families of children with learning difficulties had a family history of learning problems compared to 12% of the general population (Rutter et al 1970). Although it is difficult to dissect inherited factors from the care received from parents, there is a high correlation between the IQ of parents and children, even where they are reared away from their natural parents. We often talk about children reaching or failing to reach their 'full potential'. We describe the phenomenon of improvements in development when children's circumstances are improved, for example following a day nursery placement or more radically, by removal from a deprived home and adoption into a privileged one. However, it is difficult if not impossible to predict the 'potential' of individuals and the degree of improvement to expect with improvements in care. The extent to which these levels of development can improve, depend upon the age at which adverse conditions are removed (Rutter 1980).

Environment

Housing and children's health

	Number of symptoms/child
No damp	2.04
Damp	2.46
Mould	2.86

Symptoms: aches and pains, diarrhoea, wheezing, vomiting, sore throat, irritability, tiredness, headaches, earache, fever, depression, tantrams, bedwetting, poor appetite, persistent cough, running nose.

Source: Platt et al 1989

Housing conditions can have a profound effect upon children's health and development. Peaks of ill health and mortality in the winter months, which are a prominent feature in the UK, are probably related to dampness (Platt et al 1989), and defects in heating and ventilation. It has been well known since the earliest days of Public Health, that overcrowding and poor sanitary conditions are related to the spread of infectious disease, particularly gastroenteritis and respiratory infections (Lowry 1991). Passive smoking will add to the risks of acquiring respiratory infections and secretory otitis media. Poor housing is also associated with an increase in childhood accidents. Children living in flats or in other circumstances where there is no safe, supervised play area, such as a private garden or a playground, are likely to be at risk through playing outside on roads and other dangerous areas. Poor housing can lead to maternal depression and adverse effects upon child development. Overcrowding can lead to conflict within the home and children can suffer from lack of personal privacy, which is especially important for teenagers, and lack of space and proper conditions to do homework.

Homelessness may result in inadequate housing in bed and breakfast accommodation with very restricted facilities for play and for preparing meals. Frequent moves result in stress for families, insecurity for children and disrupt continuity of service provision in terms of changes in school, changes in medical practitioner and in social work support (Edwards 1991). Growing numbers of teenagers are sleeping in the streets of our towns. They are often the graduates of disturbed family lives or inadequate local authority care.

Neighbourhood

Community paediatricians are well aware that health is not only powerfully affected by the quality of individual houses, but by the nature of the neighbourhood as a whole. Within a neighbourhood there are often associated problems of lack of local amenities, public transport, adequate

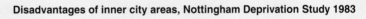

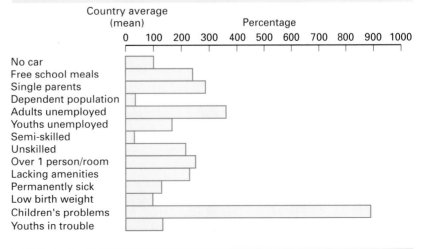

Disadvantages of inner city areas, Nottingham Deprivation Study 1983

refuse collections and shops. Blocks of flats may have particular problems with security and vandalism (Coleman 1985). Deprived neighbourhoods are also associated with increased unemployment and increases in juvenile crime (Nottingham County Deprivation Survey). Profiles of neighbourhoods, case loads or practices can be used to target resources. Health workers need, therefore, to be aware of local living conditions and the difficulties they create for parents in bringing up their children.

Income

Many indices of child health such as growth, mortality rates, respiratory infections, hospital admissions and educational attainments have been related to income. The problems of income and appropriate utilisation of income have been discussed by many. Those on low income spend 30% of their money on food compared to 12% for the average family and are more likely to provide a poor quality diet for their children with less fruit, fresh vegetables and fresh meat (Sheppard 1986, Graham & Stacey 1984).

Lack of disposable income leads to difficulties in budgeting. Skills in budgeting or getting value for money may not be sufficient to prevent families slipping into debt. For the families at the lowest income level, providing an adequate diet and remaining out of debt may be an impossibility. Debt or fear of debt puts large stresses on families. Poverty and the outward appearances of it may also have a detrimental effect on self esteem and provide an obvious badge by which they can be identified by others. Health workers, therefore, should be aware of the limitations placed upon child care by low income and of the personal sensitivities related to poverty.

Family structure

21% of live births are illegitimate, only 80% of children now live with both natural parents. One in three marriages ends in divorce, 56% of these couples have children under the age of 16. What then is the effects of these differing family structures on children? Perinatal, neonatal and postneonatal mortality rates are higher for illegitimate births. Educational attainments at age seven are poorer in illegitimate children (Crellin et al 1971). In practice, the difficulties that the children have may arise from a number of factors associated with family structure; these may be economic due to low income, secondary to the stress or depression that an unsupported parent may experience or related to family tensions and arguments. Professional help may need to be focused at all these three levels. Marital breakdown occurs more commonly in families where parents' childhoods were marked by divorce or separation. Skilled counselling is needed to explore family relationships.

Culture

In the UK, there are higher perinatal and infant mortality rates for some immigrant groups. Part of this may relate to lower socio-economic status and part to inherited disease particularly where there is consanguinity. Health workers are often faced with different child rearing practices and different family traditions (Henley 1979, Black 1990), which they need to understand before acceptable advice can be given. For example, understanding religious dietary restrictions or the contrasts between lifestyles or living conditions in their country of origin and the UK can form a basis for explaining some medical problems such as iron deficiency and appreciating the degree of adaptation required to a new environment. Interpreters and link workers recruited from the community to promote health care and explain customs are an essential part of the service to immigrant communities.

Stimulation

Children can only learn as a result of the stimulation that they receive. Lack of such early stimulation results in impaired language development and later educational difficulties. Bath (1981) found significant language delay in up to 50% of children attending social service day nurseries in Nottingham. Interventions may involve general advice to parents on the importance of language stimulation, the introduction of language programmes or help for underlying problems such as parental depression which may impair communication. Pollak (1979) found poor levels of development associated with inadequate stimulation from child minders in south London.

Nurture and affection

Bonding is a powerful, specific attachment between parents and child that enables care, protection, affection, sacrifice and empathy to take place. Its origins are in the parents' own child rearing experience. It is facilitated by early contact between mother and child and is inhibited by separations, malformations or unresponsiveness of the child or adverse circumstances such as an unwanted pregnancy. Children who do not receive affection and whose parents are consistently critical are likely to suffer low self esteem and severe emotional problems. Facilitation and understanding of positive reactions between parents and children are important in the prevention and management of these behaviour problems. Children in early life are often withdrawn (though often later having more outwardly difficult behaviour), fail to thrive and have characteristically cold extremities (deprivation hands and feet).

It is difficult to overstate the effect of parenting on the well being of children

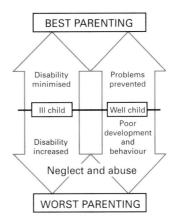

Diet

Non-organic growth delay is associated with developmental delay as shown by Dowdney et al (1987), in a study of 4 year olds from an inner-city area. Children whose weight and height lay below the tenth centile were found to have a general cognitive index of 77.1 compared to 97.7 for controls. 2% of the caucasian inner city children fitted their definition of chronic non-organic growth retardation and of these 35% had a cognitive index below 70 points. In these children an inadequate diet is the main cause of their failure to thrive. In Nottingham, Marder et al (1990), found 25% of inner city children to be iron deficient at 15–24 months with a rate of 39% in Asian children. In Birmingham, Grindulis et al (1986) found that two-fifths of their Asian toddlers were vitamin D deficient. Treatment of iron deficient children in Birmingham led to improved weight gain and 42% of the children whose haemoglobin rose by 2 g or more as a result of treatment achieved six or more new skills on the Denver scale compared to 13% in controls (Aukett et al 1986). There are conflicting claims for improvement in IQ by giving vitamin and mineral supplements to school children (Whitehead 1991).

Poor nutrition is clearly common in a relatively wealthy country such as the UK and is associated with poor development. Causes, however, may be complex and can relate to low income, inadequate knowledge about diet or, as described by Skuse (1985), a maladaptive behavioural interaction between caregiver and infant, sustained by high emotional tensions. Barker & Osmond (1986) have suggested that poor nutrition in childhood may have longterm consequences in the incidence of ischaemic heart disease in adult life.

In the Jamaican Study (Granthan-McGregor et al 1991), the effects upon development of both nutritional supplementation and stimulation were investigated in stunted children, age 9 to 24 months. The authors were able to demonstrate the relationship between these two factors. The developmental quotient improved for stimulated and supplemented children, but not in the controls. Children who received both supplementation and stimulation did better than children who received only a single intervention. Children who received both had a mean IQ 13.4 points greater than controls after 24 months; with improvements of 6.5 and 7.9 for single interventions.

Access to services

Access to adequate child welfare services is not equal. Parents in disadvantaged areas face difficulties if they do not have a telephone to contact the doctor or personal transport to bring their child to clinic or surgery. Children from disadvantaged families are certainly much more likely to be admitted to hospital for preventable causes of ill health (Wynne & Hull 1977, Carter et al 1990, Conway 1990). The cause of this may be related to the ability to prevent or recognise ill health as well as to decision making with regard to medical consultation and access to health care.

Life events

Life events in a child's family may have profound effects upon the functioning of the family overall. Obvious examples are the death of a parent or the onset of disability in a parent. Unemployment, housing problems, family separations, convictions or being a victim of crime are also important. Life events can of course, be positive as well as adverse – 'he hasn't looked back since...'. Medical records may with advantage, have life event lists, which can usefully supplement problem lists and other summary sheets.

Temperament

Children of similar levels of intelligence given the same opportunities, and the same quality of care do not always reach the same outcomes. An important factor is the individual child's temperament (Oberklaid 1991). Important characteristics of an individual child's temperament may be drive, adaptability to change, persistence, distractibility, regularity of behaviours such as sleeping and thresholds of responsiveness. The child's temperament needs to match or be compatible with the lifestyles and expectations of the rest of the family. For example a child who is quiet and thoughtful may be of concern in a family whose general characteristics are boisterous and out-going. In others an 'average' child born into a quiet and thoughtful family may be viewed as hyperactive. Our assessment of individual children and their families must take temperament into account and must also recognise that our own individual temperaments may also influence our judgement at times.

EARLY INTERVENTION SCHEMES

Here we outline examples of community programmes that are designed to prevent the consequences of disadvantage or at least to minimise its effects. These aims are central to any 'mission statements' of community paediatric services. Research to demonstrate the effectiveness of these programmes is difficult in securing sufficient numbers of children and long enough follow up to demonstrate outcomes.

Pre-school education

Osborn & Milbank (1987) in the Child Health and Education Study of a cohort of 13 000 children born in 1970, found better attainments in the children who had received preschool education. Children who attended nursery schools and playgroups did best and children from disadvantaged families did best when they had attended nursery schools. Children who had attended day nurseries had the poorest attainments in reading and mathematics. This important study supports community health workers who advocate both the availability and the uptake of preschool education. It also indicated the importance of preschool education for disadvantaged groups and the need to improve educational provision in day nurseries.

The Radford Family Centre

Family centres are designed for parents and children to attend. They provide support for parents, but also education in child care and an important element of 'parenting of the parents'.

The aims of the Radford Family Centre (Polnay 1985)

- to promote practical parenting skills
- to promote better home management
- to promote literacy
- to provide insight for parents into the needs of children, both in family life and in education
- to promote satisfaction for parents in parenting, and enjoyment of their children
- to reduce dependence on agencies for day to day care and acute problems

The centre was staffed by a multidisciplinary team which included a social worker, a nursery teacher, a playgroup leader and a health visitor. Additional help was obtained from adult literacy teachers, a cook (who also taught), a hairdresser and a paediatrician!

Some family centres work with families with severe multiple problems or those where there has been child abuse. For example of 22 parents attending the Radford Family Centre, 14 had literacy problems of which 9 received special education, 13 had court appearances, 11 had been in care as children and 7 had psychiatric problems. Work in the centre included individual reviews and counselling, a daily rota organised for tasks such as washing up and serving food and group work and practical activities including health education, budgeting, literacy, child care, play, family life, bereavement and cooking. The focus of work was on decision making, self help and personal responsibility as well as the acquisition of knowledge and skills. Improvements in self esteem and in self care and appearance were important elements in the functioning of the centre. Results are variable: some children ten years later are in care, but other families are performing much better with no special professional involvement and with their children making normal physical, emotional and developmental progress.

Perry Preschool Programme In the Perry Preschool Program in the USA, children whose mothers had been engaged in an early intervention programme when their children were infants, were found to have better educational attainments, better chances of employment on leaving school and less chance of having been in care or in trouble with the law (Schweindart & Weihart

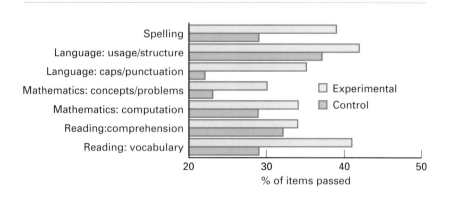

1980). The crucial features were an early start and parental involvement. It involved weekly home visits and a daily preschool programme extending over two years. The authors in this study were also able to demonstrate that their programmes were cost effective. They estimated that for each $1000 invested in the programme, $4130 would be returned to society because of the costs that would have been associated with juvenile crime, special education and unemployment. The authors conclude that the child positive attitudes and increased parental aspirations were important factors in the success of the programme.

Cope Street

In the Cope Street centre in Nottingham's inner city referrals are mainly teenage parents (Billingham 1989). The core staff are health based, consisting of a health visitor, a midwife and nursery nurses. The programmes at Cope Street centre around parents defining their own needs and groups and topics chosen by parents are set up. Increasing self-confidence has been an important theme in the work of the centre. The centre staff recognise that parents may learn more from others in the same situation than from traditional teaching by health professionals. They also stress that people learn by doing, hence the practical activities in the centre. Parents are involved in the planning, organisation and evaluation of group sessions. The groups include teenage antenatal, teenage mothers, food, Open University using the Open University Courses for parents, craft, coping with kids and a literacy summer school.

The approach of Cope Street has been most successful. Examples of achievements have been all the members of the Open University group going onto College; the teenage mothers' group giving talks in local secondary schools and featuring on a local radio programme; the food group producing their own cookery book; groups addressing meetings of health visitors and midwives; and the coping with kids group continuing to meet in each other's houses after the group at the centre had finished.

Cope Street and other similar centres break away from the mould of conventional health service provision. They provide a much more intensive service than is available from routine programmes and a message and medium which is acceptable to their target group. Short term follow up has suggested that the programmes can not only impart knowledge and skills, but also overcome the consequences of the teenagers' own deprived childhoods, their own emotional needs and the difficulty of combining adolescence with parenthood.

Bristol Programme

The Child Development Programme has been developed by the Early Childhood Development Unit at the University of Bristol (Barker). This is a structured programme carried out by specially trained health visitors. It is focused on first time parents usually during the antenatal period and the first eight months of life, but can be extended up to the age of three years. The parents receive more frequent home visits and the health visitor uses attractive cartoon style materials that encourage parents to develop their own skills rather than be passive receptacles for advice.

Important issues covered are early health, nutrition, language, socialisation, early education and parent's own health and self-esteem. The programme includes a system for monitoring of results.

The programme claims increased parental self-esteem, improved diet and immunisation rates, reduced hospitalisation of children and greater job satisfaction for health visitors. More research is needed to confirm these results and to see how much these improvements are due to more health visiting, the success of the programme or the selection of the health visitors who carry it out.

Language schemes

Language delay is a common finding among children in disadvantaged families. For this reason language programmes have been developed to prevent language delay or to manage children from these groups who are already delayed. Bath (1981), developed the use of language programmes in day nurseries by nursery nurses. She used programmes developed along the lines of the Wolfson Developmental Language Programme (Cooper et al 1978). This follows a sequence through attention control, through comprehension and symbolic understanding to expression. Assessment preceded enrolment on the programme and careful records were kept on each child. Results show rapid progress in the majority of children and maintenance of a normal rate of language development one year after their involvement in the programme ended.

The Burnley, Pendle and Rossendale Language programme was developed in 1983 by the speech therapy department of Burnley, Pendle and Rossendale Health Authority. It is designed for use with groups of children in day nurseries and comprises five daily topics covering eight weeks. The programme is prepared on two levels to meet individual abilities. It is designed for children who are linguistically deprived, rather than those who have specific language problems. Examples of the topics covered are: name and use of common objects; listening and attention (sound sequences, rhythm, stories); classification, (identifying like or related objects eg cups, spoons, books on shelf, coats on hooks, bricks by colour); action day (demonstrate use of objects, identify objects by mime); positioning (understanding use of 'on', 'under', 'in' etc); size and shape; and sequencing (eg putting objects in requested order). This programme is now used throughout the day nurseries in Nottingham.

Portage

The Portage scheme was developed in Portage, Wisconsin as a home based scheme to help the development of pre-school children with moderate learning difficulties (Cameron 1982). It is very widely used in the UK and other countries. A trained portage worker visits the family for about an hour a week. A developmental check list covering social, language, cognitive, self-help and motor skills is then filled out by the parent and portage worker. Targets are then chosen and broken down into stages with a series of activities that can be completed within the week. The portage materials include cards with suggestions for activities that will lead towards the target. The portage worker shows the parent that stage of the programme including important techniques such as reinforcement and will also observe the parent carrying it out. Progress records are kept by the parents so that skill levels before and after teaching are known. The system works well for children whose developmental delay is related to their deprived backgrounds as well as for those with intrinsic causes for their learning difficulties.

Correcting iron deficiency   Intervention programmes may also very successfully target their interventions on important clinical problems. James et al (1989) set up a programme of education and screening to reduce iron deficiency in an inner city general practice. Dietary information was provided antenatally and in the first year of life. An information sheet on foods rich in iron, including those suitable for vegetarians, was given to all mothers. Haemoglobin was measured at the time of MMR immunisation in the second year of life. Iron deficiency in the practice dropped from 25% to 8% following the introduction of the education programme. This study, conducted from general practice, is an instance of the effectiveness of a community based nutrition education programme.

REFERENCES AND FURTHER READING

Aukett A, Parks Y A, Scott P H, Wharton B A 1986 Treatment with iron increases weight gain and psychomotor development. Archives of Disease in Childhood 61: 849–57
Barker D J P, Osmond C 1986 Infant mortality, childhood nutrition and ischaemic heart disease in England and Wales, Lancet ii: 1077–81
Barker W Child development programme, School of Applied Social Sciences, University of Bristol, Bristol BS8 1HP
Bath D 1981 Developing the speech therapy service in day nurseries: a progress report. British Journal of Disorders in Communication 16: 159–73
Billingham K 1989 45 Cope Street: working in partnership with parents. Health Visitor 62: 156–7
Black D 1980 Inequalities in health: Report of a research working group. DHSS, London
Black J 1990 Child health in a multicultural society. British Medical Journal Books, London
Blaxter M 1981 The health of the children. A review of research on the place of health in cycles of disadvantage. SSRC/DHSS Studies in deprivation and disadvantage, vol. 3. Heinemann, London
Browne K, Davies C, Strattan P (eds) 1988 Early prediction and prevention of child abuse. John Wiley , Chichester
Burnley, Pendle and Rossendale Health Authority 1984 Speech therapy language programme
Cameron R J (ed) 1982 Working together: Portage in the UK. National Foundation for Educational Research-Nelson, Windsor
Carter E P, Drew A G, Thomas M E, Mohan J F, Savage M O, Larcher V F 1990 Material deprivation and its association with childhood hospital admission in the East End of London. Maternal and Child Health 15: 183–6
Coleman A 1985 Utopia on trial: vision and reality in planned housing. Hilary Shipman, London
Conway S P, Phillips R R, Panday S 1990 Admission to hospital with gastroenteritis. Archives of Disease in Childhood 65: 579–84
Cooper J, Moodley M, Reynell J 1978 Helping language development. Edward Arnold, Sevenoaks
Crellin E, Pringle M L, West P 1971 Born illegitimate. Social & Educational Implications, National Foundation for Educational Research
Crittenden P 1988 In: Brown K, Davies C, Stratton P (eds) Early prediction and prevention of child abuse. John Wiley, Chichester
Dowdney L, Skuse D, Hepstinstall E, Puckering C, Zur-Szpiro S 1987 Growth retardation and developmental delay amongst inner-city children. Journal of Child Psychiatry and Child Psychology 28: 529–41
Dowling S 1983 Health for a change. Child Poverty Action Group, London

Edwards R 1991 Homeless families, highlight no. 99. National Children's Bureau, London

Grindulis H, Scott P H, Belton N R, Wharton B A 1986 Combined deficiency of iron and vitamin D in Asian toddlers. Archives of Disease in Childhood 61: 843–8

Graham H, Stacey M 1984 Socioeconomic factors related to child health. In: MacFarlane J A (ed) Progress in child health, vol. 1. Churchill Livingstone, Edinburgh

Graham P 1988 Social class, social disadvantage and child health. Children & Society 2: 9–19

Grantham-McGregor S M, Powell C A, Walker S P, Himes J H 1991 Nutritional supplementation, and mental development of stunted children: the Jamaican study. Lancet 338: 1–5

Henley A 1979 Asian patients at home and at hospital. King's Fund, London

Idjradinata P, Pollitt E 1993 Reversal of developmental delays in iron-deficient children treated with iron. Lancet 341: 1–4

James J, Lawson P, Male P, Oakhill A 1989 Preventing iron deficiency in preschool children by implementing an educational and screening programme in an inner city practice. British Medical Journal 299: 838–40

Jarman B 1983 Identification of under privileged areas. British Medical Journal 286: 1705–9

Lowry S 1991 Housing and health. British Medical Journal Books, London

Marder E, Nicoll A, Polnay L, Shulman C E 1990 Discovering anaemia at child health clinics. Archives of Disease in childhood 65: 892–4

Murphy J F, Jenkins J, Newcombe RG, Sibert J R 1981 Objective birth data and the prediction of child abuse. Archives of Disease in Childhood 56: 295–7

Oberklaid F 1991 The clinical assessment of temperament in infants and young children. Maternal and Child Health 16: 14–7

Osborn A F, Milbank J E 1987 The effect of early education: a report of the Child Health and Education Study. Oxford University Press, Oxford

Osborn A S, Morris A C 1979 The rationale for a composite index of social class and its evolution. British Journal of Sociology 30(i): 39–60

Platt S D, Martin C J, Hunt S M, Lewis S W 1989 Damp housing, mould growth and symptomatic health state. British Medical Journal 298: 1673–8

Pollak M 1979 Nine year olds. MTP Press, Lancaster

Polnay L 1985 A service for problem families. Archives of Disease in Childhood 60: 887–90

Rutter M 1980 The long-term effects of early experience. Developmental Medicine and Child Neurology 22: 800–15

Rutter M, Madge N 1976 Cycles of disadvantage. Heinemann, London

Rutter M, Tizard J, Whitmore K 1970 Education, health and behaviour. Longman, Harlow

Schweindart L J, Weihart D P 1980 Young children grow up. The effects of the Perry pre-school programme on youth through age 15. Monographs of High Scope Educational Research Programme, no 7

Sheppard J 1986 Food facts. London Food Commission, London

Skuse D H 1985 Non-organic failure to thrive: a reappraisal. Archives of Disease in Childhood 60: 173–8

Syla K 1989 Does early intervention work? Archives of Disease in Childhood 64: 1103–4

Tudor Hart 1971 The inverse care law. Lancet i: 405–12

Wedge P, Essen J 1982 Children in adversity. Pan Books, London

Wedge P, Prosser H 1973 Born to fail. Arrow Books, London

Whitehead M 1987 The health divide: inequalities in health in the 1980s. Health Education Authority, London

Wicks M 1989 Family trends, insecurities and social policy. Children and Society 3: 67–80

Wynne J, Hull D 1977 Why are children admitted to hospital. British Medical Journal 2: 1140–2

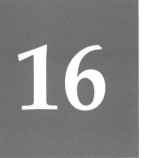

16 Accidents

Dickens' Mr Micawber observed that accidents will occur in the best regulated families. It would have been helpful if he had added that they are less likely to do so in well ordered families in well ordered environments. The elements of a healthy environment include good sources of nutrition, appropriate housing and warmth, clean air, good clothing, safe play spaces, and safe engineering built into the design of homes and their equipment, roads and public buildings. We for our part should learn how to contribute and maintain a safe environment for our children as well as ourselves.

An accident is defined as 'an unpremeditated event resulting in recognisable danger' (World Health Organization 1957, technical report No.118). Accidents are the commonest cause of both morbidity and mortality after the first year of life. In the UK there has been a gradual decrease in the total number of accidents over the past 40 years and the patterns have changed with changing behaviour. For example, in 1971 80 per cent of 7 and 8 year olds were allowed to go to school on their own, but by 1990 this figure has dropped to 9 per cent. Following the introduction of safety measures such as the flame-proofing of fabrics, burns from this cause have decreased.

Fatal accidents 0–15 years (1989)

Road traffic accidents	450
Fire, including smoke suffocation	107
Drowning	81
Choking	36
Falls	36
Mechanical suffocation	26
Poisoning	20
Electrocution	5
Other	45

Accidents in childhood per year

Fatalities	700
Hospital admissions	120 000
A&E attendances	1 320 000

1 in 6 children attended A&E each year
1 in 5 of all admissions are due to accidents

Most injuries are not severe and are thus not reflected in these statistics. The line between the near-miss minor injury and the major injury is very fine. Road Traffic accidents are only 2 per cent of the total of childhood accidents but represent well over 50 per cent of the mortality due to their severity.

Sites of accidents

Roads. Child passenger injuries have fallen since legislation required the use of seatbelts. Head injuries to cyclists are also falling following the introduction of protective head gear. However, there has been an increase in young teenager pedestrian accidents and the phenomenon of 'joy riding' is likely to increase this statistic further.

Road accidents by time of day and year

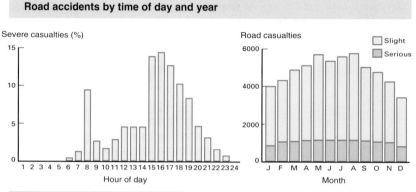

Deaths, E & W (1987)

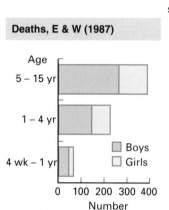

Home accidents. Home accidents are common in the under fives. They resulted in 560 000 injuries in under five year olds in 1989 and 221 fatalities overall. The total number of home injuries for all age groups is in excess of 900 000. These accidents involve particular features of the home and its equipment, for example safety of glass, stairs, window catches and hazards like kettles and saucepans.

Home accidents

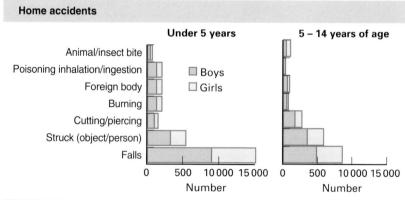

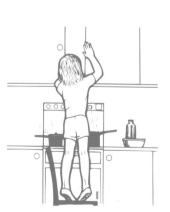

Accidents at school. Nearly 250 000 children were injured in school or college during 1988. About half of these injuries occur in the grounds of the schools rather than in the buildings.

Sports and leisure facilities. Around 150 000 children per year require medical attention because of playground accidents and a further 100 000 injuries in relation to sports facilities. These injuries are much more common amongst children of school age.

Injuries at places of work (railways, construction sites). These are due to child trespass and result every year in 25 major incidents on railway lines and 50 on building sites. They occur both within and without ordinary working hours and sometimes despite fencing and boundary restrictions.

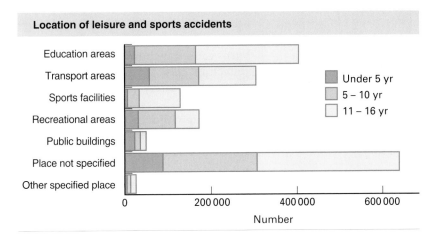

Location of leisure and sports accidents

Farms. In 1989/90 in the UK, 37 children were seriously injured on farms, including 6 fatalities. Some of these have happened when children are helping with farm machinery.

Age of child

The type of accidents that children suffer relates to their level of development in terms of mobility, agility and understanding and their exposure to risks that they are not ready to meet. The drive of children to be independent and explore inevitably involves risk taking.

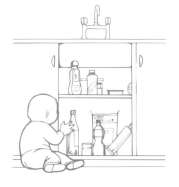

Infants and toddlers. Falls occur from three to four months of age, when infants are able to roll, and increase as locomotor skills increase. The ability of toddlers to navigate often does not match the complexity of the environment about which they must steer themselves. Choking on small objects can occur as manipulative skills develop at around 4–5 months. Plastic bags have caused suffocation. Scalds occur from about 9 months when a child is learning to stand and may reach and grab trailing objects, such as kettle flexes. Once a child is mobile he can crawl to and reach household materials including cleaning agents, medicines and garden chemicals. Drowning becomes a hazard not only in the bath but in paddling pools. Falls from stairs or windows occur from 12 years, poisoning by the ingestion of the enclosed material is a risk. Road accidents increase from 15 months of age as the child can walk independently in public. Parents often *over*-estimate the abilities of their children to cross roads. In one study 50 per cent of mothers of five years old and 19 per cent of mothers of two year olds thought that their children could safely cross a main road by themselves. Eleven to 13 years is the probable age when children have acquired this level of maturity. Cuts and bruises can occur in imitative play as children try to copy adult behaviour.

Pre-school children. Playground accidents are common, especially falls, but trauma also occurs from unsafe or misused equipment. Two-thirds of drowning accidents in the under fives occur in or around the home, for example in the bath, garden ponds and there is increasing risk with home ownership of swimming pools. 70 per cent of childhood burns occur in those under five although the numbers of these are now decreasing. Injuries arise either from smoke inhalation or from contact burns caused by burning clothing. Accidents related to breaking of architectural glass, for example in patio doors, windows and greenhouses, occur where safety glass is not used in these situations.

School age children (5–11 years). Road accidents become more common and are associated with increased freedom and street play. There are clear peaks in child road accidents according to the hour of day when children are travelling to and from school. Home based accidents are 50 per cent less common than in the under fives. Drowning in pools, rivers or canals occurs as children have wider freedom and less supervision.

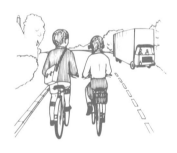

Secondary school age children. Road traffic accidents as pedestrian and cyclist remain common. The 'macho image' resulting in risk taking behaviour can lead to trespass and falls. There is an increasing incidence of sports and leisure injuries and more injuries occur away from the home and in younger age groups.

PROTECTION

The same age groups can be analysed with regard to the adult's understanding of the child's development and curiosity and the need to provide appropriate protection and supervision. As the child gets older, responsibility for this extends beyond the home to other agencies such as schools and local government.

Infants and toddlers. The infant should be protected from falls, for example off beds and from the hazards of suffocation. Burns can be prevented by an appreciation of the temperature of feeds, bath water, or the provision of thermostatic control of the water from the hot tap. Microwave ovens which reheat infant feeds unevenly are an added hazard. Children travelling in cars need to be secured by properly fitted straps. Unintentional injuries can be inflicted by siblings and choking can occur from poor design of equipment, for example cot bars or cords attached to dummies which become entangled around the baby's neck.

Pre-school. The child needs appropriate supervision within and outside the house and a safe environment with appropriate fastening to doors and windows. Secure storage of household cleaning materials and medicines is required.

School age (5–11 years). Opportunities for safety especially with regard to water and road safety are important. Supervision is still necessary and parents often have too high an expectation of a child's abilities. Responsibility outside the house is shared with the education authority and local authority.

Secondary school age. Parents and schools continue to have responsibility but peer group pressure is often in the direction of risk taking rather than safety.

PREVENTION

Accident prevention is a central pillar of our child health surveillance programme. Accident prevention involves the individual, the community, the health authority and local and central government. What is preventable is not just the accident but the subsequent emotional trauma, disability and mortality that results. Approaches to accident prevention include individual education, improvements to the environment to separate children from hazards, and legislation. Although education remains important, evidence supports the effectiveness of legislation and environmental change.

Information

Information on types of accidents – who are involved and where they happen – is necessary in order to implement local initiatives. Accurate information needs to be collected from sources such as the Accident and Emergency Department, Police, and Planning and Transportation Department. It should be collated and distributed to local health professions and to those who have influence upon the design of our road system and housing environment. In Nottingham, a multidisciplinary task force of public health and community paediatrics combined with the local authority Planning and Transportation Department, Accident Prevention Units, Community Nursing and Family Health Service Authority, has proved a highly effective network for ensuring collation of results and the implementation of joint intervention programmes.

Priorities and resources

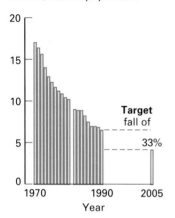

Target fall in accidents

Deaths/100 000 population

Target fall of 33%

1970   1990   2005
Year

Health Authorities need to focus their attention not only on the management of accidents and their consequences, but also upon a programme of accident prevention throughout childhood and adult life. One of the key targets in the Government's White Paper 'Health of the Nation' is to reduce the death rates for accidents among children aged under 15 by at least 33 per cent by the year 2005, that is from 6.5 per 100 000 population in 1990 to no more than 4.5 per 100 000.

Legislation by local and central government can be highly influential in preventing accidents or reducing their severity. Examples may be the use of seat belts, reduction of speed limits to 20 mph in highly populated areas, and safety built into the design of buildings and the workplace.

Accident rates are strongly related to socio-economic class. For parents with limited disposable income, safety measures may be low on their list of priorities. External stresses, parental depression or chronic illness may distract them from the need to identify and act upon risk factors. Prevention strategies have to acknowledge this.

Seasonal factors will influence some types of accident, for example burns, and play locations and their hazards are determined by the time of year. These variations in incidence need to be understood and incorporated into programmes for prevention.

Programmes

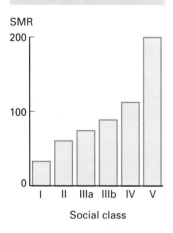

Accidents by social class

SMR

I   II   IIIa   IIIb   IV   V
Social class

Programmes for child accident prevention rest upon a number of interrelated factors. Accident prevention should be part of the training of all doctors and nurses. Programmes should be locally based and rely upon accurate local information and interdisciplinary working. Local initiatives should be based on identified risk factors and risk groups within the community. Combined approaches involving the education and active participation of the public are likely to be most successful. For example in a deprived estate in Broxtowe, Nottingham a 'traffic calming scheme' was introduced. This involved the Health Authority and the Local Authority working together. Initially public attention was drawn to accidents by erecting large black spots on lamp-posts at the site of an accident to a child. Then public meetings were arranged in schools so that the local people could identify the sites and also consider the causes of accidents and they then became involved in setting up a 'traffic calming scheme' to slow traffic in the neighbourhood.

Teaching of first-aid more widely would not prevent accidents but it could save many lives. All parents should know what to do if a baby chokes or if the child is found face down in water but very few do. 'Off the peg' safety teaching material is readily available. Examples are the Royal Society for the Prevention of Accidents Care in the Home materials, the Child Accident Prevention Trust project 'Approaches to local child accident prevention' and the BBC Television 'Play it Safe' series.

The staff of primary health care teams can be very effective in accident prevention. They have a unique knowledge of the home environment and could influence and hopefully sometimes provide resources to implement environmental change within the home. There is the opportunity to reinforce the importance of accident prevention and highlight issues such as the changing risks which relate to different stages of development. The provision of community follow-up after accidents to review safety, alert to other dangers, comfort and reassure is another important function of the primary health care team. Parents may also need counselling because of anxiety and guilt following accidents. Professionals also need to be aware of the possibilities of abuse or neglect when accidents are multiple.

Policy and planning

An effective multidisciplinary accident prevention group must start with a satisfactory database.

The Royal Society for the Prevention of Accidents 'Action for Accidents' suggested the following dataset

1 Age and sex
2 Name, GP and Health Visitor
3 External cause
4 Nature of injury
5 Severity of injury
6 Postcode of patient
7 Postcode of accident venue
8 Length of stay in hospital
9 Number of out-patient attendances

This information must be collated, analysed and disseminated in a readily understood form to field workers and managers. The outcomes that may result from such a process could include an improved basis for targeting prevention and better use of resources; subsequent data collection would indicate the effectiveness of the measures used. Health, Education, Social Services, environment and housing need to be involved collectively in the analysis of data as well as in interdepartmental groups. Written policies, for example with regard to water safety, first aid policy, teaching programmes in schools and child health surveillance programmes are often valuable if they are actively used.

Role of designers

Design has an important contribution to make in terms of safety. Design of materials for use with children, for example cots, prams, highchairs, toys, should take into account safety features. Household utilities, for example plugs, leads, tops of bottles should also incorporate safety features. Fabrics and furnishings can be made of flame proof materials. Housing designs of floors, windows, staircases should be made with the child as well as the adult in mind. Thermostatic control of hot water systems with a suggested maximum water temperature of 54°C would reduce burns. They are recommended but not legally required. Playgrounds can be made safer by better design of apparatus and attention to surfaces which absorb impacts. Public highways should provide appropriate illumination and wherever possible separate the child from the traffic. Siting of housing development and the parks, schools, shopping and leisure facilites should take account of the functional needs of children to travel between them.

Role of legislators

Legislation can be costly and improvements often require coordinated campaigns. These date back to the early days of public health where public campaigns concerning the employment of children and improvements to the safety of their workplace and factories were opposed on the grounds of cost. Successful legislation has led to decreasing car passenger injuries, decrease in burns with the use of flame proof fabrics, decrease in playground injuries and decrease in toxic effects of house fires because of legislation related to foam-filled furniture. Smoke detectors built into a house have saved lives but are not legally required. Safe areas around school entrances and fencing of swimming pools are safety arrangements which could become targets for campaigns.

The role of education

Childhood, by its very nature, is characterised by high levels of physical activity associated with impulsive behaviour, desire to fulfil the needs and curiosity of the moment, with little attention given to the sequelae of the action. Children are encouraged to be curious, to explore, to experiment and normal childhood development whilst providing some barriers and restrictions, should also allow opportunities for independence and experimentation. In such a climate children will be constantly exposed to risk and danger. Reducing the risk by targeting the child is likely to result in minimal success. Targeting the child's environment is likely to be more successful.

A number of studies have been carried out to evaluate the effectiveness of accident prevention education programmes. Such studies have shown an increased awareness, but this has not been associated with a decrease in accidents. The BBC series 'Play it Safe' originally broadcast in 1981 targeted parents and carers of children. The effectiveness of the programme was difficult to evaluate. Sibert found no difference in the incidence of reported childhood fractures. However, Colver in Newcastle found that 60 per cent of the families who were encouraged to watch and were also supported by health visitors reinforcing the education element of the programme, did take some action to improve safety measures in the home. A survey in Birmingham in 1979 following a 'Medicines Amnesty' did not produce any improvement in poisoning incidence.

Education can be targeted on the child whose knowledge may be increased but where we are unlikely to see any change in the normal risk taking behaviour of children and adolescents. Parents and carers may be influenced but the effectiveness of such campaigns will depend upon resources and priorities within the family. The belief that the family is not vulnerable is a strong factor mitigating against taking advice. Traditions such as playing out in the street are not easily changed. Teachers can reinforce the advice to parents and children and schools can be actively involved in campaigns and projects related to their immediate environment.

Role of the A&E dept

The Accident and Emergency Department can operate as a centre for quickly alerting colleagues in the community about individual accidents and clusters of accidents. It can act via Liaison Health Visitors and should communicate directly with Health Visitors about attendances.

HEAD INJURIES

All children by nature of their activity, adventurousness and impulsiveness will at some time hit their head! There is a continuum between minor head injuries and major injuries. Boys are twice as likely as girls to suffer head injuries. One in 20 children per year will have a head injury, equivalent to 600 000 children per annum. 15 per cent of deaths in children between 1 and 15 are due to head injury and 25 per cent of deaths in age 5 to 15 are due to head injury. The vast majority of children who suffer a head injury will have no adverse effects.

Indications for close observation and skull X-ray

- loss of consciousness; development of CNS signs
- fall on to a hard surface for any child under 5 years of age
- fall from a height of 60 cm to the ground.

---

5 per cent of children who have severe head injuries die at the site of the accident. 20 per cent of the survivors of severe injuries have motor difficulties and 10 per cent severe learning difficulties. Sequelae may include short term memory loss, concentration problems, language disorder, personality changes, behavioural and emotional disturbance. Improvement can take place for up to five years following the trauma. The most rapid recovery is within the first nine months.

There is a need for consistency in the management and follow-up of these conditions. It is recommended by the British Paediatric Neurology Association that every child with a head injury requiring admission should be admitted under the care of a specialist team including a paediatrician with access to paediatric rehabilitation staff.

A study in Newcastle of 255 fatal head injuries (Sharples et al 1990) occurring between 1979 and 1986 found that 50 per cent of children were playing at the time of the accident. 76 per cent sustained the injury in a road traffic accident and of these 195 children, 135 were pedestrians. Of these 120 were participating in 'unsafe behaviour' at the time of the accident. Over 60 per cent of the accidents occur between 3 pm and 9 pm and were within 2 km of the child's home. Most accidents occurred amongst children living in deprived areas and the authors concluded that these accidents could be appreciably reduced if children were supervised and protected from traffic during play.

Follow-up

Three per cent of all childhood accidents lead to some permanent or longterm disability, be it emotional, physical or in terms of disfigurement. Follow-up may be required to provide care for the individual and also protection of others in the household from the same or different dangers. The parent held child health record will provide useful information on individual accident attendances providing these are recorded and will give a broad picture of the safety of the whole family. An unacceptably high level of accidents can identify the failure to protect which requires social work intervention.

POLLUTION

> 'If you go to American city,
> You may find it very pretty,
> Just one thing that you must beware,
> Don't drink the water and don't breathe the air'
>
> (Calypso by Tom Lehrer – entitled *Pollution*)

Children need access to clean water, clean air and protection from the unseen hazards of polluting toxic substances, in order to sustain normal growth and development. Whereas many aspects of accident prevention can be placed on parental shoulders, the environmental pollution is outside their control. Contamination of air, soil and water can all be harmful to the child.

Water pollution

Infection. In the United Kingdom the incidence of water borne infection is low. It is however a major source of mortality and morbidity in the Third World. One of the triumphs of the early public health movement was to separate fresh from waste water and strict guidelines for installation exist in order to protect the public.

Lead contamination of water supplies. As old lead water piping is being gradually replaced, the risk of lead contamination is steadily decreasing. European Community Regulations govern the acceptable level of lead in household water supplies. The upper limit allowable is 50 µg/l though levels much lower than this are desirable.

Toxic substances. Water supplies can occasionally be contaminated by accidental or deliberate dumping of toxic material from industrial sites. The effects on the health of humans and the local flora and fauna can be dramatic.

Air pollution

Lead poisoning. Atmospheric lead pollution arises from the use of leaded petrol. There is a possible link between high lead levels from atmospheric pollution and poorer intellectual performance. Results of studies are contradictory and there is not general agreement as to what can be regarded as safe levels for children.

Toxic substances. These include benzine derivatives from diesel engines, sulphur dioxide and nitrous oxide from industrial development. Claims have been made about the possible harmful effects of these substances but further epidemiological research is needed.

Passive smoking. Passive smoking is associated with a much higher incidence and persistence of secretory otitis media and asthma amongst children who live in households where there are smokers.

Soil pollution

Refuse collection. In the UK the local authority is responsible for refuse collection. Refuse bins should be strongly constructed to prevent contamination by rats and other vermin. Refuse is then disposed of by either incineration or tipping. Tipping usually on 'landfills' in quarries is controlled by legislation governing the size of the tip area, depth to which refuse should be covered and the time that household refuse should be left uncovered. The regulations are designed to reduce the risk of contamination by vermin and also fire and explosions.

Industrial waste is causing increasing concern with recognition that legislation regarding its disposal is inadequate. The extent to which toxic materials are being tipped and then leaked into the soil has not been adequately investigated. Additionally there are continuing concerns regarding the disposal of nuclear contaminated material. International as well as national agreements are required on the disposal of hazardous wastes. The child who has pica will be most at risk of soil pollution.

Housing. Throughout this chapter the basic requirements for a safe and healthy home have been stressed, in addition to the requirements for warmth and protection the home gives. Individual housing and housing estates need to be designed with the needs of all age groups in mind. Design features should include safety especially for doors, windows and stairs. A safe playing space protected from the road outside and from hazards within the home is a requirement for every child. Poor housing does not provide these needs and occurs almost exclusively amongst the disadvantaged groups in our population. Indeed part of the numerous definitions of disadvantage include poor housing. Too little indoor space pushes the child outside to play where he is beyond the supervision of parents.

Poor housing also causes psychiatric morbidity particularly depression. Depression may be associated with a lowered level of vigilence in terms of child care. The increased presence of medication provides more opportunities for childhood poisoning. The likelihood of childhood poisoning relates directly to the presence of stress in adults. Highrise flats are associated with increased risk of illness, depression and accidents. Homes with multiple occupancy are also linked with increased fire risk and childhood morbidity from fires. These are also the situations where smoke alarms are less likely to be fitted.

Design of homes and estates should be planned as a dialogue between architects, occupiers and potential occupiers, local authority, education and health to ensure that the fabric of the estate is designed with safety in mind and the estate has the physical resources, shops, health centres, schools, leisure facilities, to meet the needs of the population.

REFERENCES AND FURTHER READING

Armstrong A N, Molyneux E 1992 Glass injuries to children. British Medical Journal 304: 360

Child Accident Prevention Trust 1989 Basic principles of child accident prevention. Child Accident Prevention Trust, London

Child resistant containers now. 1982. Drug and Therapeutics Bulletin 20: 5

Constantinides P 1987 The management response to childhood accidents. Primary Health Care Group. King's Fund, London

Crouchman M 1990 Children with head injuries. British Medical Journal 301: 1289–90

Deddenham A, Newman R J 1991 Restraint of children in cars. British Medical Journal 303: 1283–4

Hall D 1991 Health for all children. Oxford University Press, Oxford

Kemp A, Sibert J 1992 Drowning and near drowning in children in the United Kingdom: lessons for preparation. British Medical Journal 304: 1143–6

Levene S 1991 Coroners records of accidental death. Archives of Disease in Childhood 66: 1239–41

Lindrum J, Mason A R, Sunderland R 1988 Cost to the NHS of accidents to children in the West Midlands. British Medical Journal 296: 611

Lloyd-Thomas A R, Anderson I 1990 ABC of major trauma: Paediatric trauma: a secondary survey. British Medical Journal 301: 433–7

Lowery S 1992 Injuries from domestic glazing. British Medical Journal 304: 332

Mayer H, Adams J, Whitelake J 1990 One false move. A study of children's independent mobility. Policies Study Institute, London

Patterson E D, Chadwick E 1990 The world we live in. Lancet 336:1482–5

Pless I B 1991 Accident prevention. British Medical Journal 303: 462–4

Sharples P M, Stoney A, Aynsley Green A, Eyre J A 1990 Causes of fatal childhood accidents involving head injury in Northern Region 1979–86. British Medical Journal 301: 193–7

Sibert J R 1991 Accidents to children: a doctor's role. Education or environmental change? Archives of Disease in Childhood 66: 890–3

Sibert J R (ed) 1992 Accidents & emergencies in childhood. Royal College of Physicians of London

17 Avoiding Harm: Child Protection

Child prostitution and the use of children for sex has been documented as an accepted and normal practice at various points in written history. In terms of work and punishment too, children had usually been treated very much as powerless small adults. In the seventeenth century, religious and social changes in Europe, paralleling the rise of Protestantism, meant that children began to be seen as innocent, not sharing in original sin, and in need of special treatment, education and protection until adulthood. Incest was made a crime under church law and in the 19th century the Factory Acts and universal primary education were instituted. In 1875 the use of children as chimney sweeps was ended. In 1870 a major issue was baby farming. For a fee, unwanted or illegitimate babies were handed to an adopter who, instead of care, was free to provide a lingering death from neglect, starvation and laudanum. In 1878 Tardieu in Paris described post mortem findings of sexual abuse of children (Tardieu 1878). Incest was dealt with in ecclesiastical courts until it became a criminal offence with the passing of the Punishment of Incest Act in the UK in 1908. Various pieces of legislation followed relating to age and permitted relationships but even amongst experts the sexual abuse of children was thought to be confined to rare acts committed by perverts.

Cruelty to children. As philosophies have changed, fashions in names have changed to reflect the users' new thinking. In 1875, Mary Ellen was brought before the US supreme court wrapped in a horse blanket to test her case under animal protection laws. The adoptive parents were convicted and imprisoned. The ensuing outrage led to the New York Society for the Prevention of Cruelty to Children being formed. The concept of 'cruelty to children' was developed. It embodied the idea of deliberate and sustained mental and physical assault by an evil person, or institution, and the view that the child must be rescued. Ideas quickly crossed the Atlantic and a number of UK SPCCs were founded. The London SPCC, formed in 1884, expanded and adopted the title National Society (PCC) in 1889. One of the NSPCC's greatest triumphs was the passage of the 1889 Prevention of Cruelty to Children Act. Known as *the children's charter*, it allowed for the legal removal of a child to the care of a fit person in proven cases of cruelty. It was the first time the law had intervened in the conduct of parents to children. The NSPCC remains an independent body with statutory legal duties today.

Battered child syndrome was described by Henry Kempe, a paediatrician from Denver Colorado, in 1962 (Kempe et al 1962). It brought new medical knowledge to support previous social proofs of abuse. The concept that severe injury and death could be inflicted within a family with no externally obvious criminality or deviance was shocking and slow to be accepted by many people.

Non accidental injury (NAI) became the medically correct term used by doctors in the UK who now found themselves on the front line of an army previously staffed by police and social workers. Government circulars used the term NAI throughout the 1970s, and in 1974 recommended that each local authority set up an inter-agency committee to agree on procedures and review practice. These were named, interestingly, without any reference to their main agenda, Area Review Committees, or ARCs. Widespread public recognition of the extent of child sexual abuse swept across the USA in 1977 and 1978 and thence to the UK. Here sexual abuse was the province of the police as long as they had evidence, usually through witnesses or police surgeon examination, that a crime had been committed. Action was focused primarily on convicting a criminal and the victim was helped only to that extent.

Child abuse. Sexual abuse and severe neglect only came to acquire mandatory social work action under revised procedures in the 1980s. NAI became an inadequate description and the term child abuse was preferred, as the whole spectrum of abuse, with overlapping categories, became clear. Staff training programmes mushroomed and new jobs such as 'nurse adviser – child abuse' were created in the health service to implement child abuse procedures and work with social services and police.

Child protection. The late 1980s saw an increased emphasis on prevention and early intervention in child abuse. Child abuse was what adults did to children and not a term that described medical, social or police work. Child protection was the new title adopted by the register, the procedures and the nurse advisor. The first set of Department of Health guidelines, *Working Together*, issued following the Butler Schloss enquiry into child abuse in Cleveland in 1988, recommended that ARCs be reconstituted as ACPCs (Area Child Protection Committees).

Organised network abuse. New words for the nineties, though recognised several years earlier in the Netherlands and the USA, are Satanic Abuse and Ritual Abuse. Organised network abuse is the official title recognised in the 1991 second edition of *Working Together*, a document revised as part of the Children Act papers. In the same text the recommendation was made that emotional abuse be added to the list of registrable categories of abuse.

A GLOBAL VIEW OF THE ILL TREATMENT OF CHILDREN

A conference in Berne in 1985 agreed the following definition.

'Child abuse is any intended or unintended act or omission which adversely affects a child's health, physical growth or psychosocial development, whether or not regarded by the child or adult as abusive.'

In the UK as in all industrial countries there has been a huge rise in the numbers of documented cases of child abuse and neglect in the last 20 years (Bankowski & Carballo 1986). In developing countries there has been much less reported abuse, but children's problems have been seen as a symptom of the economic and social state of the country, with widespread malnutrition and up to 20 per cent mortality in the first five years. Even here specific abuse patterns are seen. For example, the practice of child marriage in Bangladesh, child pawning and the use of children as beggars, prostitutes and street hawkers. In Latin America, poverty, urban drift and the abandonment of children has led to vagrant gangs of street children ruled by a brutal subculture of violence. In the Far East a whole industry exists supplying the demands of a paedophile tourist trade (Anon 1987).

War is another great abuser of children through physical injury and death and through the psychological stress of the survivors. Today's war children become tomorrow's militiamen and freedom fighters at very tender ages. Military spending as a priority directly reduces the investment in maternal and child health and education (Woolhandler & Himmelstein 1985).

Origins of UK opinions

In this century opinions about child abuse in the United Kingdom have been shaped by three major forces.

Social and political change. The work of reformers in legislating for improved education, work, social and health conditions. For example Lord Shaftesbury, and Benjamin Waugh, first director of the NSPCC. EPOCH (End Physical Punishment of Children), the campaign to end physical punishment of children, is a modern example.

The women's movement. As women have gained power over their work and home lives they have been able to speak about their childhood experiences of abuse. This has enabled people to look at the lives of today's children in order to identify abuse early and attempt to intervene.

Child abuse enquiries. One after another, starting with Lord Monckton's enquiry into the death of Denis O'Neil in foster care in 1945, these have galvanised public outrage and driven the passage of new legislation. The enquiry into the death of Maria Collwell (HMSO 1974) and into child abuse in Cleveland (HMSO 1988) are mandatory reading for any community paediatrician. Original reports are now hard to get hold of.

The Department of Health has published an excellent digest of twenty enquiries over the decade 1980–1989 (HMSO 1991). Some problems persist in spite of recommendation after recommendation but gradually others improve.

Numbers of children on child protection registers in England (31 March 1990)

	Under 1	1–4	5–9	10–15	16+	Total
Boys	1400	7400	7100	4700	500	21 200
Girls	1300	7000	6900	6400	1100	22 700
Total	2700	14 400	14 000	11 100	1600	43 900
Rates/1000 population						
Boys	4.27	5.77	4.62	2.73	0.75	3.80
Girls	4.15	5.67	4.75	3.90	1.77	4.30
Total	4.21	5.72	4.68	3.30	1.24	4.04

Source: NCH factfile, quoting data from DoH of CP registers

DEFINITIONS

Though books are written to describe the range of abuse, brief definitions are necessary for the purposes of research and communication and the framing of legal and criminal procedures. The following definitions are used for the purpose of the registration of abused children and have recently been updated as part of the 1989 Children Act guidance.

A child or young person. People under 18 years old (previously younger than 17) are now covered by the act unless they are married.

Physical injury. This is: Actual or likely physical injury to a child, or failure to prevent physical injury (or suffering) to a child, including deliberate poisoning, suffocation and Munchausen's syndrome by proxy.

Sexual abuse. This is not defined in the act but the most widely used definition originates again from Henry Kempe:

'The involvement of dependent developmentally immature children and adolescents in sexual activities that they do not fully comprehend, to which they are unable to give informed consent or that violate the social taboos of family roles.'

Neglect. This is: The persistent or severe neglect of a child, or the failure to protect a child from exposure to any kind of danger, including cold or starvation, or extreme failure to carry out important aspects of care, resulting in the significant impairment of the child's health or development, including non-organic failure to thrive.

Emotional abuse. This is: Actual or likely severe adverse effects on the emotional and behavioural development of a child, caused by persistent or severe emotional ill treatment or rejection. All abuse involves some emotional ill treatment. This category should be used where it is the main or sole form of abuse.

The following categories are not defined as part of the 1989 Children Act.

Grave concern. This was a separate and large registration category prior to October 1991. It consisted of children who were considered at risk in the above categories, for example siblings of abused children. Now these children are registered according to the nature of the perceived risk.

Ritualistic abuse. This may be defined as repetitive, bizarre, sexual, physical, and psychological abuse of children that includes supernatural and/or religious activities (Snow & Sorensen 1990). Three forms have been typified (Finkelhor et al 1988).

True cult based, type 1, involves child abuse as an expression of an elaborate belief system.

Pseudo, type 2, has the sexual abuse of children as the primary motivating factor.

Psychopathological, type 3, includes abuse as part of an obsessive or delusional system of an individual or group.

Child sex rings. Organised networks of abusers may not use ritual. A study of 11 such rings (Wild & Wynne 1986) showed that most perpetrators used child ring leaders to recruit victims. Others became a 'family friend' or obtained a position of authority over children. Secrecy was encouraged and bribery, threats and peer pressure used to induce participation in sexual activities. Detection is difficult, and conviction of such a ring, particularly when extra-familial, is often the subject of public approval and much media interest. Many early cases in the USA revolved around children's day care nurseries.

Inter-familial rings, particularly with a ritual element, are even harder to detect and act upon. Several large sex abuse rings alleged in Nottingham, Rochdale and the Orkneys have had such bizarre details as to be beyond general public credibility and understanding. Matters are even worse when agencies cannot agree, and instead of going forward together sharing the difficulties, retreat to opposing professional moral high ground. The police say 'where is the material evidence?' Social services say 'listen to what the children say' (Report of HM Inspectorate of Constabulary and Social Services 1991).

THEORIES OF CAUSATION

Psychopathic

Early research focused on mentally disordered parents as a cause of the problem. Kempe reported only 10% of the parents of abused children as mentally ill, however other personality traits were noted in some abusing parents. These included a distorted perception of their own children, impulsive behaviour which could also be extremely aggressive, depression and preoccupation with self and lack of empathy with the child. Many were also either victims of, or witness to, abuse themselves. Another feature was transference from parent to child. The child was seen as hostile, manipulating or persecuting and as the cause of parental problems and a focus for anger. Other features were low self esteem, isolation and lack of social support and problems of alcohol and drug abuse (Kempe et al 1962).

Social and environmental

These look at external factors causing stress which are clearly not accounted for in the psychopathic model. These are low wages, unemployment, marital breakdown, overcrowding and poor housing. Violence is seen as an adaptation to stress. Extreme violence must be seen against the general background culture. Is violence an expected part of child rearing, either in institutions or in the home? How much of what happens inside the home is open to public interference?

Abusing and neglecting families (after Crittenden)

	Neglecting families	Neglecting and abusing families
Skills	Illiteracy common Depression common Unemployment common	Wider range of skills Unemployment or frequent job changes
Family structure	Young family Partner present 'Empty' relationship	Unstable, partner changes Violent relationships
Parents' childhood	Neglected	Maltreatment
Expectations	Low	Very high or nil 'Just want peace and quiet'
Network support	Poor	Poor relationships Isolated
Parental coping strategies	Withdrawal	Violent outbursts or withdrawal Punishment is an expression of frustration
Children	Passive in infancy Can be very active, when older Developmental delay	Out of control
Prognosis	?Poor Limited skills and 'vision' of change	Variable

Special victim

In contrast, work in the 1970s looked at how much factors in the child might be responsible in making them vulnerable or an attractor of abuse. When abused children were compared with their unharmed siblings they were found to be more likely to have had an abnormal pregnancy, to have experienced neonatal separation and to have suffered illness in the first year of life. Disability has also been associated with increased finding of abuse.

An integrated model of child abuse and neglect

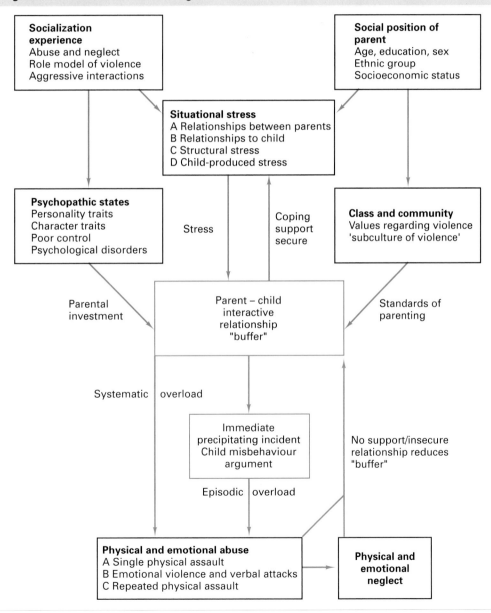

This integrated model assumes that violence in the family is influenced by situational and structural stress but that whether this stress results in violence depends upon a family buffer in the form of the strength of interpersonal relationships within the family. Insecure and anxious relationships will fail to buffer the family during stress and episodic overload may result in a physical or emotional attack. From Browne et al (1988).

Psychosocial

This combines simpler explanations in suggesting that certain stress factors and adverse background influences may serve to predispose individuals to violence which will occur in the presence of precipitating factors such as a child misbehaving. Rather than seeing 'abusers' as distinct from 'non abusers' it is more helpful to think of a continuum of behaviour and outcome.

Model for sexual abuse

Finkelhore (1984) outlined four preconditions:

The perpetrator needs to be motivated to abuse. Motivation may derive from one or more of three distinct sources.

1) *Emotional congruence,* whereby relating sexually to the child satisfies some important emotional need. This may be due to arrested emotional development, or the need to feel powerful and controlling. It may be a re-enactment of childhood trauma or a narcissistic identification with self as a young child.

2) *Sexual arousal,* where the child becomes a potential source of sexual gratification. In an individual perpetrator this may be due to: childhood experiences that were traumatic or strongly conditioning; modelling of sexual interest in children by someone else; misattribution of arousal clues; biological abnormality. On a social and cultural level it may be due to: child pornography; erotic portrayal of children in advertising; the male tendency to sexualise all emotional needs.

3) *Blockage,* where alternative sources of sexual gratification are not available or are less satisfying. This may be true of an individual who: has an Oedipal conflict; has a castration anxiety; fears adult females; has had traumatic sexual experiences with an adult; suffers marital problems; has inadequate social skills. There may be blockage in societies with repressive norms about masturbation and extra-marital sex.

Whatever the motive, he needs to overcome inhibitions within himself. In the individual, inhibitions are lowered by alcohol, psychosis, senility, impulse disorders, and by failure of incest inhibition mechanism in family dynamics. On a social or cultural level inhibitions are weakened by: social toleration of sexual interest in children, weak criminal sanctions against offenders, ideology of patriarchal prerogatives for fathers and by social toleration for deviation committed while intoxicated.

He needs to overcome inhibitors beyond himself. In the individual these environmental protections are lowered when the mother is absent or ill, or the mother is not close to or protective of the child. They are also reduced if the mother is dominated or abused by the father or the family is socially isolated. Other risk factors are: unusual opportunities to be alone with the child, ie babysitting, lack of supervision of the child and unusual sleeping or rooming conditions. At a social and cultural level, environmental protective factors are overcome by: child pornography, male inability to identify with the needs of children, lack of social supports for mothers, barriers to women's equality, erosion of social networks, and the ideology of family sanctity.

He needs to overcome resistance by the child. Though the perpetrator is completely responsible for the abuse there is no doubt that children themselves play an important part in whether or not they are abused. This goes beyond the ability to shout 'no' to an abusive approach. Subtle aspects of behaviour, personality and *front of invulnerability* may cause an abuser to select an alternative victim.

On an individual level a child's resistance is lowered when the child is emotionally insecure or deprived or lacks knowledge about sexual abuse, where there is a situation of unusual trust between perpetrator and child, or there is bribery or coercion.

On a social and cultural level resistance is lowered by the social powerlessness of children and the unavailability of sex education for children.

This model is useful in that it is as applicable to family system models for father-daughter incest, as it is to abuse by the stranger paedophile, or abuse between children. It can also serve as a guide to work with abusive families and individuals, analysing the weak areas and serving as a guide to intervention.

This model assumes a male. About five per cent of perpetrators are female. These divide into those who cooperate with an abusive male partner and those whose behaviour can be framed as above, but with differences. Women have much greater access to children, and because they are usually the protectors, precondition three does not apply. Society has an ambivalent attitude and is less likely to perceive that a woman who seduces a boy might harm him.

RECOGNITION

Acceptance

Recognition first needs an acceptance by society that physical and sexual abuse occurs, and support for the work of professionals who make the diagnosis. Acceptance occurs in stages at different rates in different societies.

Knowledge of risk factors

The following should raise suspicion.

> **Risk factors**
>
> - Injuries in very young children. Immobile children are at the mercy of others. Head injuries in the first year of life should not pass without a thorough checking of the explanation.
> - Explanations for injuries which do not match the appearance of the injury.
> - Multiple types and age of injury.
> - Finding injuries of 'classic' abuse site and character.
> - Delay in presentation of injury. Here the doctor must be realistic about how

> injuries are perceived and the reasons why people take the treatment actions that they do.
> • Things the children themselves may communicate during examination.

Child protection registers All staff need to be alert to children who have already been abused. Their names may be on registers held by social services. When families move to different counties elaborate systems have been set up by health and social services in many areas to pass this information forward. There are systems, manual and computerised, in many A & E departments to tag the hospital records of children on the local register. There may be a time lag in transfer of data and so it depends upon the skill of medical and nursing staff to recognise suspicious circumstances and lift up the phone to check with the register. The register custodians operate a 'call back' system to secure the register against unauthorised enquiries.

CLINICAL FEATURES OF PHYSICAL ABUSE

Torn labial frenulum This can be caused by a blow to the upper lip or by a feeding bottle rammed hard into the mouth. Along with other injuries inside the mouth it can occur after forced penetration with a spoon or penis. However it is also a common accidental injury in children of early walking age who hit their faces when they fall.

Hidden head injuries must be searched for carefully, in the scalp, behind the ears and in the ear canals. A burst ear drum occurs on the side of the head which is struck due to transiently increased pressure. The eyes may have conjunctival bleeding. Retinal haemorrhages may indicate other brain injury such as sub-dural haematomas. The brain may sustain widespread injury from shaking without any external bruising. The term *gently battered child* was coined to describe a presentation with prolonged unexplained lethargy, vomiting or poor feeding. Skull fractures can be present without obvious external injury just as a normal skull x-ray does not exclude brain injury.

Patterns of bruising characteristic of inflicted injury. Bilateral cheek bruises may be due to a facial squeeze. Slap marks show the pattern of four or five stripes of bruising or abrasion in the shape of a hand. Linear grip marks may be found around wrists, shoulders and ankles. Grip on larger body parts such as thorax and pelvis may produce isolated small round marks known as fingertip bruising. Stick and belt marks characteristically leave traintrack marks of parallel lines. Children are hit with all manner of objects which may be usefully compared with the shaped marks they leave. *Petechial haemorrhages* are rashes of tiny discrete bruises which may be found on many body parts after pressure, particularly through clothes. After strangulation they may be found on the face and particularly the eyelids. Here there may also be symmetrical grip marks around the neck.

Ageing of bruises. This is not easy. The bruise is a collection of free blood cells undergoing degradation and resorption with a characteristic haem colour change sequence. Blood may track along tissue planes to show up days later in a different site. For example a blow on the top of the head may show as colour changes under the eyes. The rate of resolution depends on the site and the amount to be resorbed.

A general guideline to bruises

- Initially red or violet.
- Changing to blue purple or black after one to three days.
- Becoming green yellow or brown after three days.
- Yellowing and fading between seven and fourteen days.
- Resolving in two to four weeks.

Easy bruising. Clotting disorders may not show until the child is several months old and should always be excluded in cases of unexplained bruising. Other children who are said to bruise easily prove to be hyperactive or beyond the control of their parents. Still others seem to develop bruising unaccountably more severe than siblings following trivial trauma without any measurable abnormality of blood, skin, blood vessels or connective tissue. Here diagnosis is not usually a problem when site, distribution and explanation for the injury are evaluated.

Lack of bruising. A widespread myth used by those unwilling to accept that parents can severely damage their children is that the absence of bruising means the injury occurred with minimum force, and here a brittle bone hypothesis becomes attractive.

Bruising in black children. At one time the myth that bruising would not be visible in Afrocaribbean or Asian children meant that diagnoses were missed. In fact with skins of varying depths of brown, bruises are quite clear to see in all but the faintest and oldest lesions. Injuries may also be raised, tender or accompanied by breaks in the skin. These children often react to inflammation with a deepening of skin pigmentation which can be quite marked, for example after chicken pox.

Conditions which may be mistaken for child abuse. *Striae* in various parts of the body associated with obesity, adolescence or steroids may resemble stick marks. *Specific ethnic practices* such as hot cupping , coin rubbing and tribal tattooing need understanding in their correct context. *Mongolian blue spots* are patches of blue/black pigmentation classically found on the lumbar and sacral regions of Afrocaribbean children at birth. They continue to be mistaken for the marks of inflicted injury. What is less well known is that the markings can also be found in caucasian children of every skin tone, more commonly in Indian and Pakistani children, less commonly in Mediterranean children. The marks may be on other parts of the body, for example shoulders and hands.

Fractures

These need to be looked for and their interpretation is definitely the realm of the experienced paediatric radiologist. Skull fractures are particularly difficult and words can hardly describe the interdisciplinary chaos when what seemed like a firm diagnosis by one doctor is contradicted by another. The characteristic *bucket handle* and *metaphyseal chip* x-ray appearances are now thought to be due to fractures through the growth plate, the weakest part of a child's bone. Most doctors will agree that spiral fractures of normal long bones result from great violence. The difficulty in interpretation comes in judging whether that explanation, eg a particular description of a fall down stairs, is sufficient. Could such force be reasonably expected from a clumsy father attempting to dress his child in a babygrow two sizes too small?

Conditions that may lead to spontaneous fractures in infancy. The false accusation of abuse in these cases is extremely upsetting for families. A full family history, an examination of sclera and teeth, and review of x-rays should prevent error (Taitz 1991).

Profound prematurity. This is usually babies born weighing less than 1500 g. They are likely to show evidence of rickets and/or osteoporosis on x-ray. There will probably be a raised alkaline phosphatase.

Osteogenesis imperfecta (Paterson & McAllion 1989)

Type 1. This is the commonest form. The sclera are always blue, and in 90% of cases one parent will have blue sclerae and a history of multiple fractures. Some normal infants have blue sclerae, which become white at about one year of age.

Types 2 and 3. These are very severe autosomal recessive conditions with either death or gross deformity in early infancy.

Type 4. This is usually quite severe but with normal sclerae. There is controversy as to whether the condition may occur with normal radiological appearance. Most cases have a family history of multiple fractures, odontogenesis imperfecta and deafness. It is very rare.

Copper deficiency. Fractures have been described only in preterm babies fed copper deficient formula or given parenteral nutrition lacking in copper, or full term infants over five months suffering from severe malabsorption and fed copper deficient diets. It does not occur in normal healthy infants. All affected babies with fractures have had severe haematological abnormalities and radiological evidence of osteopenia.

Burns and scalds

These are common accidents where the precautions which protect children fail. There may be negligence on the part of the carer. More rarely they may be deliberately inflicted, perhaps as a form of punishment. They are found in 10 per cent of physically abused children and 5 per cent of sexually abused children. Of all children presenting at hospital with burns between 1 per cent and 16 per cent receive inflicted injuries; however the differentiation from accidental aetiology is very difficult and abuse certainly goes underrecognised, particularly where the burns unit doctors are not paediatrically trained.

Scalds have a shape which is related to dripping or splashing and are often altered to follow the contours of clothes. They most commonly occur when a toddler pulls a container of hot fluid from a high kitchen surface causing irregular burns on face, arms and upper trunk. Similar patterns can occur if, for example, a cupful of hot tea is thrown over a child. Scalds on the extensor surfaces are more likely to result from abuse. Symmetrical glove and stocking burns are also suspect. One characteristic pattern is the doughnut burn which results from forced immersion of the buttocks in a sink of hot water. Extensive burns occur but spare the centre of the buttocks which is cooled by contact with ceramic.

Dry contact burns cause a well defined mark of uniform depth in the shape of the object that touched the skin.

Cigarette burns produce characteristic superficial elliptical and usually solitary marks when accidental. The marks of inflicted burns are deep circular ulcers and their coincidence with other injuries is quite significant. They are not common and the lesion the doctor is likely to be asked about will usually come from the long differential diagnosis including impetigo, old chicken pox, insect bites, eczema, psoriasis and excoriated spots.

Bites

Produce bruises in the shape of a dental impression which can be forensically useful. An adult can produce quite a small bite by nipping.

Suction bruises (lovebites) may be found in sexually assaulted or physically abused children.

Ligature marks

These must be distinguished from the marks of tight clothing. Finding them around wrists or ankles should arouse worry about children being tied up either as a punishment or a form of confinement or possibly as part of a ritualised abuse. The tying up of children can be controversial. Three examples are a canal family in Yorkshire who came into conflict with social services over their practice of lashing children to the longboat rail; a travelling family who kept their young children on a long leash whilst camped; and a Vietnamese family working in a restaurant found to have tied a child to the foot of the stairs to keep him out of the kitchen.

'Munchausen' by proxy

This is a bizarre psychiatric condition. A parent fakes an illness in a child, for example by spiking urine samples, with blood causing prolonged hospital admissions with all tests negative. The parent may go further by poisoning or suffocating the child to produce episodes of apparent illness such as seizures or apnoeic episodes. The diagnosis can be made by having the child in hospital and excluding the parent or involving the police with video monitoring whilst a suspect carer is with the child. A small number, possibly 2 per cent of children, who die an apparent cot death may have been smothered. Great sensitivity is needed for the implication of this line of thought for the 98 per cent devastated by a cot death. Signs that infanticide should be considered are: previous episodes of unexplained apnoea; an infant over six months old; previous unexplained disorders affecting the child; and other unexplained deaths of children in the same family.

NEGLECT AND EMOTIONAL ABUSE, SIGNS AND CONDITIONS

Frozen watchfulness

This is the apt description of a child who has become emotionally damaged from prolonged abuse. The face is expressionless and the child is motionless and afraid to speak. The eyes are wary that the next adult encounter may be painful. *Radar gaze* describes the searching eyes of a neglected child hungry for any human contact. *Pick me up and cuddle me someone* describes the behaviour of the neglected child who by toddler age has not developed close bonds with family adults and therefore shows no wariness for strangers.

Failure to thrive (FTT)

This implies both a failure to grow and a failure of emotional and developmental progress. There are many medical causes for this but when due to parental neglect and abuse the term *Non Organic Failure To Thrive (NOFTT)* is used. The diagnosis of NOFTT is synonymous in many health visitors' minds with the presence of severe social deprivation.

There has been considerable debate as to whether emotional deprivation in the presence of adequate calories may cause abnormal growth in children under two. The current feeling is that the lack of calories is the cause. The problem is that this is often difficult to prove. Maternal dietary histories are notoriously unreliable and families quickly learn what answers health professionals wish to hear. The food may have been offered as stated but studies have shown that poor weight gain may be associated with a number of poor feeding practices: irregular and unpredictable meal times; very rapid spoon feeding; lack of age appropriate supervision; lack of interpersonal contact during feeding; distraction such as television during feeding; inappropriate seating (Skuse & Wolke 1992).

Hospital in-patient investigation is often arranged to confirm the diagnosis by showing a continued poverty of growth and development in the face of adequate calorie intake. A positive diagnosis of NOFTT may also be made when there is a very rapid weight gain whilst in hospital. Similar catch up of both weight (and height over the longer term) is also seen in children moved away from abuse and neglect into a substitute family environment, for example with relatives or foster parents.

Often FTT is applied loosely to growth measurements alone where use of the term *Failure To Grow* is more accurate. This is understandable as height, weight and head circumference are easy and objective data to gather. In very young infants particularly, weights are the most sensitive indicator of well being and may change quite rapidly.

Certain growth changes should make people consider a risk of FTT: a child falling away from a previously maintained percentile; a child whose weight percentile drops well below its length percentile; any child below the third percentile. Older children may show fall off in linear growth, *deprivation dwarfism*. Because the main growth is in the long bones, such children tend to maintain relatively infantile proportions of trunk to limbs. Wasting of muscles and frequent infections and reduced activity levels are further signs of protein energy malnutrition. In extreme starvation the picture may be of frank marasmus. The weight loss and muscle wasting may be somewhat masked by ascites and peripheral oedema in the child whose diet is protein deficient though adequate in fluid, carbohydrate and fat, for example a diet of sweets, juice, bread, butter, chips and tea. Other features which make this similar to the kwashiorkor of developing countries are thin pale weak hair, iron deficiency anaemia and general apathy.

Deprivation, hands and feet

Cold purple and red swollen extremities are found in children subjected to severe neglect. The cause is not known though it may be a form of disuse atrophy. It improves when the children's needs are met again.

CLINICAL FEATURES OF SEXUAL ABUSE

Normal anatomy

This must be familiar to any doctor attempting to interpret signs of possible abuse. This chapter does not attempt to duplicate the excellent colour atlas illustrations now available (Meadow 1989, Chadwick et al 1989). The paediatrician should take every opportunity to learn by examining normal children when the presenting medical conditions, such as urinary tract infections and perineal irritations, permit. Several general points should be understood.

Anal continence is preserved by the internal sphincter which is under autonomic control, and by the external sphincter which is part of the *levator ani* and under voluntary control.

Hymenal tissue has never been reported as absent in a newborn child (Jenny et al 1987). Hymenal tissue is oestrogen sensitive and has a pale pink convoluted appearance from birth until about the age of two. It then develops a thin red and shiny appearance similar to oral mucosa until the age of nine or ten. With the onset of puberty the epithelium becomes thickened and cornified once more. The tissue sits in a ring or partial septum across the lumen of the vagina. It is posterior to, but sometimes confused with, the exterior fold of skin at the fourchette known as the vestibule. It has many shapes but the most common appearance is a crescentic orifice measuring up to four millimetres transversely in the under fives, increasing gradually up to one centimetre before puberty. The ring is elastic and size alone is not a useful indicator of normality as it varies from moment to moment depending on the relaxation of the perineal muscles and also upon the technique of the examiner. Contrary to popular myth hymenal tissue can heal without scar tissue after being torn, leaving only a changed vascular pattern or a notch.

External injuries

Grip marks on the thighs and pelvis, and bruising or other signs of peri-anal, oral or genital trauma are particularly suspicious. It is said that 10% of physically abused children are also sexually abused.

Anal signs in abuse

Perianal erythema. This may result from the friction of unlubricated or intracrural intercourse but it is non-specific. Commoner causes are: infection with monilia or threadworms or streptococcus, poor hygiene and faecal smearing.

Lichen Sclerosus et Atrophicus is a very rare condition and its silvery friable appearance can be mistaken for trauma in both anus and labia.

The *tyre sign* is a ring of perianal oedema associated with penetrating trauma and said to resolve within 36 hours.

Anal fissures vary from superficial cracks to full thickness tears of the anal verge. The causes are either the passage of a large object in or out as in constipation or abuse, or unusual friability of the anus such as occurs in nappy rash, eczema or lichen sclerosus. Healing is rapid leaving radial scars or in the most severe cases permanent defects in the anal margin. It is very difficult to link findings with causes. The presence of *circumferential perianal bruising* as well as the presence of multiple fresh deep fissures have been well documented following anal rape. In other cases where a description of anal penetration seems undisputable there may be no findings at all.

Perianal venous distension has been reported in many cases of abuse but a causal mechanism is not known. It is not a specific or useful sign.

Anal dilatation is currently felt to be supportive but not diagnostic of anal abuse. The child is examined lying in the left lateral position and the buttocks are gently separated. Dilatation of both sphincters may be present allowing the rectal mucosa to be visible through the anal orifice of one cm or greater. This phenomenon may be seen regularly in children who are about to defaecate or who are chronically constipated or who have sacral neurological abnormality or who are undergoing a general anaesthetic. It is also seen in sick and ventilated children and may be a normal post mortem finding.

Reflex anal dilatation (RAD) refers to the finding that the anus, at first , relaxes and dilates as the examiner waits up to 30 seconds. There have been conflicting opinions as to the cause of this phenomenon. One is that it is a learned response to gluteal traction in a chronically ano-receptive child who can thereby avoid pain during penetration. Another is that it is the result of a traumatised internal sphincter, where continence

Anal signs

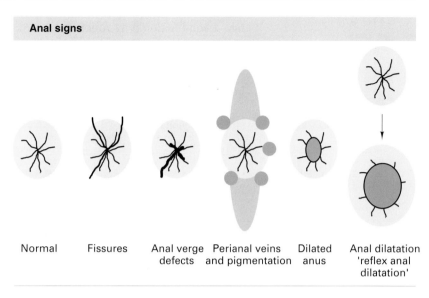

| Normal | Fissures | Anal verge defects | Perianal veins and pigmentation | Dilated anus | Anal dilatation 'reflex anal dilatation' |

is maintained by a deliberate but temporary tightening of the external sphincter. Others have explained it as an unusual but normal finding. It is certainly not a true reflex in the neurological sense. It has clearly been linked with abuse (Hobbs & Wynne 1986) but the exact causal relationships between what the child suffered and what the examiner finds are yet unclear.

Anal funnelling is the finding of external sphincter weakness said to be supportive but not diagnostic of chronic buggery in older children.

Vulval and vaginal signs in abuse

It is usual in the UK to examine the child in a supine, frog-leg position using gentle traction of posterior labia between the thumb and forefingers. Bruising, swelling, erythema, abrasions and tears of the external genitalia and introitus may result from attempted penetration. In addition there may be damage to the fourchette, peri-urethral structures, hymen and vaginal mucosa. Accidental injuries such as the classic straddle fall onto a bicycle or gymnasium cross bar usually cause superficial and anterior damage. Typical findings would be a linear bruise or laceration across the labia and swelling and bruising in the clitoral area. With the specific and rare exceptions of falls onto a sharp object, damage to the hymen and other internal vaginal structures are not accidental. Though children may in experiment or in imitation of abuse insert objects into the vagina they avoid hurting themselves. Masturbation in young girls is common but clitoral stimulation cannot be used to explain abnormality of the hymen.

Diagnostic signs of penetrating trauma are: hymenal tears and deficits and tearing or scarring of the fourchette or vaginal wall. Also longstanding and gradually escalating abuse may produce a one sided or generalised attenuation or absence of the hymenal tissue.

Other significant findings, not in themselves diagnostic, are thickening and various bumps and notches of the hymen, adhesions between hymen and adjacent tissues, and in extreme cases size of hymenal orifice. Labial fusion may follow labial inflammation both from infection and from trauma. Its presence often complicates interpretation.

Penile bruising and laceration may be due to sexual abuse but the distinction from accidental causes may be difficult. Oral injury should be specifically excluded.

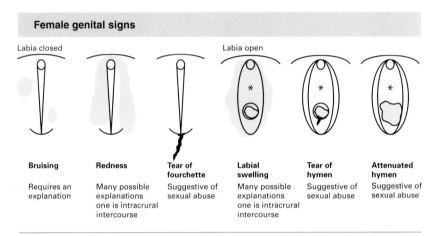

Female genital signs

Labia closed

Bruising	Redness	Tear of fourchette
Requires an explanation	Many possible explanations one is intracrural intercourse	Suggestive of sexual abuse

Labia open

Labial swelling	Tear of hymen	Attenuated hymen
Many possible explanations one is intracrural intercourse	Suggestive of sexual abuse	Suggestive of sexual abuse

Frequencies of signs

These are based on recent Nottingham figures where all sexually abused children are seen and examined by one system and an ascertainment of close to 100% can be assured (Hutchison & Mackay 1992). There were 605 examinations in 3.5 years up to September 1991 and thus the examination rate for sexual abuse is 1 per 1000 population per year. Within this population 74 per cent were female and 26 per cent were male. Only 5.6 per cent had anal signs, and 2.2 per cent had anal dilatation. Of the 436 females 18.3 per cent had vaginal signs. Looking only at the subgroup of these examined children who presented with a strong allegation of penetration, the percentage with positive findings rises to 13 per cent with anal signs, 4.2 per cent with dilatation and 51 per cent females with vaginal signs. Detailed examination of children with strong histories of penetrative abuse yields diagnostic findings in 39 per cent but fails to find significant signs in 61 per cent.

SEXUALLY TRANSMISSIBLE DISEASES

Genital warts

These in adults are caused by human papilloma virus. They are usually sexually transmitted and thus there is serious reason to be concerned about abuse when children develop genital warts. Recent research has shown that transmission in children is more complex than in the adult. Congenital infection is well recognised, and due to the prolonged incubation period may not show until the second year of life. Whole fields of tissue may incorporate virus material by passage through the vagina and only some children go on to present with a ring of warts around the anus, a presentation which could also be interpreted to suggest direct inoculation. Horizontal transmission from a carer's hands and also auto-inoculation from hand to genitals has been documented (Fleming et al 1987). The reported correlation with sexual abuse in children over age two is too high to ignore but not high enough to be useful in its own right. It was hoped that advances in DNA typing might help tracing of route of infection (types one to four are usually found in skin whilst 6,11,16 are typically genital), but this remains a research tool. The diagnosis will depend on the presence of other indicators such as a known offender in the household or other physical or behavioural signs such as a second STD or a direct disclosure of abuse. The possible implications of the diagnosis should be discussed with the family prior to referral for surgical or dermatological treatment.

Neisseria gonorrhoea

Outside living human cells this is a fragile bacterium surviving only in mucus and wet epithelium. Congenital infection is into the conjunctiva of the newborn eye. All other documented infection is by direct sexual inoculation into for example, urethra, cervix, anus or oropharynx. Non-sexual transmission remains a technical possibility but has never been demonstrated in vivo. The incubation period is 3 to 7 days and both adults and children may be asymptomatic. Neonatal eyes apart, gonorrhoea in childhood makes sexual abuse almost certain.

Chlamydia trachomatis

This is an intracellular bacterium that can be acquired congenitally and sexually. It needs special culture techniques and if present over the age of two is likely to be due to abuse, particularly if the alleged abuser is also infected.

Trichomonas vaginalis

This is a unicellular flagellate thriving only in the genital tract of humans. It can be congenitally acquired but does not persist. If found in older children sexual contact is almost certain and in the pre-pubertal child the contact will have been within the previous three weeks because the organism does not survive very long in the alkaline pre-pubertal vagina.

Genital herpes

This may cause vesiculated and ulcerated genital lesions and is likely to be due to sexual contact. DNA typing may help to identify the perpetrator.

Bacterial vaginosis

This is one of the commonest adult infections. It is due to colonisation with a mixture of *Gardnerella vaginalis* and vaginal anaerobes. Sexual abuse should be suspected.

Syphilis

Fortunately syphilis is very rare in pre-pubertal children in the UK and if not congenital should be presumed to be the result of abuse.

HIV

HIV infection in children in the UK to date has been acquired congenitally or by infected blood products, and not from sexual activity.

GOOD MEDICAL PRACTICE GUIDELINES

Clinical standards are accepted parts of a quality service. Good practice in relation to child abuse examination should now be overt. Sometimes guidelines stand alone and sometimes they are wholly or partially imbedded in area procedure manuals.

A version of the following description of a standard paediatric examination has been given to magistrates at their request for use when emergency protection orders are sought. It was agreed by a group of paediatricians in three Nottinghamshire health districts as a *guideline* for good practice, to ensure that all reasonable indicators of abuse may be noted and may be properly interpreted in the context of the child's general health and circumstances.

The paediatrician's role

A doctor's role in the diagnosis of child abuse entails not only an examination of presenting signs such as bruises, burns and fractures but also the careful consideration of these symptoms in the context of the child's general, physical and emotional condition and his/her social history and circumstances.

The examination

It is therefore essential that a doctor conducts a comprehensive examination with as full knowledge as possible of the child's personal and family circumstances. It follows that it is not appropriate for a doctor to perform a limited examination in restricted conditions without access to clinical and social information. (This particularly relates to requests that doctors assess suspected abuse in a child's home – see procedures.)

Consent

When legal caretakers present a child to be seen by a doctor, there is implied consent that the doctor will examine as much of the child as is felt necessary. Failure to do so may be regarded as negligent. It is the custom of paediatricians to carry out a full examination of the child. It is also customary to seek the consent of the child if of a maturity to understand the reasons for the examination. Parental consent is not necessary under an emergency protection order. Furthermore examinations not specifically ordered by the Court may not be admissible in evidence. A Court Order does not allow a doctor to proceed against the informed wishes of a child who does not consent. The rules of consent may be altered in the case of a medical emergency.

INTERVENTIONS

Positively no smacking. Most parents in Britain were smacked as children (Newson & Newson 1989). Many continue as they were taught but increasing numbers in all parts of society choose not to. There is a growing pressure for legal change in the UK to make the physical punishment of children a civil offence (Cook et al 1991). This was done in state schools in 1987.

The arguments against smacking children are:

- That children are entitled to the same rights as all other members of society; the freedom from assault. This includes emotional assault.
- Even mild physical punishment may be dangerous.
- Physical punishment is an ineffective form of discipline and often escalates. It is on a continuum with physical child abuse.
- Interpersonal violence breeds violent attitudes and behaviour.
- Alternative forms of control and discipline improve the self esteem of both parents and children.

Practical ideas to avoid smacking are available from many sources (eg EPOCH address in Appendix B). Paediatricians need to review their own attitudes as health visitors are doing. To help all parents to move their relationships with their children onto a non violent footing is also to support families who abuse.

Voluntary and self help groups. These provide essential resources which cannot and perhaps should not be provided by the statutory agencies who provide the legal and professional general framework for child protection. Most districts will have a *Rape crisis centre* and one or more *Abuse survivors groups*. These can provide confidential help by people who have had similar experience. *Homestart* works directly with families having difficulties in parenting. *Childline (0800 1111)* is a confidential free telephone counselling service started in October 1986 for those worried about abuse. By 1988 the London desk had helped over 43 000 children and was receiving 8000 calls a day. It has now set up regional lines to cope with the demand. There are many others and a local directory of voluntary groups is as useful to a community paediatrician as a stethoscope.

An example of hospital and community medical staff procedures

Hospital and community medical staff working within the health authority for the protection of children must be committed to full co-operation in working together with other Agencies. Every attempt should be made to:
1) Accommodate the child's wishes in relation to the gender of the examining doctor wherever the service allows.
2) Meet the needs of the child and the family in providing a worker of the same race/culture and in terms of communication, a person who speaks the first language of the family.
3) Have sensitivity to any special needs of the child, e.g. learning or physical difficulties.

Physical abuse

Where there is any suspicion that a child has suffered physical abuse, the child should be referred immediately for the specialist opinion of a paediatrician.

Where the paediatrician's conclusion is that there has been physical abuse or the child is at risk of abuse:
1) The duty officer for the social service department in the area where the child resides, or hospital social worker, should be informed immediately (Out of office hours ring emergency duty team).
2) The parents must be kept informed of the proceedings being undertaken in the interests of the child.
3) In the hospital units, in the unlikely event of the child being removed against advice whilst waiting to be seen, and before a paediatrician has seen the child, the matter should be discussed by telephone with the paediatrician who will decide if it should be referred immediately to the duty social worker in the area where the child resides, or hospital social worker. (Out of office hours ring emergency duty team.) The senior nurse on call should be informed.
4) The paediatrician should be available to present medial evidence in court after 72 hours should an emergency protection order be sought or challenged.

Where sexual abuse is suspected

Either as a result of the child physical abuse examination or as a result of an examination for some other purpose or for other reasons such as a child's behaviour or symptoms: the social services department should be contacted as above. The circumstances, such as the child being in A&E, or the police holding a suspect may make the medical examination urgent and precede joint interviews.

If there is uncertainty as to whether particular behaviour or appearance relates to sexual abuse refer to a paediatrician. Where there is a clear allegation or disclosure of Child Sexual Abuse:

1) Accurate recordings should be made of the account of the allegation or disclosure and by whom and any comment offered by the child, or the account of any other concerns.
2) The child's demeanour should be noted, but the child should not be exposed to direct questioning regarding the allegation.
3) The social services department should be contacted.
   Sexual abuse procedures differ from physical abuse procedures and consist of:
a) A joint initial assessment interview by police and social services in order to prevent the child from being exposed to repeated interviews.
b) A medical examination where appropriate.
c) The subsequent calling of a Child Protection Case Conference

Neglect and emotional abuse
Where there is concern about adequacy or appropriateness of parenting

1) The Doctor should obtain further relevant information from: nursing colleagues from within the department; health visitor, school nurse, general practitioner in the community; hospital paediatrican, accident and emergency department, and should re-assess the initial concern in the light of any information received.
2) If the concern remains apparent the information should be pased to the Duty Social Worker in the area where the child resides, or Hospital Social Worker. The Emergency Duty Team may need to be informed if the situation becomes urgent.
3) Accurate notes should be made of all concerns in the child's medical records, including interpretation of weight, growth and development charts, good quality photographs should be obtained, if appropriate.

Case conference
Wherever possible doctors involved in seeing the child should attend the Child Protection Case Conference. A written report should be prepared and sent to Social Services regarding any incident and relevant aspects of his/her knowledge of the child and family.

Case reviews
Whenever a case involves an incident leading to the death of a child where child abuse is confirmed or suspected, or a child protection issue likely to be of major public concern arises, there will be an individual review by each agency and a composite review by the Area Child Protection Committee. Medical staff involved in such cases must co-operate with a Health Authority Review and with any Inter-Agency Review required by the Area Child Protection Committee.

History and circumstances
History of family.
Place in family tree.
Composition of household.
Other professionals involved with the children.
Family medical conditions.
Family accommodations and suppports.
School circumstances.
History of child (best from someone who knows the child well).
Age, medical and developmental history.
Significant life events.
Previous injuries/hospital admissions.
General health, recent symptoms or illness, medicines.
Is child on child protection register?
Have there been other register enquiries about the child?
Circumstances.
Adequacy and completeness of explanation for injuries or assault.
Any delay in seeking medical help.
Changing explanations or different explanations from different people.
Recurring injuries in child or sibling.
Injuries that could not have occurred simultaneously.

Standard examination will normally include:
Examination of the whole child with comments on:
General appearance, cleanliness, state of clothes.
Length/height, head circumstance and weight plotted on percentile charts with previous measurements, if known.
Interactions with parents and staff.

General emotional state and development.
In particular, scalp and hair where injuries may be hidden.
Behind ears, ear canals and drums.
Eyes for conjunctival haemorrhage and ophthalmoscopic search for retinal haemorrhage.
Mouth, particularly for gum or tooth damage, torn frenulum.
Face and neck for fine bruises.
Ribs for bruising, swelling, tenderness of fractures.
Arms and legs for grip marks, ligature marks. Palms and soles.
Abdomen for bruises or internal damage.
Genitalia inspection of penis, scrotum, anus, vulva, urethra and hymen.
Document the child's injuries in precise detail: length, widths, positions, colour, definition, character, age. Use diagrams, plus photographs of injuries where possible.
Arrange for any X-rays or blood clotting tests that are necessary.
Contemporaneous legible hand written notes with date and signature. Summary and conclusions that agree with verbal reports.
Typed or hand written report for social services within 72 working hours.

Where sexual abuse is suspected:
The medical examination is often done jointly by a paediatrician and police surgeon where staffing permits, so that any forensic evidence can be preserved and repeat examinations avoided. However the essential feature is that the doctor performing the examination should have experience and training in the examination of sexually abused children.
A complete examination will be done as described in the physical abuse section with the difference that the child will not usually be asked to repeat the story of abuse if this information has already been gathered in police and social work interviews.

In addition:
1) The examination of the genitalia and anus will be undertaken in more detail.
2) Swabs may be taken to check for infection.
3) Forensic samples may be taken.
4) Instruments are only occasionally needed to inspect beyond the anus or hymen. This might occur in a post-pubertal child. A pre-pubertal child needing internal examination (eg after injury or rape) may necessitate special arrangements for a general anaesthetic.

Time-scales. Once physical abuse is recognised all agencies may need to make swift decisions. The police may need to secure evidence and consider whether there are grounds for arrest or criminal prosecution. They may be particularly short of time if they have a suspect in custody and need to either press charges or release him. Social services equally may need to take immediate steps to ensure the safety of the child with the backing of criminal and civil law if the family is felt to be unable to protect its children. Health services need to provide authoritative interpretation of any measurable harm the child has suffered and institute necessary treatment. Health and social services and police must work cooperatively, passing on necessary information and not hindering each other's task.

There may be need for swift action in sexual abuse, but often a more measured action is best. It may be the role of the doctor to insist that immediate physical examination is not appropriate.

The time-scales in cases of neglect are inevitably long and often the situations are so chronic that it is hard to be clear when an intervention should happen. Frequently an otherwise small physical injury or a new suspicion of sexual abuse will be the trigger for interventions in what are essentially neglected children.

Legal status of the child

The legal framework for child protection with its various court orders is outlined in chapter 7. If the child is the subject of a court order this should be clearly recorded on the child's medical record. Any contact arrangement ordered by the court must be co-ordinated and supervised by the designated social worker. The child must not be discharged from hospital without the agreement of the social worker. If there is a danger that a child, who is the subject of a court order, may be removed, the police should be called immediately and the responsible paediatrician, social worker and hospital manager informed at once.

Case conferences

The case conference is central to child protection procedures. It is not a forum for a formal decision that a person has abused a child: that is a matter for the courts. It brings together the family and the professionals concerned with child protection and provides them with the opportunity to exchange information and plan together.

Initial child protection conferences. These are normally convened by either social services or NSPCC and held within eight working days, but not before all parties have had a chance to complete and write up initial investigation. Reports are essential from any person unable to attend, and even if attending a written report may save misunderstanding or wrong minuting. Conferences are not democratic. The main decision, whether to register the child or not, rests with the social service Chair. When a child is registered a key worker must be appointed and recommendations will be made for work to be carried out by each agency. A date will be decided for a **child protection review** which is the second type of case conference.

Participation in case conferences by parents and young people is required by the 1989 Children Act. Initial professional reaction opposed this and there were a number of worries. These included: inhibiting effect on those attending; problems of confidentiality; conflict of interest between parents and children; the conference as a pseudo court of law; the family not coping with the situation or becoming abusive or emotional; the prejudicing of future legal action.

Following the success of pilot studies (Shemmings 1991) there has been a sea of change in opinion. The crux of the issue is not really what happens on the day of the case conference, but centres on all the work which has to be done before and after it to establish trust and honesty between family and workers. Nothing said at the conference should surprise because it should all have been shared before hand. 'This is what is going to be said, how would you like to reply. Let us write that down'. The conference should be delayed long enough for police to have completed their initial investigations.

The views of the children themselves should be sought and if of a sufficient maturity they should be invited to contribute directly. There are a number of exceptional situations in which one or other member of the family might have to be excluded, for example where the child's welfare is really at stake.

Considerable skills are needed to chair these conferences effectively. There is no point in having 'pre conference conferences' or in inviting parents in for part of the proceedings as all trust will be undermined.

Family members may need to be accompanied by advocates during the conference. Professional workers will have to be clear and honest about what they are saying and be willing to say it to the parents' face.

It remains to be seen whether these changes will swing the pendulum too far in favour of parents and whether in reality social service departments will have enough resources to train staff and do the extra work necessary for the success of this way of working.

Protection Committees Area Child Protection Committees (ACPC) are the inter-agency cooperative forum for developing, monitoring and reviewing child protection policies. ACPC members should be accountable to their own agencies and have sufficient authority to speak on their agency's behalf. Much of the nitty gritty work of the ACPC is delegated to subgroups. These may have specific tasks such as updating of procedures, or specific functions such as the coordination of training. Other subgroups provide inter-agency forums within small geographic areas.

Membership of Child Protection Committees

- Social Services and often NSPCC.
- Management and professional members of the Health Service.
- A GP and manager from Family Health Services Authority.
- A head teacher and education officer.
- Members from police and the probation service.
- Armed services where there is a local base.
- Links with voluntary agencies, religious and cultural interests, housing departments, dentists and social security offices are recommended.
- Local variations such as the inclusion of an academic are common.

Child protection procedures All staff must be familiar with the child protection procedures. These are influenced by government guidelines. They are written locally with general sections and specific staff sections, so contents vary.

DISABILITY AND CHILD ABUSE

Any child whose progress to autonomy is delayed or has to rely upon caretakers becomes more vulnerable to all forms of abuse. Congenital abnormality such as cleft lip increases the risk of assault. In sexual abuse the issue is power and dependency, and the extent of the problem has been hampered by a mistaken belief that the disability might somehow make abuse less attractive to abusers (McCormack 1991).

Muscular problems in cerebral palsy may make feeding extremely difficult. Faced with a child which is failing to grow there is a question of what is good enough parenting when huge demands are placed on the family.

Problems of mobility may prevent escape. Problems of communication may prevent disclosure. Problems of intellect or the fact that the child is subjected to intimate personal care, for example because of chronic constipation, may mean that the child is not aware that abuse is even taking place. The view of the parents of a severely disabled child as 'saints' may hinder recognition. A child with moderate learning difficulties is likely to have the validity of her testimony questioned and disallowed in court.

There are also difficulties around the chronically sick or terminally ill child. It may be very hard for parents to apply normal discipline and so difficult and challenging behaviour may result. The situation may be further complicated by the effects of the illness or the treatment producing bruises or other skin appearances similar to the appearances of abuse.

SEXUAL ABUSE IN ASIAN COMMUNITIES IN THE UK

A general principle is that minority communities must be expected to obey the laws of the country in which they live. However the protection of the child needs to be placed inside the protection of the whole family's standing in the community. Here agencies can create more problems than they solve. For example, to shield the family from stigma the transfer of a child within the extended family may be preferable to a placement in a (usually white) foster home. The practice of co-opting religious or community leaders as intermediaries in child abuse cases should be avoided because of the issues of confidentiality and vested community interests .

On a case level many western *indicators* of possible abuse need to be given different weight. For example the role of an older female child as *little mother* is frequently normal in families with traditionally distinct gender roles. The white model of the incest family where skewed children's roles extend to a sexual role with the father cannot be applied.

The figure of the *collusive mother* needs to be reinterpreted. An Asian mother may be disadvantaged when it comes to disclosure. She may be isolated and have poor English. She may have no experience or confidence in dealing with the welfare bureaucracy. The child who is known to be violated may have no marriage prospects and this stigma may cross several generations.

Poverty also plays a large part. The perpetrator may be a sole breadwinner for a large extended family both in the UK and abroad. It is not so much that the abuse is condoned, just that the whole family is trapped in it.

It is hard to generalise because Asian communities across the UK are quite diverse. The employing of Asian link workers and social workers is in principle good but may cause conflicts if they are drawn from the communities they serve. It is important to recruit and train more Asian foster carers and in some areas family group homes staffed by Asian social workers have been established and are particularly useful for Asian women who need a refuge from domestic violence.

PRACTICE ISSUES

The following themes recur in child death enquiries (HMSO 1991)

1) Poor documentation and communication with the added problem of multiple sets of notes in each health district, none of which has complete information. There is still the bogey of confidentiality. Child protection information is wrongly regarded as too sensitive to be kept with the main record with the result that important information is missing when it would most serve the child.

2) A problem of too much weight being given to doctors, both to their opinions which may be based on little evidence; but also to the value of intermittent medical examination as a method of monitoring child care.

3) The lack of professional support given to doctors in the field who may carry weighty decisions and responsibilities.

REFERENCES AND FURTHER READING

Anon 1987 Ill treatment of children. Leading article. Lancet i: 367
Bankowksi Z, Carballo M (eds) 1986 Battered children – child abuse. WHO and Council for International Organisations of Medical Science, Berne
Browne K, Davies C, Stratton P (eds) 1989 Early prediction and prevention of child abuse. John Wiley, Chichester
Chadwick D L, Berkowitz C D, Kerns D, McCann J, Reinhart M A, Strickland S 1989 Colour atlas of child sexual abuse. Year Book Medical Publishers, Chicago
Cook A, James J, Leach P 1991 Positively no smacking. Health Visitors Association, London
Crittenden P 1988 Family and dyadic patterns of functioning in maltreating families. In: Browne K, Davies C, Stratton P (eds) Early prediction and prevention of child abuse. John Wiley, Chichecter
Finkelhore D 1984 Child sexual abuse, new theory and research. Free Press, New York
Finkelhore D, Williams L, Burns N 1988 Nursery crimes, sexual abuse in day care. Sage, Newbury Park, California
Fleming K, Venning V, Evans M 1987 DNA typing of genital warts and diagnosis of sexual abuse in children. Lancet 2: 454
HMSO Report of committee of enquiry into care and supervision provided in relation to Maria Colwell 1974. HMSO, London
HMSO Report of the inquiry into child abuse in Cleveland 1988. HMSO, London
Her Majesty's Inspectorate of Constabulary and Social Services Inspectorate 1991 Report on Joint Police and Social Services Investigation of Child Sexual Abuse in Nottinghamshire. Home Office and Department of Health, London
HMSO Child abuse, a study of inquiry reports 1980–1989 1991. HMSO, London
Hobbs C J, Wynne J M 1986 Buggery in childhood – a common syndrome of abuse. Lancet 2: 792–6
Hobbs C J, Wynne J M 1993 Child abuse. Clinical Paediatrics. International Practice and Research. Vol 1(1). Balliere Tindall, London
Hutchison T, McKay M 1993 An analysis of child sexual abuse findings in Nottingham. In press

Jenny C, Kuhns M L D, Arakawa F 1987 Hymens in newborn female infants. Pediatrics 80: 399–400

Kempe C H, Silverman F N, Steel B F, Droegmueller W, Silver H K 1962 The battered child syndrome. Journal of the American Medical Association 18: 17–24

McCormack B 1991 Sexual abuse and learning disabilities. British Medical Journal 303: 143

Meadow R (ed) 1989 ABC of child abuse. British Medical Journal, London

Mtezuka M 1989 Towards a better understanding of child sexual abuse among Asian communities. Practice Autumn: 248–60

NCH 1991 The National Children's Home factfile, children in danger. NCH, London

Newson J, Newson E 1989 The extent of physical punishment in the UK. London Approach Ltd

Paterson C R, McAllison S J 1989 Osteogenesis imperfecta in the differential diagnosis of child abuse. British Medical Journal 299: 451

Porter R (ed) 1984 Child sexual abuse within the family. CIBA Foundation. Tavistock Publications, London

Royal College of Physicians 1991 Physical signs of sexual abuse in children. Report of working party. RCP, London

Shemmings D 1991 Family participation in child protection conferences. Report of a pilot project in Lewisham Social Services Department. University of East Anglia

Skuse D, Wolke D 1992 The nature and management of feeding problems and eating disorders in young people. Monographs in clinical paediatrics. Harwood Academic Publications, New York

Snow D, Sorenson T 1990 Ritualistic child abuse in a neighbourhood setting. Journal of Interpersonal Violence 5: 474

Taitz L 1991 Child abuse: some myths and shibboleths. Hospital Update May: 400

Tardieu A 1878 Etude medico-legale sur les attentats au moeurs. Balliere et fils, Paris

Wild N J, Wynne J M 1986 Child sex rings. British Medical Journal 293: 183

Woolhandler S, Himmelstein D U 1985 Militarism and mortality. Lancet i: 1375

Working together under the Children Act 1989, a guide to arrangements for inter-agency co-operation for the protection of children from abuse 1991. HMSO, London

Special Needs

'Special needs' is the term used in the 1981 Education Act to describe those **educational needs** of a child which cannot be met by the ordinary resources of that child's local school. It has become customary to use the term to describe the children themselves, as **'children with special needs'**, and this is useful in that it looks to the child's future progress. The medical label that defines the child's handicapping condition can be a static one and is sometimes unhelpful. Nevertheless the identification of impairment, disability and handicap as defined by the World Health Organization is useful in the description and understanding of the effects of disabling conditions, and recognising the distinction not only assists in the provision of services but may also help both the affected child and the caring family.

An impairment is any loss or abnormality of physiological or anatomical structure.

A disability is any restriction or lack of ability (due to an impairment) in performing an activity in a manner or range considered normal for a human being.

A handicap is a disadvantage for a given individual resulting from a disability or impairment, that limits or prevents the fulfilment of a role that is normal (depending on age, sex, and social and cultural factors) for that individual.

So if someone breaks a leg, they have an impairment. This impairment prevents them from walking and that is their disability. The handicap to them which flows from that disability will depend on what they do, it will be different for a secretary and a professional footballer. The disability and resulting handicap might have been avoided by primary prevention measures. The disability will be modified by treatment or the provision of a supporting cast and a pair of crutches. The handicap will depend very much on the availability of supporting services from family and friends. Thus the disability caused by any impairment, and the handicap resulting from that disability are modified by medical, educational and social interventions.

Prevalence of handicap

It has been estimated that 20% of children will have special educational needs at some stage during their school lives.

Prevalence of handicap (per 1000 children)	
Severe learning difficulties	3
Moderate learning difficulties	20
Physical disability	3
Visual handicap	0.3
Severe hearing loss	1
Moderate hearing loss	2
Autism	0.4

In this chapter we are considering those children with more long lasting and complex needs. It is useful to consider how and when the child who may have special needs is recognised and by whom. Impairment may be recognised in:

The antenatal period by a variety of health professionals.

At birth, when a handicapping syndrome, or CNS abnormality is recognised, or when a baby has such severe and continuing problems that neurological abnormality seems inevitable. These conditions are most frequently recognised by the hospital paediatric staff.

In the first year deafness, motor handicaps, and profound and severe handicap may become apparent. Often it is the parents themselves who first raise the possibility of a problem. A variety of health professionals, family doctor, health visitor, or community paediatrician are likely to be consulted.

In the pre-school years. Moderate or even severe handicap, language disorder, and autism, may not be recognised until the child is in the second or third year or even later. Parents and close family are usually the first to recognise a problem though others like health visitors and experienced nursery staff may be the first to question the child's progress.

Causes of handicap		
Prenatal	Perinatal	Postnatal
Genetic	Effects of prematurity	Infection
Chromosomal	Birth asphyxia	Other severe illness
Single gene	Perinatal infection	Trauma
(Molecular)		
Multifactorial		
Infection		
Rubella		
Toxoplasma		
Cytomegalovirus		
Herpes simplex		
Other infections		
Environmental		
Poisons – drugs, smoking, alcohol		
Malnutrition, social class gradient		

After disasters, for instance head injury, encephalopathy, or other life threatening illness. Parents, and health care staff alike can be slow to recognise permanent impairment after such events.

Children are therefore identified by a combination of child health surveillance, parental suspicion and referral and in response to concerns from other professionals. All three are important.

Reaction to handicap

Whether the news of handicap comes suddenly or after a period of anxiety, no one is really prepared to hear the news that there is something wrong with their child. Parents' dreams are shattered and they find it difficult to make sense of what is happening or to plan the future. Professionals need to understand, not only the classical stages of bereavement reaction, but also the variability of the reaction, from family to family, and from parent to parent, and from day to day and week to week in the same family.

Model reaction to disclosure of handicap		
Parent is told	Manifestations	Needs
Shock phase	Emotional disorganisation, confusion, disbelief	Sympathy and support
Reaction	Sorrow, grief, anxiety, aggression, denial, guilt, defence mechanisms	Listen to parent with sympathy but also honesty
Adaptation	"What can be done?"	Reliable information on medical and educational treatment and future
Orientation	Parents start to plan and organise future	Provide regular help and guidance

The first reaction of numbed shock may last a few moments or for weeks. Many people take in only a tiny proportion of the first disclosure made to them, but others seek out help and information from the beginning. Following this, parents become overwhelmed with feelings of fear and loss, anger and blame for themselves or others. It is not unusual for parents to want physically to get away from the situation, and sometimes from the child. Others avoid thinking and talking about it, arguing it must be a mistake. Many parents describe how they hoped their child would not survive. The feeling that 'This isn't happening' has survival value giving parents space to get thoughts into some sort of order which makes sense to them. Gradually they accept diagnosis and try to work things out. It is at this stage that parents seek more information to help them get things into perspective.

Parents, and other relatives, swing between times of calm when they feel more organised and of intense sadness. Sometimes their strong feelings of protectiveness cause them to over-react to any hint of criticism about the child by others. Parents can also feel very threatened or even revolted by the thought of handicap or disability. Many describe how they feel confused in themselves between loving the child and hating the diagnosis. Their feelings see-saw.

Gradually most families settle down to the reconstruction of their lives, which we call the process of adjustment. They may become keen members of a parents' organisation, or throw themselves into a campaign they see as constructive; on the other hand they may integrate the care of their handicapped child into their ordinary family life, and avoid 'special' facilities as much as possible. This variability of parental feelings emphasises how difficult it can be to give parents the right information at the right time.

However, all studies report that parents do not wish for any delay in being told of the concerns of those attending their child or of what their child's special needs might be. Cunningham et al (1984) showed that a 'model procedure' for giving parents the information that their child has Down's syndrome led to a much greater rate of satisfaction.

When and how to tell parents about their child's problem

- By a consultant paediatrician (if possible with the health visitor who is to be involved in early intervention present)
- As soon as possible after the birth of the baby
- Both parents being told together
- The information given privately, with no nurses or students present
- With the newborn infant present, unless seriously ill
- The information to be given directly, and the parents given time to ask questions
- They are told that the health visitor will see them again soon. The parents are given adequate privacy immediately after the interview.
- 24 hours after disclosure, a further interview is arranged with the consultant paediatrician and the health visitor

---

The situation in which handicap becomes apparent only gradually is more difficult to handle. When do we share our fears with parents? Sometimes in an effort to be kind, we hold back until we are certain of the diagnosis but, again, retrospectively parents tell us that they would far prefer to be involved from the moment that there are any doubts in the doctor's mind.

Management of handicap

The practical ways in which help is provided will differ according to the time at which special needs are recognised, and whether that recognition is gradual or sudden. The role of the community paediatrician in the management of handicap in childhood is not only to be involved in the direct provision of services, but also to plan and develop services, and to be responsible for training. The doctor traditionally finds himself in a central and powerful position in the services for handicapped children; however much of the work is done by other disciplines. To be successful the doctor must understand their contribution to the total management. Paediatricians, in addition to their role in diagnosis,

Services provided by different agencies

Health services:	Education services:
Medical diagnosis and treatment, nursing care, physiotherapy, occupational therapy, speech therapy, parent support, relief care	Preschool home teaching services, educational assessment, nursery schooling Education, whether in mainstream or special schools and colleges
Social services:	**Voluntary bodies:**
Child protection, opportunities for nursery care, relief care, advice about benefits Assessment for services needed after leaving school	Parent support, play facilities, educational opportunities, sitting services

assessment and management, have a duty to provide understanding and continuity of care. The practice of regular review, where a parent may see a different doctor every visit, has little to offer the family or the child with long term special needs.

Multidisciplinary assessment of the child with special needs. District handicap teams and assessment centres have been set up to coordinate services for handicapped children and their families and to provide continuity between assessment and day to day management. Assessment Units or Child Development Centres are usually part of hospitals, led by paediatricians and the referrals come from doctors, so whilst they may be multidisciplinary, they are a Health Provision.

The functions of a district handicap team (Committee on Child Health Services 1976)

1 To provide investigation and assessment of certain individual children with complex disorders and to arrange and co-ordinate their treatment
2 To provide parents, teachers, child care staff and others who may be concerned in their care with the professional advice and support that can guide them in their management of the children
3 To encourage and assist professional field work staff in their management and surveillance of these and other handicapped children locally, by being available for consultation either in the district child development centre or in the local premises
4 To provide primary and supporting specialist services to special schools in the district
5 To be involved with others at district level in epidemiological surveys of need; to monitor the effectiveness of the district service for handicapped children; to present data and suggestions for the development of the service; to maintain the quality of its institutions;
6 To act as the source of information within the district about handicap in children and the services available
7 To organise seminars and courses of training for professional staff working in the district

Source: Fit for the Future, HMSO 1976

The basic staff of the district handicap team as planned by the Court committee consist of a consultant community paediatrician, a nursing officer for handicapped children, a specialist social worker, a principal psychologist and a teacher. In addition there may be a physiotherapist, occupational therapist, speech therapist, and consultant in mental handicap.

In 1984 Bax and Whitmore studied district handicap teams and found that the membership and function of the teams was very varied. Most

Members of district handicap teams	
Community health doctors	100%
Nurses	100%
Psychologists	100%
Social workers	88%
Consultant paediatricians	83%
Speech therapists	64%
Physiotherapists	63%
Occupational therapists	39%
Teachers	38%

teams expected to see children from birth or soon after, but the upper age limit varied from five years to well after school leaving age. Some were concerned with children suffering from asthma and cystic fibrosis as well as more usual diagnoses such as cerebral palsy and developmental delay.

District handicap teams have been set up largely by health services and do not really represent the tripartite service recommended by the Court report. This is understandable insofar as health services play the dominant role for the younger handicapped child, education is involved predominantly with the older child, and social services most important as the child enters adult life.

Full multidisciplinary assessment is a costly process and may take several weeks. It puts a heavy strain on parents and at its conclusion may still not answer all their questions. Assessment usually consists of examination and testing of the child by several members of the team, followed by a case conference, aimed at putting together the information from each discipline, with that of the family to produce a complete picture of the child and make recommendations for future management. The questions that seem to remain unanswered most often are those of aetiology and, in the early stages, prognosis. An in depth understanding of the problems of a handicapped child does not necessarily bring with it any greater chance of improvement. Counselling and parent support are just as important as actions more directly concerned with helping the child.

The educational approach

During the time in which district handicap teams were being established, important developments were taking place in education services for children with special needs. First the 1974 Education Act brought all children into the education system. Previously children with mental handicaps had been considered 'unsuitable for education in school' and provided for either in long stay hospitals, or in Junior Training Centres.

The 1981 Education Act brought in terminology which radically changed the concept of assessment and provision for children with handicaps. The thrust of the Act was towards integration of children into mainstream schools. The Act abolished the categorisation of children according to their main disability, for instance, 'Physically Handicapped', 'Educationally subnormal, severe or moderate' and introduced the concept of a continuum of special needs. Children were no longer to be described in terms of their impairment or disability, but a description was to be given of the facilities needed to teach them.

It was assumed that most children's special needs should be met within the ordinary school, but that some children required additional facilities and resources. Children who were thought likely to have most need for additional provision because of their severe and complex difficulties were to be the subject of a special assessment. At the end of this assessment, the Education Authority might decide to issue a document which is legally binding known as **the statement** of special educational needs.

It became a statutory duty of District Health Authorities to inform the Education Authority of any preschool child who they consider may have special educational needs. It is then the job of the Education Authority to consider whether an assessment should be made. Parents may also ask for an assessment.

Assessment under the Education Act includes asking for reports from the child's nursery or school, from social service departments, and from any other professionals known to be involved with the child and from the parents. This assessment is initiated and coordinated by the Education Authority. It must include a medical report, which is coordinated by the school health service, who are responsible for collecting reports from therapists and collating medical and nursing advice. The provisional statement drafted by the education authority, after it has gathered advice from all sources, together with all the reports must be seen by the parents before it is passed. Parents have a right of appeal if they are not satisfied.

The Local Education Authority makes the decision as to how and where to provide for each child's special needs. No one may preempt this decision, and it is very important for doctors not to say in an unguarded moment 'such and such school would be just right for your child.' This can cause parents unnecessary anxiety when teachers and psychologists suggest other schools. Doctors can however, put forward strongly their views on a child's health needs.

Parents, teachers and others (including paediatricians) hold strong views on the merits of mainstream and of specialised schooling. The main points about either option can be summarised as follows:

Special schools provide

Expert teaching in smaller classes.
Teachers have developed their understanding of handicapping conditions.
Transport to and from school will be provided.
Health service support in the form of medical and nursing care, and help for pupils and staff from therapists.

Mainstream schools

Have comparatively large classes.
May have much or little extra educational and health service support.
Buildings may be poorly adapted.

But they provide:
A local environment.
Normal role models and expectations.
Local contacts for parents.

For the child it is an introduction to the real world at an early age. For parents mainstream schooling forces on them an understanding of the reality of disability and handicap. If their child goes to a special school, mixing only with other disabled children, they may put off for a long time the realisation of how his disability limits the roles he can play, thus masking the true extent of his handicap. For the teachers and children within the school it is a demonstration that people with a disability are actually around in the community.

The 1981 Education Act also provides that the needs of all **statemented pupils** (a clumsy adjective), whether in special or mainstream school, should be reviewed with their parents annually, and that there is a statutory reassessment of all statemented pupils between the ages of 13 years 6 months and 14 years 6 months. The process is similar to that of the original assessment.

Progress towards the integration of pupils into mainstream schools has been uneven in different localities, depending on political will and on the finances available. The 1989 Education Reform Act has provided that all pupils shall have access to the national curriculum, and great efforts have been made to adapt the different strands of the curriculum to pupils' needs. Local management of schools must have an effect on the process of integration of pupils with special needs; just what this will be remains to be seen.

Social services 'needs'

Under the Children Act 1989, social service departments are expected to identify **'children in need'** in their area. Children who are, or may be, disabled are included in the definition of children in need, and departments are expected to keep a register of such children. Social services departments are expected to be aware of other bodies providing services for children in need, and have a duty themselves to provide a range of services.

Services to be provided for disabled children by social service departments

- A named person who is to act as assessment officer, and to be the first contact within the Department.
- Help with day care including day nursery provision.
- Respite care facilities.
- Help in the home.
- Advice about benefits.

This is new legislation whose effect is to give social service departments an increased statutory responsibility for services to children with special needs from an early age. The effects of its provisions are not yet clear, and financial constraints are likely to limit setting up of any new services.

Disabled Person's (Services Consultation and Representation) Act 1986 and the disabled school leaver. Sections 5 and 6 of the Act, relating to assessments for school leavers, were implemented in 1988. These sections lay responsibility on social service departments to assess the needs of disabled school leavers. The purpose of the assessment is 'to ensure a smooth transition, for a disabled child between full time education and adult life'. This fits in well with work which the paediatrician caring for disabled children in the community will be undertaking to attempt to smooth the path from paediatric to adult health services.

The start of the process occurs when the social service department makes a decision as to whether a pupil is disabled. This is usually at the time of the 13+ reassessment, and paediatricians may be asked for health advice in coming to this decision. The definition of disability is the outdated one used in the 1948 National Assistance Act. 'Persons who are blind, deaf, or dumb, or who suffer from mental disorder of any description, and other persons who are substantially or permanently handicapped by illness, injury, or congenital deformity.' Local authorities have added their own guidelines to this definition; most refer to the wishes of the young person and their carers, and to the likelihood that the young person will have a need for locally provided services.

The social service department must make its assessment of needs for statutory services when informed of the young person's school leaving date. They should also give advice about the welfare of the disabled person, and his family, and make referral to other agencies regarding employment, education, health care and benefits.

So far, the sections of the Act requiring local authorities to make provision to meet the needs of these disabled young people have not come into force.

At this time health advice should contain a description of the young person in broad terms including the medical cause of disability if known, together with an account of medical care needed in adult life including important causes of concern. The report should make clear who is to provide health care, whether the family doctor or specialised adult services. The report should also contain the date and result of latest hearing and vision tests, and advice about future surveillance.

Many working parties have been set up to consider the problems of transfer of care from paediatric to adult services. There is no clear agreement about the age of transfer, the best way to approach the transfer, nor the type of service which should be provided for adolescents. Paediatric services for the child with a handicap and their family are best described as holistic, because many paediatricians caring for children with long term conditions are basically general paediatricians who also have a speciality. Adult services are far more specialised, for example, the psychiatrist in mental handicap caring for a person with multiple handicaps, would not expect to be asked to give an opinion about the state of the patient's hips. Children and young people in schools receive much of their treatment in the school setting, and are reviewed regularly by their school doctor. There are corresponding adult services in only a few areas, and opinions differ as to whether adults with handicap should use services different from those available to the general population. Current legislation surrounding community care for people with disabilities may help to bring added urgency to this debate.

Voluntary agencies

A number of voluntary agencies are concerned with the welfare of children with special needs and their families. Some are large national agencies with numerous local branches, others are smaller groups concerned with a local issue, or with a single diagnosis. Such bodies are usually readily available for consultation regarding the perceived needs and opinions of parents. Voluntary bodies have an important part to play in the dissemination of information, in parent support, and in the setting up of both local and national services. By their nature they are able to set up innovative services in areas of need, and to adapt themselves to changing situations and changing priorities.

Multiprofessional 'service'   Any account of provision for children with special needs demonstrates the complexity of the services provided. Voluntary agencies, health, education, and social services each provide services, each with a somewhat different agenda. Despite or perhaps because of the bewildering array of professionals involved, some families miss out on services which would have been invaluable to them, while others can barely call their time their own.

A truly multiprofessional service needs to be conceived at three levels: at the political level, where legislation and the organisation of funding should recognise the interaction of statutory services; at the management level, where service heads should sit down together to integrate their policies rather than sending one another ready made policy documents for comment and thirdly at casework level, where the needs and wishes of families should as far as practicable mould the service they receive.

Special needs registers   The Court report recommended that every health district should maintain a register of children with handicap. Previously many areas had run 'Observation' registers of categories of children thought to be at high risk of handicap; these had proved cumbersome and of varying use. There has been no uniform format for what have been called special needs or special conditions registers and districts have developed their own models. Some (Colver & Robinson 1989) have been developed on microcomputer systems, and others (Woodruffe & Abra 1991) linked to District child health systems.

The purposes of registers are:

- To improve and coordinate the care of individual children.
- To facilitate planning of services.
- To provide epidemiological data.

All schemes register those children who have a statement of educational needs, and those with serious handicapping conditions. Difficulties arise in deciding just where to draw a line for children with such conditions as epilepsy (all?, those on medication? those whose fits seriously affect their schooling?), congenital heart disease, or asthma. It is even more difficult to decide inclusive criteria for young preschool children who have developmental delay without reverting to the observation register of former times. Blair (personal communication) suggested those children requiring either (a) above average input from one or more services involved with the professional care of the child, i.e. health, education, social services (excluding cases of child abuse), or (b) prolonged (more than eight months) specialist treatment or supervision, for a defined list of conditions.

Problems of registers

The upkeep of a special needs register is an onerous task, for field workers, clerical staff and for the paediatrician in charge of the register, especially if large amounts of data are entered. Unless a register is seen to be a useful tool staff are unlikely to continue feeding in data, and a downward spiral is established.

It has been suggested that registers should be shared between health, education and social service departments. However there are problems, not only of confidentiality, but also of the rather different requirements of the different professions. Health Authority registers contain many diagnoses irrelevant to educational provision; social service registers of disabled children are to be based on the prediction of 'Substantial and permanent disability' and will exclude many children with medical and educational special needs.

Inputs to special needs register include:

- Registration and demographic data.
- Diagnoses using ICD9, and associated local codes for disability and aids to daily living.
- Listing of health service personnel involved.
- Current educational provision including whether the child is statemented.
- Social Service involvement.

Outputs from a register are:

Regular reports required for the management of children on the register, for example:
- Data sorted by GP or hospital paediatrician to enable joint discussion of cases and coordination of medical care.
- Sorted by school to facilitate school based reviews: by health visitor to help enable both the health visitor and the community paediatrician to target individual children needing help, and to alert the schools of preschool children with special needs.
- Sorted by disability, to help plan adaptations both to homes and schools; by diagnosis, to look at trends over time and over geographical areas.
- For processing of ad hoc enquiries of varying complexity. A researcher may wish to look at the different ages at which a specific condition was diagnosed before carrying out a detailed study about how the diagnosis was made. Educational authorities may wish to enquire how many children in certain schools require extra help with various aspects of daily living.

Resources

The resources that should be provided for children with special needs and their families divide into a series of 'menus':

- people and skills
- places where those skills are delivered
- equipment
- financial help (benefits)

The resources may be needed for medical diagnosis and treatment, education, recreation and family support. The latter two are important for quality of life for the child and his family. The limits of provision are determined by funding (contracts), local policy both within and between agencies, access which may be limited by geography, transport and mobility and of course the wishes of the child and family. The possible combinations of people and places is very large and a district service often develops as a series of best buys rather than an ideal that provides a made to measure service for every child. There are sadly always children for whom the off-the-peg service is not adequate. Under the 1989 Children Act, the local authority now has the duty to identify need and provide services for all children in need, including those with disabilities.

Purchasers

- Health authorities
- GP fund holders
- Local authorities
- Voluntary organisations
- Private individuals

Purchasers must assess need and plan the most effective use of resources. Because children with special needs often require a broad range of services from different purchasers, inter-agency cooperation is essential.

Providers

- Primary health care team
- Community paediatric team
- Child development team
- District handicap team
- District mental handicap team
- Child & family therapy team
- Hospital paediatric & surgical teams
- Clinical genetics team
- Hearing assessment team
- Visual assessment team
- Special education team
- Social work team
- Welfare rights team
- Voluntary organisations

Each team may contain at least five, and many contain more, different professionals with different skills. It is easy to see how coordination is essential and someone, often the community paediatrician, must act as network controller.

Places

- Home
- Assessment centre
- Schools
- Nurseries
- Community clinics
- Hospitals

Equipment

Equipment may be needed in a variety of settings and more than one set may be required, for example at home and at school. Some equipment may be very expensive, e.g. computers, wheelchairs, stairlifts, high tech hearing aids; other aids and appliances, e.g. walking aids and magnifiers are relatively cheap and effective. Funding may be difficult and voluntary bodies and charities often prove useful.

Investigation of children showing delayed development

History

- Family history of learning problems
- Social history
- Developmental history, ? any regression
- Past medical history from birth

Clinical

Look particularly for:
- growth problems (small or disproportionate)
- evidence of neglect, poor nutrition
- dysmorphic features (face, hands, skin)
- cardiac defects
- hepatospelenomegaly

Laboratory tests

Commonly carried out investigations are:
- FBC and ferritin
- Chromosomes
- Creatine phosphokinase
- Thyroid function test
- Urine metabolic screen
  - amino acids
  - mucopolysaccharides
  - organic acids
- Serum amino acids
- Blood calcium
- Blood lead
- Serology for congenital rubella, toxoplasmosis, cytomegalovirus, herpes simplex

Other investigations:
- Skull x-ray
- CT scan
- EEG
- Liver biopsy & enzyme estimations
- WBC enzymes
- Nerve and muscle biopsy
- Nerve conduction studies

REFERENCES AND FURTHER READING

Committee on Child Health Services (Chairman Court D) 1976 Fit for the future. HMSO, London

Colver A F, Robinson A 1989 Establishing a register of children with special needs. Archives of Disease in Childhood 64: 1200–3

Cunningham C C, Morgan P, McGucken R B 1984 Down's syndrome, is dissatisfaction with disclosure of diagnosis inevitable. Developmental Medicine and Child Neurology 26: 33–9

Jones H L 1988 Smith's recognisable patterns of human malformation. W B Saunders, Philadelphia

Stephenson J B P, King M D 1989. Handbook of neurological investigations in children. Wright, London

Woodruffe C, Abra A 1991 A special conditions register. Archives of Disease in Childhood 66: 927–30

World Health Organization 1980 International classification of impairments, disabilities and handicaps. WHO, Geneva

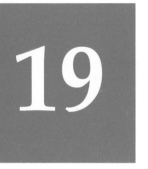

Physical Handicap

Young people with a severe physical handicap will need lifelong involvement with many professional services. As well as this they need continuous support from parents, family, friends and their local community. The transition into adulthood will not be smooth without a considerable amount of motivation and hard work on the part of everyone, not least the young person himself. The aim of management during childhood and adolescence is to produce an adult who can be as physically independent as possible, within the limitations of their disability and who has the emotional independence to enjoy adulthood. They should leave the paediatric services with a full knowledge of their disability. Along with this, they should know what services they should be requesting and how to seek them.

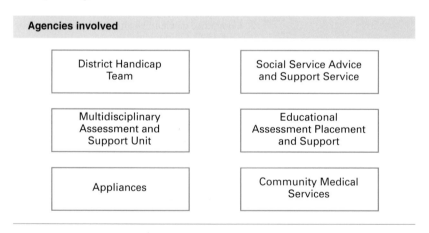

Agencies involved

District Handicap Team	Social Service Advice and Support Service
Multidisciplinary Assessment and Support Unit	Educational Assessment Placement and Support
Appliances	Community Medical Services

There are many causes of physical handicap, but the principles of management are similar. In many children the medical problems are manifest at birth or within the first few months of life, e.g. spina bifida or cerebral palsy, whilst others have an acquired handicap such that the child and family may experience some years of normal life before their problems begin. The acquired handicaps may be static as a result of a traumatic or infective incident like head injury or encephalitis or progressive such as with a neurodegenerative or inflammatory condition, for example Duchenne muscular dystrophy or juvenile arthritis.

Children whose diagnosis has been made during their early life are likely to have a multidisciplinary assessment in the context of their local district handicap team, but for those with acquired problems the services may not be so well organised. The parents of children with cerebral palsy and spina bifida often have intense support and counselling at the time of diagnosis. The infant is too young to be involved in this and without positive efforts to counsel them as they mature, it is easy for them to reach adolescence without knowledge of their condition or involvement in their management decisions.

Children whose diagnoses become manifest during their childhood are more likely to be involved in discussions about their illness from the outset, so hopefully will be better informed and more able to be involved in planning their management from the start.

The emotional aspects of progressive disorders need to be considered not only for the young person but also for their families and carers. Many conditions have a genetic component and more than one member of the family may be deteriorating. The younger children sometimes have to cope with the death of their sibs or peers knowing that their life is following the same downhill path. The community paediatrician may be in a key position to provide the appropriate support, not only after a death has occurred but also in educating staff, so that the dying child is supported by people around them who have been able to come to terms with their deteriorating disease. Parents, siblings, extended family, therapy staff and teachers are usually involved but school transport staff, dinner ladies and teachers of the unhappy brothers and sisters must not be forgotten.

EPIDEMIOLOGY

The prevalence of physical and multiple handicap amongst school children is approximately 10–20 per thousand. Until recently all of these children would attend special schools; now increasingly they are going to their local schools, especially in the primary years. Some of the schools for children with physical handicap will have their roll almost entirely consisting of children with cerebral palsy and neurodegenerative problems and are not at all a reflection of the prevalence of handicap but of the philosophy of their local education department. There are few epidemiological studies looking at the prevalence or changing prevalence of physical handicap in childhood. Hopefully special needs registers will be able to produce this information in the future.

The commoner causes of physical handicap include cerebral palsy at 2.5 per 1000, spina bifida 0.3 per 1000 and muscular dystrophy 0.2 per 1000. The incidence of spina bifida has fallen significantly recently, in part because of an unexplained reduction in natural incidence and in part because of the antenatal screening services. The remainder consists of rare central nervous system and orthopaedic abnormalities.

EDUCATION

It is recommended that wherever possible, handicapped children should be integrated within their local schools. This gives them access to a broader based curriculum and permits social contacts with their able bodied peers. The decision on schooling must depend upon the wishes of the young person and their family, as well as the level of handicap of the child, the learning ability of the child, communication and toileting problems, special resources which are needed, the geographical access to the school building and the attitude of the education authority of the individual school. Work has to be done within the school to ensure that both staff and pupils accept the handicapped child within their peer group. The children who are most likely to succeed in their local school are those who are self motivated, without learning problems, with outgoing personalities and where the school and parents are committed to integration. Difficulties tend to arise with children who have communication and continence problems and those with poor self esteem.

Children in mainstream schools can be deprived of the services, facilities and expertise which special schools have developed, in particular opportunities for regular therapy, independence training, sport and leisure, access to computer hard and software, overcoming perceptual problems and counselling both for themselves and their carers. Some children will have partial integration where special schools liaise with the neighbouring schools so that children can spend time benefiting from each. Successful integration requires staff in many schools acquiring expertise in the management of children with physical handicap and is time consuming for both therapy and support services visiting each school. Unless authorities develop mainstream focus schools for the children with a physical handicap, it is likely that many schools will

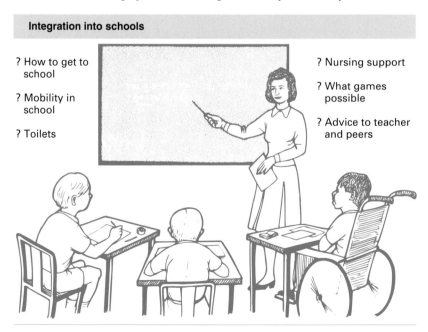

Integration into schools

? How to get to school

? Mobility in school

? Toilets

? Nursing support

? What games possible

? Advice to teacher and peers

have just one such child resulting in feelings of isolation for pupils, parents and staff.

Some schools for children with physical handicap are run on 'conductive education lines' with staff from different disciplines working together within a classroom with equal roles. Conductive education has arisen out of treatment methods used at the Peto Institute in Hungary. Conductors are trained staff who are involved in every aspect of the child's education. They combine the roles of teacher, physiotherapist, speech therapist, occupational therapist and carer. Conductors have a multidisciplinary training and this is being piloted in Britain. Children with spina bifida and cerebral palsy may benefit from this approach, whilst some people feel that it is less suitable for children with neurodegenerative disorders and that the latter may fit less well into their local school for children with physical handicap, if they are using this conductive education approach.

ASSESSMENT AND MANAGEMENT

All children with a physical handicap will need repeated assessment and appraisal of their needs so that a management plan can be initiated. The most important people are the young persons themselves and their parents and family. Many professionals are likely to be involved even if the physical handicap is not complicated by sensory impairment, learning difficulties or other medical problems. It is important that these professionals liaise not only with each other but with the family. A multidisciplinary case review should occur repeatedly and especially at key times such as initial diagnosis, planning for pre-school needs, school entry, transfer to secondary schooling, planning for school leaving and at the time of transfer to higher education, employment or day care.

Review of personnel involved with a child with a physical handicap

Doctors	General Practitioner, Hospital Paediatrician, Community Paediatrician, Specialists
Paramedical Staff	Occupational Therapy, Physiotherapy, Speech Therapy, Health Visitor, School Nurse
Educational	Parent Teacher Counsellor, Educational Psychologist, Peripatetic Teacher for the Visually Impaired
Social	Social Worker, Local Authority OT, Voluntary Society Social Worker, Link Family
Family	Grandparents, Aunts, Uncles, Step Families
Friends	Neighbours, Support Groups, Leisure Clubs

It is useful at review meetings, if everybody can produce current reports so that written plans can be produced for circulation to all those involved. Nowadays, parents are invariably participating in such review meetings and increasingly the young people themselves. The review meetings are best held at the place where the child has most involvement, which may be at the hospital, the child development centre, the nursery, the local health centre or the school. In some areas child development centres and schools for physically handicapped children are working as places of excellence from which the resources, both staffing and equipment, are then disseminated into the community with day-to-day management based within a more personal and local setting.

Role of the community paediatrician. The role of the community paediatrician will vary, depending upon the strengths of the other staff involved in the care of the child. Many would perceive the task as being that of co-ordinating the medical care, identifying and reviewing the child's multiple needs, along with other members of the team. In reality, few teams are fully staffed since the turnover of personnel is high and there are frequent vacant positions. At a medical review, there are three aspects to be considered; identification of personnel involved with the family, consideration of medical needs and review of the child's activities of daily living. The emphasis placed on different aspects will depend upon the work of others within the team. If there is no occupational therapist actively involved then the latter needs to be discussed so that appropriate referral is made.

Involvement of other team members. It is important to identify everybody involved with the family, not only the professionals. In some families, a grandparent may be the key person in the family dynamics whilst in others, lack of family support may be a real problem. Some families will have an abundance of people involved and restricting these to those most essential at one point in time, may make a family feel more in control of their own life, and not 'swamped' by time consuming appointments. Other families may not have been in contact with an important agency and since a maturing child's needs vary, services develop and family needs change, the contacts have to be repeatedly appraised. Parents can obtain considerable support from workers employed by voluntary societies or other families in support groups. They should be welcomed as part of the team sharing information, depending upon the family's wishes.

MEDICAL REVIEW

Mobility

The child's mobility will not only depend upon their functional ability, but also upon the environment in which they are living and the appliances with which they are equipped. The physiotherapist will be promoting motor development as well as encouraging functional development at the same time as trying to prevent deformities. The latter will occur more frequently when there is neuromuscular imbalance.

Hand function

A child's hand function is assessed by an occupational therapist who can help with the provision of appropriate equipment. As a preliminary to this, a child's seating has to be optimal so that they can see and reach and interact with their environment so that play and learning can begin. Older children may need assessment for typing with appropriate keyboards, i.e. key guards or microwriters.

Growth

Many children with a physical handicap will be short. This in itself may be the main functional problem, such as in achondroplasia or osteogenesis imperfecta. The occupational therapist may need to provide suitable equipment for height access. It is equally important to assess the symmetry of growth, muscle imbalance, immobility and unsatisfactory posture which all compound the problems of kyphoscoliosis and hip subluxation. The development of obesity may turn a walking child into a wheelchair child. Transfers will become difficult, skin care will become harder, personal hygiene poorer and self catheterization in those children with a neurogenic bladder may become impossible. Some children, i.e. with cerebral palsy, may have problems with their body awareness and may ignore their ill functioning limbs. Their body image can be distorted along with their ideas of self esteem. Anxieties about puberty and sexuality frequently occur in parents and young people and early open discussion can minimise fears. Advising on methods of menstrual control in girls can often allow anticipated problems to be dispelled.

Vision

The testing of visual acuity can be difficult especially in the young child with a physical handicap who has additional learning or communication problems. Many children with spina bifida and cerebral palsy will have perceptual and visio-spatial problems, some of which only become apparent as the child grows older and can more easily be tested. Awareness of these problems is important but planning ways of overcoming them is very difficult. Some children will have problems with scanning and initiating gaze movements like those with nystagmus or ataxia telangiectasia.

Hearing

As with visual testing, audiometry can be equally difficult in these children. Sensorineural deafness may be present from diagnosis as occurs with cerebral palsy or may develop, for example following mumps. Conductive deafness needs to be managed promptly to maximise the child's sensory input. Balance disorders such as may occur in cerebral palsy can be detrimental to mobility.

Dental care

All children with a physical handicap need regular dental review. Oral hygiene can be poor and regular brushing difficult either by the child or carer. Electric toothbrushes can be very helpful. Fluoride coating and fissure sealing is sometimes advised. Abnormal dentition and malocclusion can occur as part of the primary diagnosis i.e. osteogenesis imperfecta and juvenile arthritis.

Food and oral problems

A balanced diet should be offered to prevent nutritional deficiencies. The appropriate consistency of food is given to ensure the correct amount can be swallowed. A high fibre diet may be needed to overcome problems of constipation which may result from the child's immobility or neuromuscular problems in the bowel. The speech therapist can help with oral desensitization programmes for children with cerebral palsy and can improve upon dribbling. Children with progressive bulbar problems, i.e. progressive spastic paraparesis, can find these aspects of their disease quite distressing.

Medical review of a child with a physical handicap		
Every occasion		Sometimes
Vision	Communication	Immunisations
Hearing	Oral problems	Genetics
Growth	Sleep	
Continence	Behaviour	

Communication

Speech and communication problems can be difficult to assess in the young multiply handicapped child who may also have various general or specific learning problems. Children with progressive bulbar involvement have equally difficult but different problems. The combined assessment by the speech therapist, occupational therapist and teacher is important. Significant communication problems can lead to serious frustration, behaviour problems, social isolation and under estimation of intellectual function. Simultaneous problems with hand function such as in the child with athetoid type cerebral palsy, may mean that a communication signing system like Makaton is inappropriate. A manual board with symbols or words which can be pointed at, may be the most functional form of communication. The board can be personalised for the child and the child's vision and hand control can dictate the picture size.

Portable communication aids with computer links and voice synthesizers are a rapidly improving field. They are either based on pre-recorded speech with limited output or on simulated speech with endless combinations produced. The user needs to be highly motivated in communication, to have adequate manual dexterity and to have receptive listeners.

Continence

The development of a regular bowel regime should be started early. The immobility of a child with a physical handicap may lead to constipation and neuromuscular problems can also impair bowel control. Bulbar involvement may mean a low fibre diet is eaten and this may also increase these difficulties. Bulking agents and bowel stimulants often have to be used together and for emotional reasons, suppositories and enemas should be avoided whenever possible. Urinary continence is often easier to achieve than bowel control. Constipation in itself can often lead to poor bladder function so both aspects have to be investigated together. Children with spina bifida often have urodynamic problems and need a clear regime which is rigidly adhered to. Intermittent catheterization can be commenced with young children and with motivation and support, some can achieve this alone prior to school entry.

Children with a physical handicap may wet because of problems with communicating their toileting needs to their carers or because of delay in physically reaching the toilet. These should to be clearly separated from the problem of lack of sensation or control. Some children wet or soil as part of their behavioural problems, associated with their physical handicap.

Behaviour

Physical handicap can lead to frustration, isolation and unhappiness. The problems can be different for the child with an acquired handicap who has lost his previous skills whilst the child who has never known normality has missed many early experiences and may have been treated as 'being handicapped' all their lives. The children with progressive conditions may see their hard earned skills lost as they deteriorate, in spite of much work to retain their functional abilities. The prospect of early death may also have to be faced, as in the child with progressive muscular dystrophy.

The children's reaction to their physical condition will be coloured by their family's emotions over their disability. A supportive environment with positive encouragement can lead to a healthy emotional development rather than a multiply handicapped child and family.

The daily life of a child with a physical handicap – weekday or weekend

- Routine of waking   : Toileting
                         : Dressing
- Going for breakfast   : Eating
- Other meal times   : Drinking
- Leisure time
- Preparing for bed   : Bath time

Behaviour problems may be compounded by a primary neurological diagnosis, e.g. head injury or encephalopathy. These in turn may be worsened by uncontrolled epilepsy. The side effects of some medication can lead to mood changes, e.g. salbutamol for asthma, indomethacin for arthritis and promethazine for eczema.

Immunisations

Children with a physical handicap should not be denied their protection from infectious diseases without a careful consideration of the risks involved in either giving or withholding immunisations. The problems rarely arise in those with acquired handicap, whilst those older children with cerebral palsy may not have received what younger children are being offered in the light of current recommendations.

Genetics

The need for genetic counselling has to be repeatedly re-assessed. This can be directed to the child with the handicap, the parents or the siblings. A re-appraisal of the diagnosis may mean a genetic cause has become apparent, like progressive spastic paraparesis from a previous diagnosis of cerebral palsy. Change in family circumstances with either parent acquiring a different partner, may mean that the new couple need counselling. Advances in medical knowledge need to be relayed on to families so that they are aware of new antenatal screening tests.

Older children may need the opportunity of discussing their sibling's diagnosis. Many parents find it hard to objectively discuss their child's handicap with their able bodied offspring. The siblings may have distorted views of the genetic implications for themselves, which simple counselling can easily dispel.

Play and leisure

The normal child through play acquires fine motor and gross motor skills and knowledge of the world around. The child learns through imitation and imaginary play, and with other children learns to socialise. Although play is primarily for pleasure, children learn considerably from their experiences. Those with physical handicap should be encouraged to play, not only for the fun but also for the education. Suitable play equipment needs to be provided and many child development centres have Toy Libraries which will lend out not only small items such as posting boxes but also larger equipment.

All children should be encouraged to enjoy leisure activities. These may involve joining local or specialist clubs. Many cub or brownie packs will take children with varying handicaps. Many towns have PHAB Clubs (Physically Handicapped and Able Bodied Clubs) or other youth groups that not only have evening and weekend activities but also organised holidays, whilst some packs are aimed at those with a disability. There are an increasing number of sports groups aimed at the physically disabled such that most activities can be appropriately adapted. These can include swimming, horse riding, wheelchair sports, angling, archery, table tennis and, for the more adventurous, outdoor pursuit centres will teach wheelchair abseilling, yachting and skiing. Involvement in such activities can not only give pleasure, but also a feeling of achievement and increasing self confidence. Many people however do not like joining group activities and individual hobbies should be encouraged. However, it is very easy for a physically handicapped child to be offered the 'company' of a television, video or computer games, without considering that most leisure pursuits can be modified if the interest is there.

EQUIPMENT FOR THE PHYSICALLY HANDICAPPED CHILD

When considering equipment for a child with a physical handicap, the requirements not only of the family, therapists and teachers but also those of the child must be considered. Supplying something which a child does not want is of no value, it will not be used and will be a wasted expense. Some splints, supports and seating can worsen a handicap so that a child's total requirements need to be assessed **before** providing any gadgets. Resource centres increasingly allow equipment to be tried out if not borrowed before a decision is made as to what is best for a child at any one point in time. When equipment is ordered, it should arrive promptly for a child to achieve maximum benefit, as otherwise the needs may be outgrown before it comes. Sadly this is often a frustrating problem and increasingly so as budgets become tight.

Equipment to prevent deformities and allow development

Seating. Correct seating can both open up the handicapped child's world and prevent deformity. For the multiply or physically handicapped child very soft seating is perilous and bean-bags are absolutely contraindicated as they lead to the wind-swept deformity. Seating must be firm and promote an upright posture. Some useful seats are: corner seats, moulded seats, activities tables with inset, saddle seating for adductor spasms, self propelled chairs and Matrix body supports.

Position

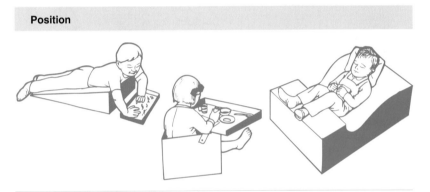

Prolonged sitting keeps a child's hips flexed for too long a period. Some time spent standing is useful and is achievable in all but the most handicapped child by use of a standing frame. It would however be wrong simply to select a chair from the above 'shopping list'.

Each child needs individual assessment by a therapist. When placing a child in a seat his posture must be considered critically, particularly that of the hips and spine. A fixed deformity may need surgical intervention before adequate seating is achievable.

The seated child's feet should be flat to provide security. They are also vulnerable to deformity, especially when the child is beginning to stand. For younger children firm slippers (e.g. Shoos-Shoos) and for the older child Piedro boots are useful.

Splints and supports. Ankle-foot and knee ankle-foot orthoses are useful in holding joints in positions which are not possible naturally due to spasticity or weakness. Although they appear simple in design, their use is a highly specialised subject. Most centres are now using rigid plastic orthoses which are cosmetically much preferable to the older metal braces. Much more straightforward are gaiters which will keep arms, legs or bodies straight; they are especially useful for arms that insist on flexing back towards the child.

Wedges and rolls are excellent in helping the floppy child develop spinal and head control.

Mobility equipment. The handicapped child's world opens up when he becomes mobile. Some useful appliances are: Cell Barnes Walker, crawlers, trundle toys, rollators, prone boards (for very floppy children).

Mobility

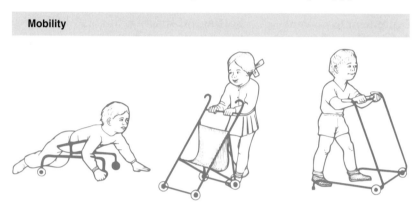

Equipment that help with skills

Wheelchairs. There is no perfect buggy or wheelchair, again individual assessment by a therapist is essential. The advantage for the parent or child is that they get you quickly and efficiently from A to B. Unless, of course, getting from A to B involves climbing into a bus or car. Buggies and wheelchairs are bulky.

Feeding. Dycem mats (sticky mats that stop plates sliding about) are extremely useful. Feeding dishes and beakers have been designed for children with poor motor-skills. 'Prior and Howard' spoons are plastic but malleable such that they will not break even with children who have pronounced bite reflexes. Heated dishes (from Boots and Mothercare) into which hot water is put before feeding are valuable. They are heavy enough not to slide about and keep food warm during long feeding sessions.

Bathing. Bathing the handicapped child always seems perilous but can be helped by different equipment. The Western Medical Bath seat which is like a baby-relax but waterproof and sits in the bathwater, is good for babies. Non-slip bathmats increase safety, as do whole bath inserts which reduce the depth of water so the parents do not have to bend double over the side of the bath. For older children the Safa-bath seat and Suzy-Air chair both fit inside a normal bath.

Toileting. For any success at toileting it is essential that the child feels secure on the toilet. A number of devices are available. For babies there are built-up potties. An older child can use the Watford Potty chair or insert seats into the family toilet. Most mobile physically handicapped children over 5 will need substantial home alterations including a toilet with handrails, and provision for a wheelchair if necessary. Such substantial adaptions need a lot of forward planning with therapists and parents.

How to obtain equipment   When all the relevant parties have decided on the equipment and preferably when a short term loan has demonstrated its usefulness, it then needs to be obtained. Usually the therapists will be known in local channels but they may need medical support for an application. Where to apply and who pays will depend on the equipment, the age of the child and where it is to be used. For the more expensive items a number of options often have to be explored.

Department of Health. The Department has rulings over the substantial items it will and will not supply. Many pieces are in a 'grey' area and it is always worthwhile applying.

Handicap/Rehabilitation Centres often have a certain number of items for loaning out, especially if they have a resource centre.

Social Services Departments will provide many home and personal appliances. Contact the social services department's occupational therapists who also can advise on home alterations.

Local Education Authorities will provide equipment for educational purposes. How broadly this definition is interpreted depends on the authority. Most will allow such aids to go to the home, but often this is not practical, e.g. with bulky wheelchairs.

Local charities if approached will sometimes pay for equipment and will welcome guidance as to what is needed.

Businesses. Some companies will loan out equipment on a short or long-term basis.

Family Fund. When other channels have failed this government financed agency can help out for substantial items.

Manpower Services Commission. This will sometimes provide equipment (e.g. typewriter) if it will enable a person to gain employment. Enquiries should be made to a disablement resettlement officer.

The family. Parents and extended family members can be very resourceful in providing home-made equipment. This is to be encouraged as they know their child's needs best. However, they should not be expected to pay out large amounts as the financial burden of a handicapped child is considerable.

COMMUNICATION

Delay in the development of language and communication skills is a critical problem in the care of the handicapped. Lack of understanding of expressive language raises barriers to further learning with immense frustration for both parents and children.

Language development programmes demand careful observation of the child to record current abilities. This means paying attention not only to comprehension, expression and articulation but also to other more basic skills of symbolic understanding and attention control. From these initial observations an individual language programme can be constructed, based on the child's ability. Each step in the programme is structured so that the progress of the child can be easily monitored. Opportunities to acquire language skills should be available throughout the day as well as concentrated in therapy spells. The use of carefully chosen toys to encourage growth of attention and symbolic understanding is most useful.

Speech therapy

The specialised speech therapist is essential to the team assessment of the child and in directing therapy. They must be involved early and not just as an afterthought because speech has failed to develop. The speech therapist has a number of roles, the first begins very early in the handicapped child's life. In their initial assessment they evaluate tongue, palate and mouth movements and advise over feeding problems. At a slightly later age they can assess the child's inner language, the essential prerequisite to expressive language. They will see what concepts of language have developed and how this development can be enhanced through play. The therapist will not be confined to verbal communication but will concentrate on functional communication by all means so that the child's needs can be met. In the pre-schools years, the therapist works with and through the parents and carers of the child (e.g. nursery nurses in a day nursery). As in physical development, the development of communication may not be automatic. Often a considerable amount of therapy through play is necessary. Hence it is doubly important that parents and carers understand concepts of early language development and enact the development programmes themselves. Once at school the child's communication therapy is again more likely to be directed by the speech therapist via the work of teachers and parents than given directly. The therapist will advise on alternative communication systems. Throughout the child's life the therapist and community paediatrician will check his hearing.

Communication systems

Multiply handicapped children often have considerable communication problems which can result in frustration, social withdrawal and under-estimation of their abilities. Physically handicapped children also can have problems if their speech or hand function is affected. The possibility of using alternative communication may therefore arise. A communication signing-system like Makaton, or communication equipment such as an electric typewriter may be used. Parents are often afraid that using such a device may inhibit normal speech development and as a result they tend to be introduced too late rather than too early. On the whole, alternative systems and equipment encourage rather than inhibit language development. Sometimes they are used at a young age and abandoned later as natural communication takes over. In practice such devices are helpful in a minority of multiply handicapped children only. It is not easy to decide which children will benefit. Three questions should be asked.

What is the child's ability and motivation? The child needs to want to communicate and to have a cognitive ability of at least 12 months, preferably 18 months. Sometimes verbal comprehension is the only means by which one can assess the child's cognition. If the child has severe mental handicap chronological age is rarely important.

How is the child communicating? If the child is already communicating all his needs as much as he apparently wants, a device will not be successful. However, if he is not, the type of communication he and his parents are using will give a clue to what sort of equipment is appropriate. Is the child using any speech and if so, how much? Is he using direct pointing or associative pointing, that is pointing directly to food or to plate meaning 'I'm hungry'. Is the child using symbols like pictures in a book? Can the child cope with delay in communication? Is he using gesture or mime?

What are the limitations for the parents/carers/school? For any device to work, the parents have to be committed to it, the school similarly. If a family takes an alternative system all or almost all those dealing with the child have to use it, which can be a considerable strain. Families often cope very well but schools and other institutions have problems if only one or two children are using a particular sign system.

Types of systems

Sign languages. These have the advantage over other systems in that they are immediate in their communication. Their disadvantages are that they demand a lot of parents and school staff and require a certain level of hand function.

British sign language for the deaf. This was developed from spontaneous gestures into a formal language. The gestures are equivalent to ideas not spoken language and it has its own grammar. There is a finger-spelling supplement and communication is aided by facial expression and body language. It is rarely suited to the multiply handicapped because it needs good cognition and reasonable two handed function. Details are available from the RNID, 105 Grosvenor Street, London WC1E 6AH.

Makaton vocabulary. This takes 350 of the most useful and easier hand signs from the British sign language. It was developed for the deaf, severely mentally handicapped and is now used widely by severely handicapped children and adults in schools and adult training centres. Parents and carers talk while they sign. It is possible to start with a few basic signs and build up to a larger collection. Makaton is less successful for children with severe motor problems and two-handedness is needed.

Paget-Gorman. This needs more cognition than Makaton and the hand movements are complex. Parents often find it hard because of its complexity. It is a translation of spoken English and you talk as you sign. Hence it is much used in schools for the speech impaired.

Total communication. This is a manual, auditory, and oral system of communication, recognising signs as an essential reinforcement to oral and auditory aspects of communication for deaf persons. While it is rarely formally used for multiply handicapped children, many parents are naturally using all those modalities of communication.

Non-sign languages

Direct pointing picture or word boards. The BLISS symbol board was developed in Canada and uses a mixture of pictograms, abstract symbols and ideograms usually representing an idea or concept rather than a 'word'. Arrays of symbols are displayed on a board or TV screen for children to point to. The English equivalent words are displayed above each symbol so training is less necessary. Details of courses are available via BLISS Symbolics Communications Resource Centre (UK). Children need only limited motor skills for this system. It is rather laboured for the parents and the child needs cognition above a 2.5 year level.

Physical devices. There are a variety of these being developed in parallel with advances in micro-electronics. But as yet few are available widely. There are 'direct accessing' devices, for example head pointing apparatus for those with poor hand function and specialised typewriters for those with limited but usable hand function. 'Indirect accessing' equipment such as scanning devices which run a pointer or light over a list of letters, symbols or words and the child halts the scanner when he chooses, are also being developed.

Many of these devices are heavy and are often only usable in one place, thus a child using a computer can only communicate where that equipment is located. There are currently problems getting this equipment supplied and paid for. The DoH only recognises the POSSUM and PET computer and children must be assessed by a DoH representative before they are issued. Education Authorities may pay for adapted typewriters if it can be proved they are essential to education; usually the typewriters are restricted to the school and cannot be used at home.

CEREBRAL PALSY

Cerebral palsy is a persistent disorder of posture and movement appearing in the early years and due to a non-progressive disorder of the brain. It is by far the commonest cause of physical handicap in childhood. As well as the motor disability children have associated communication and learning problems - epilepsy, visual disorders and hearing loss (both conductive or sensorineural). There is enormous individual variation in the pattern of disability and multiple handicap invariably occurs.

Early diagnosis is not always easy since there is such a wide variation in normal motor development. It is important not to rush into an early, incorrect diagnosis in children with transient neurological abnormalities in the neonatal period, but persistent problems with failure of developmental progress should be appropriately assessed. Cerebral palsy may present in infancy as feeding difficulties, crying, unsettled behaviour, seizures or apathy. Once the diagnosis has been made, appropriate multidisciplinary assessment and management needs to be initiated.

Patterns of involvement

Cerebral palsy may be classified according to neuromuscular tone; spastic, hypertonic, rigid, hypotonic, athetoid, ataxic or dystonic. It can also be grouped according to the pattern of the limbs affected; monoplegia, hemiplegia, diplegia, quadriplegia and bilateral hemiplegia. It is important to realise that these patterns are not static and that during the course of neurological maturation children may go from a hypotonic phase through a dystonic phase to a spastic phase.

Initial assessment

Clues about aetiology may be obtained from the ante-natal, peri-natal and post-natal history. A family history can also be relevant. Physical examination will show delay in motor development. Tone may be increased or decreased according to the patterns described above and primitive reflexes may be unduly persistent. Tendon reflexes are often very brisk and increase or imbalance in muscle tone may cause abnormal posture or deformity. Voluntary movements are poor and lack precision. Where the cause is not obvious, further investigation should be considered. This may include investigations for congenital infection (rubella, cytomegalovirus, toxoplasma, herpes simplex), aminoacid chromotography, skull x-ray, CT scan and chromosomal analysis.

Management problems

Vision may be affected in a variety of ways. There may be partial sight, refractive errors, a squint, hemianopia and other field defects. The latter may impair left-right sequencing in reading or writing.

Circulation to arms and legs is sometimes poor, making them susceptible to cold injury. Advice on warm clothing can be helpful.

Deformities are common but are often preventable when they result from muscle imbalance, immobility and incorrect positioning.

Toilet training can usually be achieved. Firm, comfortable seating in which the child feels secure is vital and training is easily upset by anxiety. Behavioural approaches are often useful.

Persisting primitive reflexes particularly the asymmetric tonic neck reflex and the tonic labyrinthine reflexes may interfere with postural reactions and the development of voluntary hand movements. Central head positioning is vital in inhibiting those reflexes.

Deafness is common both conductive and sensorineural. The latter is particularly frequent with high tone loss in children with athetosis.

Perceptual problems relating to identification of shapes, directions in space and body image, produce practical problems in self help such as undressing and in acquiring reading and writing skills. In some intel-lectually-able children, these problems may only become apparent when they are struggling with mathematical concepts such as the conversion of a table of numbers into a linear graph or pie chart or in geography with the conversion of a flat map into a three-dimensional picture.

Children with spastic diplegia are often of normal intelligence with few perceptual problems. They invariably cope in their local school if the problems of mobility can be overcome. Children with hemiplegias are often also managed within ordinary schools though perceptual dif-ficulties and visual field defects need to be carefully looked for. The child with spastic quadriplegia often has more complex needs both in terms of therapy, posturing and learning problems. The greatest chal-lenge to education is often the child with athetosis who may have a combination of communication difficulties and involuntary movements but who may also have the intellectual ability to greatly benefit from advanced and complex electronic equipment.

SPINA BIFIDA

In the United Kingdom there is currently a natural fall in the incidence of this condition. The number of infants with severe handicap due to spina bifida has fallen significantly, following the alpha fetoprotein screening programmes, the greater availability of genetic counselling and selective surgical management of the newborn. Folic acid supple-mentation starting pre-conception is recommended for mothers with a high risk of having a child with spina bifida. Its recommendation for all women contemplating a family is not yet resolved.

The individual needs of children with spina bifida depend upon the level and extent of the spinal lesion and the degree of CNS abnormality secondary to hydrocephalus. The falling prevalence of the condition means that multidisciplinary expertise may diminish. Co-ordination can be difficult when the doctors involved – neurosurgeons, orthopaedic surgeons, paediatricians, paediatric surgeons, work in different centres.

Management problems   **Mobility.** With lesions above T12 there is little hope of walking. Between L1 and L3 walking may be achieved, but only by extensive use of calipers and with tremendous muscular efforts of trunk and arms. However, most children resort to the use of a wheelchair as this enables more mobility, independence and dignity to be achieved. With lesions between L3 and S1 children usually manage with short calipers with or without sticks. Children with lesions at S2 or lower can manage without calipers but muscle imbalance may require orthopaedic operations to maintain the feet in a good functional position. For young children, a variety of trolleys are available in which the child can sit with their legs extended on a base, to give them some independence.

Urinary continence. In some children there is a flaccid paralysis of the bladder and in others there are strong unco-ordinated bladder contractions likely to produce back pressure. Bladder pressure studies can help decide on the appropriate regime for each individual child. Possible approaches include the use of drugs, bladder expression, intermittent catheterisation, penile appliances, ureterostomies and ileal loop diversions and simple toilet training regimes.

Hydrocephalus and shunt. Of those who develop hydrocephalus, one third will settle spontaneously and two thirds will require shunt procedures. Shunts may become infected or blocked and this may be suspected by changes such as drowsiness, pyrexia, personality or visual changes. Rapid action is therefore essential.

Orthopaedic problems. Kyphosis and scoliosis are common and surgery may be required. Immobility may give rise to dislocation of the hips and leg and foot deformities.

Puberty and adolescence. Menarche is often early in girls with spina bifida. A combination of immobility, incontinence and menstruation can cause considerable distress. Anxieties about sex and fertility are common and counselling needs to cover not only these aspects, but also the fact that their children have a higher risk of inheriting the condition.

Educational problems. Learning difficulties are common in children with spina bifida and many lack motivation. Characteristically, many of the children get 'cocktail party' speech in which the child has deceptively precocious expressive language with very poor comprehension. There may also be significant fine motor problems and visio-spatial difficulties. Careers have to be chosen with these problems in mind.

MUSCULAR DYSTROPHY

Muscular dystrophy is a genetic term covering a variety of types of muscle disorder. The most common form is Duchenne muscular dystrophy (incidence 0.3:1000 boys). The condition should be suspected in any boy with delayed or progressive difficulty in walking. Prominent hypertrophied but weak calf muscles are an important sign. Diagnosis is by a blood test for the muscle enzyme creatinine phosphokinase, electromyography and muscle biopsy. Even allowing for individual variation, the disease is relentless with motor skills being lost progressively. The boys are rarely walking unaided beyond 12 years and death from cardio/respiratory failure usually occurs before the mid twenties.

Inheritance is by an X-linked recessive gene with a considerable number of spontaneous mutations. Carrier mothers, aunts and sisters can be detected once a case is identified. Genetic counselling for all the family should be offered as soon as a diagnosis is made. Recent advances enable diagnosis to be made antenatally with the option of termination for an affected fetus.

Educational implications

With a lot of help most boys are able to start in an ordinary school, but as they get older and the handicap progresses, more help is needed with toileting, dressing and mobility. Many secondary schools are built on two or more levels and are not designed for wheelchairs, though hopefully this will not be the case in the future. Some schools have provided the means to get round all these difficulties and boys have been educated with their peers throughout their school life. However, integration is not the ideal for every boy, each case has to be considered individually. Some boys become more depressed at the gap in ability between them and their peers. Loneliness is common. These two problems may be expressed aggressively. The boys may be happier in a physical handicap (PH) school where there are other boys with similar problems and in such a physical handicap school the 'Duchenne' boys often stick together.

In the special school awareness of long term prognosis often leads to depression, especially following the death of one of the boys. Such an event affects the staff as well as the boys. Treatment facilities and expertise are more readily available in a special school, but the school itself may not be near to home. For rural children the nearest school for children with a physical handicap may be many miles away and boarding is the only option. A normal part of adolescence is 'kicking over the traces' of adult control, like sneaking into an 'X' film. This is much harder to do in a wheelchair and can lead to a lot of frustration. Some special schools have found ingenious ways round this.

This disease has such a relentless and predictable course that it is quite easy to predict future needs of the boys and their families; house conversions, ramps for wheelchairs, adjustable beds for night-turning, toileting aids, lifting facilities. Delays abound. It is vital for professionals and parents to anticipate the needs and develop a relationship with the local authorities so that facilities are provided when they are needed.

REFERENCES AND FURTHER READING

Association for Spina Bifida and Hydrocephalus 1983 Sex for young people with spina bifida or cerebral palsy. ASBAH, London
Bowley A H, Gardener L 1980 The handicapped child. Churchill Livingstone, Edinburgh
Brocklehurst J C 1976 Spina bifida for the clinician. Spastics International Medical Publications, London
Dubowitz V 1978 Muscle disorders in childhood. W B Saunders, London
Finnie N 1974 Handling the young cerebral palsied child at home. Heinemann, London
Hewitt S 1970 The family and handicapped child. Allen and Unwin, London
Jeffree D M, McConkey R 1976 Let me speak. Souvenir Press, London
Jeffree D M, McConkey R, Hewson S 1977 Let me play. Souvenir Press, London
Levitt S 1982 Cerebral palsy and therapy. Treatment of cerebral palsy and motor delay, 2nd edn. Blackwell Scientific, Oxford
McCarthy G T 1984 The physically handicapped child. Faber & Faber, London
McGovern S 1982 The epilepsy handbook. Sheldon Press, London
O'Donohoe N 1985 Epilepsies of childhood, 2nd edn. Butterworths, London
Riddick B 1982 Toys and play for the handicapped child. Croom Helm, London
Royal College of Physicians 1986 Physical disability in 1986 and beyond – a report of the Royal College of Physicians. Journal of the Royal College of Physicians 20: 160–194
Russell P 1978 The wheelchair child. Souvenir Press, London
Smith D 1976 Recognisable patterns of human malformation. W B Saunders, London
The good toy guide 1983 Toy Libraries Association and Inter-Action
Thomas A P 1989 The health and social needs of young adults with physical disabilities. MacKeith Press, Oxford

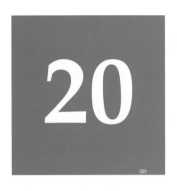

20 Vision

Disorders of vision are common. Impaired vision can result from malformation, injury or malfunction of any part of the visual pathway from the eye to the visual cortex.

Incidence

Four per cent of school entrants will be found to have a reduced visual acuity and 8 per cent of those leaving school will be found to have a reduction in visual acuity. However severe visual handicap is rare in the UK with the prevalence of 1 in 2500 children. This would give rise to fewer than 3000 children attending special school because of visual handicap. In tropical countries blindness is a much more common condition resulting from keratomalacia secondary to vitamin A deficiency often exacerbated by infection with measles or trachoma.

Children with a visual acuity of 3/60 or less in the better eye are registered as blind. Those with a corrected visual acuity in the better eye of 4/60 to 6/24 are registered partially sighted. Official estimates of the numbers of children with visual handicap may be underestimates especially as children with other associated severe handicaps may not be registered.

The recorded incidence of children with visual defects rises with age. This is partly due to abnormalities not being detected early on as vision

Causes of blindness

% of blind and partially sighted children

Optic atrophy
Congenital cataracts
Choroido-retinal degeneration
Malformation
Retrolental fibroplasia
Myopia
Albinism
Retinoblastoma
Uveitis
Other causes

Total
Genetic

testing in young children is notoriously difficult and the tests, even in the best hands, may prove unreliable. It is also due to the effects of growth of the eye causing abnormalities to appear later on. Muscle compensation will act to postpone diminished visual acuity due to an error of refraction. For this reason, vision testing in children cannot be a once and for all process. A significant proportion of those found to be normal on testing at age 7 and 11 will be found to have severe unilateral or bilateral problems by the age of 16 years.

Many other aspects of development are highly dependent upon normal vision. More than 70 per cent of early learning is visually dependant. General development, particularly language and later progress in school, will be greatly impaired in the presence of an undetected visual defect. Visually received information depends upon normal visual acuity and visual discrimination in terms of depth, colour and three dimensional perception. The ability to recognise symbols in the written word (in a variety of styles), and to relate these to meaning and the spoken word is essential for the skill of reading. A fixed reference (dominant) eye is thought to be important for the reading process.

OPHTHALMOLOGY SERVICES

Children may receive ophthalmology services either through hospital eye departments, through local opticians or through school eye clinics which are closely associated with community paediatric services. Wherever the children are seen communication is vital with community paediatricians so that the child's visual problems can be properly related to provision in school. Increasing use is being made of orthoptists for vision screening because of the acknowledged difficulties in testing younger children and those with other problems. Problems with vision

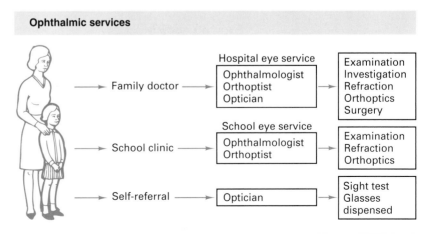

Ophthalmic services

are often not freestanding but reflect a component of a wider paediatric syndrome and hence the need for a full paediatric assessment of children with eye problems. The high incidence (50 per cent) of inherited conditions in children with severe disability makes it important for the ophthalmologist to liaise with the clinical genetics service.

The work of the medical team is complemented by that of education and social services' specialist teams. They may be involved in educational support within mainstream or in special units. They may be involved in mobility training or in general support for the family.

NORMAL VISUAL DEVELOPMENT

In the newborn visual attention can be assessed when the child is in an alert and quiet state. Babies will usually fixate on an object from the age of 33 weeks gestation. Most newborn babies fix their gaze and follow an object if it is moved slowly horizontally. Vertical tracking is usually first seen between four and eight weeks of age.

Preferential looking can be seen in pre-term infants from the age of 31 weeks gestation. In this the infant prefers to look at a more interesting object and patterned, moving or blinking targets are preferred to unpatterned static ones. This behaviour has been used to assess newborn visual function and may provide a good screening test for the future. The newborn infant has poor contrast sensitivity in that he can only discern clearly contrasting objects such as the eyes and mouth of the human face. This ability improves rapidly but does not reach adult levels until the age of three years.

The visual acuity of the newborn is only about 6/200. This improves rapidly to 6/60 by three months and is beginning to approach adult levels by the age of six months. This follows maturation of the visual pathways in the brain. Some children who turn out to have normal

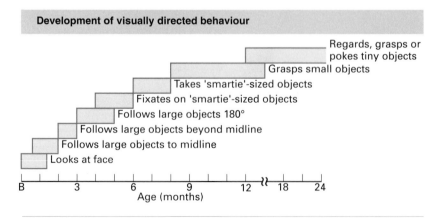

Development of visually directed behaviour

Regards, grasps or pokes tiny objects
Grasps small objects
Takes 'smartie'-sized objects
Fixates on 'smartie'-sized objects
Follows large objects 180°
Follows large objects beyond midline
Follows large objects to midline
Looks at face

Age (months)
B   3   6   9   12   18   24

vision have delayed maturation and a much slower progress towards normal visual acuity.

Binocular single vision may be seen as early as two months of age but will develop normally provided that both eyes are used equally to give clear images that are aligned and can be fused. In the newborn the attention of the infant is held mainly within a short distance of around 10 inches from the child's face. During development the child becomes aware of the wider and wider sphere of visual material being extended to around 4 feet at four months and 6 feet at five months. In order to do this the eyes must develop the abilities of accommodation and convergence by which visual information is taken in at an increasing variety of distances. Growth of the eye will result in changes in the refractive properties of the eye and hence there needs to be a continuum of adjustment in the control of the eyes if normal vision is to be maintained. Adult colour vision is probably obtained by the age of five months.

Binocular function

Monocular visual acuity is dependant upon the production of a clear image on the retina and its detailed transmission to the cerebral cortex. Binocular vision gives the advantage of distance judgement and the slightly enlarged visual field. In order for this to develop three criteria must be met: both eyes must be looking at the same object; both images must be clear; and the brain must be able to join these images to produce one visual impression (sensory fusion). From around six weeks of age the eyes begin to fix on the same object and normal binocular vision can be established. If the eyes are not both fixated at the same point then a double image will result. However, feedback of the double image will cause the extraocular muscles to realign and hence fuse again into single image. This process is called motor fusion and the range of angles over which it is possible to maintain normal binocular function is called the fusion range. If the tendency for the eyes to turn out of alignment is greater than the central nervous system's ability to control it, then a squint will develop. Thus the tendency for an eye to turn in (esophoria) becomes an esotropia or convergent squint. If the tendency for the eye to turn can be controlled by motor fusion then there is a latent squint; if it cannot, then a manifest squint will occur. There are three possible responses to a manifest squint. Firstly, the child can suppress one image and if this is allowed to occur for long enough the squinting eye becomes amblyopic and no longer able to function normally. Suppression will normally occur in children under the age of six. In other children the development of an abnormal head posture may occur. Thus a head tilt may move the eyes into a position in which binocular function can be maintained. The third response would be to keep one eye covered or closed.

Failure to develop normal fusion, ie a congenital squint, may occur for a number of reasons. In many children this is because one eye is producing a blurred image due to a unilateral refractive error or opacity. The lack of clear information reaching this eye means that the brain cannot accurately point it in the right direction and the eye usually becomes convergent. In some children there is a congenital inability to fuse and this is often seen in families with a family history of squint. In other children there are abnormalities in the control mechanism for the extraocular muscles by the cranial nerves resulting in their inability to move together within the exacting limits required for fusion. Children with congenital squints do not develop normal binocular function even with optimal treatment but those with an acquired squint can recover binocular function as a result of treatment.

Squints can be acquired when the normal coordination of accommodation and convergence does not occur. In the person with normal vision, when the eyes focus upon a near object, the focusing and convergence that are necessary take place in a coordinated manner so that both eyes remain in focus and fix on the same object. If a child is longsighted he must accommodate (focus) in order to see clearly in the distance, but he must not converge at the same time as the visual axis must remain parallel to fix on a distant object; however as accommodation and convergence are linked the child must either focus and develop a convergent squint, or keep the eye straight and then see things indistinctly. Hypermetropia (longsight) is the commonest cause of an acquired squint. Children with unequal refraction in the two eyes (anisometropia) do not always develop a squint and may appear to have two normal eyes. However on testing the eyes separately it is found that one eye is weaker than the other but has become amblyopic.

VISUAL SCREENING

Visual screening forms part of our child health surveillance programme. Justification of visual screening is the early detection of severe visual abnormalities sufficient to cause visual handicap, the detection of moderate visual problems of sufficient severity to cause difficulties with reading and the prevention of amblyopia. There are however problems with these assumptions. In the identification of children with severe visual defects Hall and Hall discovered that in 111 of 189 children the defect was discovered by parents and in only 3 was the child health surveillance programme following the neonatal examination responsible for finding a previously unsuspected defect. In practice children with amblyopia, particularly those who do not have a manifest squint present late, the major reason being the current lack of a reliable test that can be applied to young children when detection could be potentially most valuable. Hence many children are not discovered until school age testing at age five. Even in those children who are detected early, so-called optimal treatment can give discouraging results and some treatment strategies may be poorly tolerated by children.

People have advocated different methods of screening in the first year of life using techniques such as refraction or through screening methods developed through research on preferential viewing or through the use of a refraction camera which uses photographic techniques to

Summary of vision screening programme

Age	Test	Notes
Newborn	Red reflex.	Inspection for congenital abnormalities.
6 weeks	Red reflex. Inspection Interest? Fixates? Follows?	Importance of family history and parental concerns. Parents who are concerned about vision or squint should be referred not 'reassured' by crude screening tests.
6–8 months	History. Observation.	Cover test very difficult and unreliable.
18 months	History. Observation. Visual performance with small objects.	Cover test remains very difficult. No specific tests at this age.
$2\frac{1}{2}$ – $3\frac{1}{2}$ years	No specific test of visual acuity recommended for all children. ? High risk only. Linear chart more reliable than single letters. Orthoptists used in some areas.	6/9 – retest in six months. 6/12 – refer. Watch for children who have obvious difficulty with one eye and those who 'peer' or move their heads – refer. 4 out of 5 children should be able to perform the test at this age.
School entry	Acuity using linear (Snellen) chart at 6 metres. A few authorities carry out near vision test too.	Repeated at age 8,11 and 14 as myopia develops as the child gets older.
11 years	Colour vision using City Plates or Ishihara test.	Ishihara very sensitive and picks up children with trivial defects who will pass City Plates.

identify unequal or abnormal light reflections. Vision testing in young children is notoriously difficult even in very experienced hands. In some districts orthoptists have been used in preference to health visitors or doctors because of their more specialised skills in this area. However the need for correcting lesser degrees of impaired visual acuity for educational purposes does not arise until school children are required to cope with progressively smaller print.

Some children at high risk of vision problems may require special attention. These include preterm babies who have received intensive care, children where there is a family history of squint, amblyopia or visual impairment and children with other disabilities, eg cerebral palsy, where there is a much higher incidence of eye problems.

Vision testing programme This is part of the surveillance programme (chapter 8). In the younger age group the important elements are informed parental observation supplemented by professional observation of visually directed behaviour and observation of the eyes. In the older age group tests for visual acuity can be applied; they require cooperation, concentration and the ability to match symbols. For these children the use of linear charts is preferable to the matching of single letters as the latter can over-estimate visual acuity by as much as 2–3 lines compared to a standard chart. This is known as the crowding phenomenon in which single letters are seen more easily than those in rows of letters. Some of the tests designed for use with younger children, such as rolling balls and toy tests are very poor at picking up children with moderate defects and indeed will miss some with severe defects.

Near vision is tested at a distance of 25 cm using standard type equivalents to those used for distance testing. In young children, it may be better to let them choose their own distance rather than insist on 25 cm. N4 size is that found for entries in the telephone directory.

The performance of visual screening programmes can be improved by providing appropriate training and review of skills to those carrying out the tests. Attention to detail in test procedures, eg distances, lighting, full occlusion of the eye not being tested so that the child cannot see round the patch, can all lead to improved performance of the screening programme. Audit of the results of screening programmes and efficient administrative systems are required to ensure that all children are tested and that children who require it are referred or re-assessed.

Colour vision testing

Colour vision testing is usually carried out in the first year of secondary school but can be done earlier. Up to 10 per cent of boys may have a defect in colour vision with problems being very rare in girls. The commonly used tests are the Ishihara test in which numbers have to be identified from a matrix of small coloured dots and the City University Plates where the colour of the central dot needs to be matched to one of four other dots surrounding it. Both these tests give reliable results only when carried out under appropriate lighting conditions as the colours of the test materials are dependant upon the light in which they are observed. The significance of colour vision defects is that they would be a barrier for certain occupations, for example some grades in the armed forces, electrical work and airline pilots. The table below shows common types of colour vision problems which may be detected.

Types of colour vision defect

	(%) Boys	(%) Girls	Grey confused with	Common confusions
Protanopia	1	0.02	Blue, green or red	Brown/black/red Blue/purple
Protanomalous	1.5	0.03	Pale red	Yellow/orange
Deuteranopia	1	0.01	Reddish purple	Green/tan Green/brown/red
Deuteranomaly	5	0.4	Pale purple	Greenish Blue/purple Yellow/green
Tritanopia	1: 13 000 –	1: 65 000	Violet, olive or yellow	Green with blue

ABNORMALITIES OF REFRACTION

Hypermetropia

In hypermetropia the eyeball is slightly shorter than normal so that parallel rays of light are brought to focus behind the retina. This is the normal state in the infant and diminishes with growth. Minor degrees are overcome by the normal powers of accommodation but difficulty will be experienced in more pronounced cases when distance vision is tested. In severe hypermetropia near vision is usually quite good though the child may need to bring his eye very close to the object he is looking at. Distant vision is impaired. Hypermetropia may produce frontal headache or convergent squint. It may be associated with astigmatism. It is treated with glasses using convex lenses to aid convergence of the light source.

Hypermetropia and myopia

Hypermetropia (long sighted)   Myopia (short sighted)

Myopia

In myopia the eye is marginally too long and parallel rays of light are brought to focus in front of the retina. The myopic child has difficulty with distant vision. Myopia usually develops between the ages of 5 and 15 due to excessive growth of the eye. There is often a family history. The condition is treated with glasses and the defect is corrected by concave lenses. Rarely congenital myopia occurs and may be associated with retinal detachment.

Astigmatism

This arises when the curvature of the cornea and lens is different in the horizontal and vertical planes. Minor degrees of astigmatism have no significance but greater degrees produce difficulties in focusing horizontally and vertically simultaneously and will give rise to difficulties in reading and a dislike of prolonged close work. Some children screw up their eyes in an attempt to improve acuity.

Refractive error

In most of the defects in visual acuity it is necessary to measure the degree of refractive error causing that diminution in acuity in order to apply appropriate correction. In young children this is generally done by retinoscopy following the use of drops to dilate the pupil and paralyse accommodation. With the eye in this condition the underlying properties of the lens may be determined. If there is no error of refraction parallel light entering the eye will emerge as parallel light. If the eye is hypermetropic the rays are divergent, if the eye is myopic the rays are convergent and if the eyes are astigmatic the rays emerge in a band. Trial lenses are then applied in front of the eye until the rays emerge parallel, indicating that refractive error has been corrected. This method is generally used for children under the age of six. Older children may be assessed using a trial frame and a chart. The strength of lenses is measured in dioptres: convex lenses have positive values, concave lenses have negative values. It is the reciprocal of the focal length measured in metres.

Acceptance of glasses

Children frequently do not wear the glasses that have been prescribed for them. A few of these may have been prescribed for minor defects but there are still a significant group of children for whom the wearing of spectacles for near or distant work is important. In these cases close cooperation from doctors, parents, teachers and the children themselves is required. Attempts at educating all children about the value of spectacles will probably be more successful than putting pressure on individual children.

Squint

The majority of squints are due to refractive errors. However a minority are caused by neurological disorders affecting the innervation of the extraocular muscles or by eye disease affecting the cornea, lens or retina. Squints may result from conditions such as cataract, retinoblastoma, cerebral palsy, meningitis and hydrocephalus.

Descriptive terms for types of squint

- Alternating : either eye can take up fixation
- Accommodative : influenced by accommodation or wearing glasses
- Concomitant : deviation is constant
- Incomitant : deviation depends on angle of gaze

Squint may be detected by observation where there is a pronounced manifest squint. In other children asymmetry of the corneal light reflections from a distant source may be seen. Limitation of ocular movements in one direction gives a paralytic cause of the squint. The cover test illustrated in the diagram is often difficult to carry out. Gross deviations in a cooperative child are easy but small eye movements in a difficult child require expert observational powers few of us have.

In a few children abnormal head posture may be observed. An alternating squint is sometimes seen. This tends not lead to amblyopia, but binocular vision is not developed.

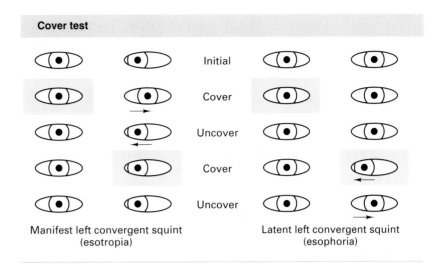

Cover test

		Initial		
		Cover		
		Uncover		
		Cover		
		Uncover		

Manifest left convergent squint
(esotropia)

Latent left convergent squint
(esophoria)

Management of squint

The aim of treatment is to prevent amblyopia, which remains the single most significant vision problem in childhood. Occlusion is the mainstay of therapy for squint but many children will not tolerate this. Occlusion encourages the use of the squinting eye with development of fixation. Glasses may correct the refractive error and this may be all that is required in many cases. The orthoptist will be able to assess binocular function and some children benefit from orthoptic exercises. Surgery will correct the appearance and for some children may be beneficial in the development of binocular function.

VISUAL HANDICAP

So far we have been concerned with visual disorders which, although important in their recognition and treatment, do not leave a residue of handicap significant enough to affect education and everyday life. This section covers the problems of blindness and partial sight. In 1977 in the UK, there were 2196 children registered as blind, and 2635 registered as partially sighted. Of the causes of blindness reported in a sample of 100 blind and partially sighted children in 1975 in the UK, 45 per cent were genetic. Important pre-natal causes include cataract, optic atrophy, glaucoma, retinopathy, and congenital infections. Blindness is frequently associated with other handicaps. Fifty per cent of visually handicapped children have no additional handicap, but 37 per cent are mentally handicapped, and others have hearing losses, cerebral palsy or epilepsy. Up to a third have serious social problems.

Clinical features

The suspicion of visual handicap by parents or professionals requires a prompt response as some children, for example those with opacities, can have their vision restored by surgery and all children will receive the benefit of early and appropriate developmental guidance.

Enquire about photophobia and look for nystagmus and visual field defects. Photophobia is experienced with congenital glaucoma and albinism, and with achromatopsia, in which there is an absence of retinal cones and thus reduced visual acuity and total colour blindness. Keratitis and iritis also give rise to photophobia. Nystagmus may occur when central vision is poor, for example in albinism, congenital cataracts, optic nerve and macular abnormalities. It is usually pendular. There may be tunnel vision, a loss of central vision or other field defects. Children with hemiplegias may have a homonymous hemianopia. Electrophysiological tests can check the intactness of the visual pathways (visual evoked responses, VER), and the retinal responses to light (electroretinogram, ERG).

Registration of people as blind is done by the Director of Social Services on the advice of the consultant ophthalmologist.

Development

Deprivation of vision affects many aspects of learning, behaviour and development. Bonding is facilitated by eye contact between the mother and the child. The development of fine motor skills starts with hand regard. The size of the environment that the child can see is reduced to that immediately around him. Sound is a poor substitute for vision in terms of understanding distance. Objects are named by attaching a verbal label to a particular object that is seen. The labels have no meaning or significance if the child cannot understand the nature of the object to which they are attached. Language comprehension is often delayed by as much as 9 to 12 months and expression by 1 to 2 years. Gross motor development is delayed because the child does not have vision to guide him. Obstacles are unexpected and frightening.

Social development, feeding, dressing, and play are also impeded by lack of vision. The child needs to develop a sense of touch and hearing to compensate for the deficit in vision. He needs to be spoken to constantly so that things around him can be explained, which the sighted child discovers for himself. Examples are doors opening and closing, footsteps, the chink of bottles being picked up, the sounds of curtains being drawn. He needs to be shown these objects, and encouraged to explore and feel them. Toys need to be robust, bangable and chewable and such that the child can perceive his effect upon them. For instance, mechanical toys or a dolls house would be unsuitable. Water, rattles, a collection of objects differing in size, shape, texture, etc, are useful in developing fine motor discrimination. Talking, explaining, encouraging the child to handle and feel objects and helping the child to use any residual vision are the keys to learning. Nearly all blind children do have some residual vision and the child must make the best use of this, just as a deaf child must use his residual hearing. The child with visual handicap must be physically strong to deal with the unperceived obstacles and falls which he may have. His personality must also be able to deal with the problems of coping with an environment which he cannot always understand or perceive. He needs the confidence to move about in this environment, to deal with others and to ask for help. We have only to imagine ourselves deprived of our vision, trying to go through our daily lives or our journey to work. Our awareness of these

Management of blind or partially sighted child

Ophthalmic	Assessment of vision Management of eye disorder	Registration Aids for vision
Child Health	Effect of visual handicap General health	Parent counselling Genetic counselling
Education	General and special education	Teaching aids
RNIB		
Social	Family support	Benefits

needs of the visually handicapped, and the effects on gross motor, fine motor, language and social development enables appropriate advice to be given to parents on care and education. In older children, failure to read 'body language' and facial expression may be a disadvantage in social interaction.

Children with visual handicap have to learn to use their existing vision to an optimum effect and to develop their use of hearing and tactile senses. These have to be learned and an early start is needed.

Assessment

Assessment of the visually handicapped child must include paediatric, ophthalmic, psychological and social assessments. Ophthalmic assessment involves the clinical assessment of vision and the underlying pathology.

General paediatric assessment is required, for visual handicap is often associated with other handicaps or may be part of a wider clinical syndrome. The need for genetic counselling must be considered. It is important to ensure that the hearing is normal. Although visually handicapped children do not as a rule have a high incidence of deafness, because hearing is so important to the education of the visually handicapped child, it is essential that adequate information on hearing is available. Psychological assessment is needed to determine the level of ability of the child and any particular problems in learning. Social work support is important to enable the family to come to terms with the handicap and to deal constructively with the problems that it presents.

Management

Medical management involves the clinical follow-up of the child's visual and other associated conditions. Specific management may be required with regard to surgical problems such as cataracts or corneal opacities. Glasses must be prescribed as needed. As many of the conditions giving rise to impaired vision are inherited, genetic counselling will be indicated in many cases.

Education needs to provide the child with the confidence to act in his environment and to make decisions. He may need to be taught living skills which other children just pick up. He needs opportunities for real experience of the world around him.

Numerous classroom aids are now available. The simplest of these are large type books for partially sighted readers. School resource centres should be able to reproduce standard texts in larger form. Special desks of an easel type to hold the written work are most valuable in allowing the child to get nearer to the text. Good illumination is essential. Low vision aids, for example magnifiers, may also enable the child to use more standard classroom material. Tactile maps and other technological advances are often used in the classroom. Some authorities still separate blind and partially sighted children into different groups as the former group may require Braille teaching methods. However, some partially sighted pupils will also benefit from Braille teaching as a 'backup' especially if the child's condition is progressive. Tape recorders can be used as a substitute for reading, and typewriters as a substitute for writing. Blind people may make excellent audio-typists and typing is a skill which can be taught early. Other low vision aids of great value are closed circuit television to magnify type up to the size of a TV monitor. Talking calculators are also available. The curriculum in schools provides a broad range of subjects not only English and mathematics, but languages, home economics and in some schools, sciences. Physical fitness is important, and sports, such as rowing and swimming, are applicable. Mobility training is an important part of education and the child needs to learn the route to school just as he would need to learn the route to work. Visual handicap can limit the child's understanding of the layout of the town and he may need to learn routes as sequences. He may not realise, for example, that one corridor is parallel to another.

Essential for the child's progress are space, a safe environment, more time to acquire concepts and the development of self confidence.

REFERENCES AND FURTHER READING

Bolger P G, Stewart-Brown S L 1991 Vision screening in children: A comparison of orthopists and clinical medical officers as primary screeners. British Medical Journal 303: 1291–4
Fielder A R, Moseley M J 1988 Do we need to measure the visual acuity of children? Journal of the Royal Society of Medicine 81: 380–3
Gardiner P A 1982 The development of vision. MTP, Lancaster
Hall S M, Pugh A G, Hall D M B 1982 Vision screening in the under fives. British Medical Journal 285: 1096–8
Hyvarinen L, Lindstedt 1981 Assessment of vision in children. SRF Tal & Punkt, Stockholm
Ingram R M 1988 Review of children referred from the school vision screening programme in Kettering. British Medical Journal 298: 935–6
Jarvis S N, Tamhne R C, Thompson L, Francis P M, Anderson J, Colver A F 1990 Preschool vision screening. Archives of Disease in Childhood 65: 288–94
Shaw D E, Fielder A R, Minshull C, Rosenthal A R 1988 Amblyopia – factors influencing age of presentation. Lancet ii: 207–9
Stewart-Brown S L, Haslam M 1988 Screening of vision in school. Could we do better by doing less? British Medical Journal 297: 1111–3
Stewart-Brown S L, Haslam M, Howett B 1988 Pre-school vision screening: a service in need of rationalisation. Archives of Disease in Childhood 63: 356–9

21 Hearing

Much effort is rightly directed to the early detection and management of hearing losses. For the severely deaf child, early detection and appropriate education are essential for producing the best results. Mild and moderate hearing losses are also important and far more common. Their importance in respect of delayed language development, often combined with other problems such as poor education performance and behaviour problems, is not always appreciated.

Incidence

About 3/1000 children have sensori-neural hearing loss, of which 1/ 1000 is congenital, severe or profound loss and should be detected in the first year of life. A further 1/1000 will require hearing aids for high tone deafness or moderate sensori-neural loss which is more difficult to diagnose in the first year of life. An additional 1–2/1000 will have some degree of sensori-neural loss which may require a hearing aid or develop late onset hearing loss.

Significant conductive losses will be found in 5–10% of children at some time in childhood, but probably a higher incidence occurs in younger children.

Causes of deafness

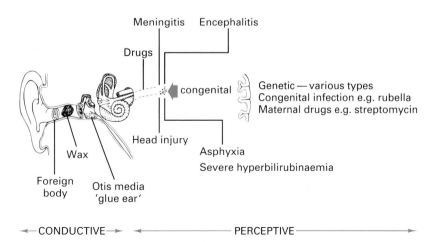

Meningitis   Encephalitis

Drugs

congenital

Genetic — various types
Congenital infection e.g. rubella
Maternal drugs e.g. streptomycin

Head injury

Asphyxia
Severe hyperbilirubinaemia

Wax

Foreign body

Otis media 'glue ear'

◄─ CONDUCTIVE ─►   ◄─────── PERCEPTIVE ───────►

Causes

Sensori-neural losses can have a wide variety of causes. In a variety of studies 20–50% are described as being inherited, either autosomal dominant, autosomal recessive or X-linked. Some of these will be part of an identified syndrome. Autosomal recessive syndromes include Usher's syndrome with retinitis pigmentosa causing visual loss in later childhood or early adult life, Pendred syndrome with associated thyroid problems, Jervell-Lange Neilson syndrome with cardiac rhythm abnormalities leading to sudden collapse. Autosomal dominant syndromes include Waardenburg's syndrome manifested by a white forelock, heterochromia irides, Stickler syndrome with severe myopia, Pierre Robin anomaly, and joint problems. Other syndromes are thought not to be inherited (CHARGE syndrome). Other causes of sensori-neural deafness are neonatal problems (birth asphyxia, prematurity, hyperbilirubinaemia), congenital infection (rubella, cytomegalovirus), drugs (gentamicin). The first deaf child in a family with no apparent cause for the deafness has a high chance of having an autosomal recessive inherited deafness. Late onset sensori-neural loss can be a result of meningitis, encephalitis, mumps, or head injury.

Conductive loss may be associated with a congenital abnormality of the middle or external ear. This may be associated with a syndrome such as Treacher Collins, or Goldenhar's. It may be an isolated abnormality of the ear which is often manifested by an abnormal pinna. In later childhood, serous otitis media is far and away the commonest cause of conductive hearing loss, though obstruction of the ear canal by wax or a foreign body can cause hearing impairment. Some children are at increased risk of serous otitis media such as those with Down's syndrome or cleft palate.

Prevention

Hereditary forms of deafness may be prevented by appropriate genetic counselling and all affected families should be offered this. Deaf adults may be quite happy to go ahead with a family despite a high risk of a hearing impaired child, because they do not see their deafness as a handicap. Some hearing parents of a deaf child are reluctant to risk having another deaf child, but may be less concerned if they see their deaf child doing well. Gene linkage is developing rapidly and it may not be long before more accurate genetic counselling can be given by identifying carriers. It should also help to clarify the situation where there is a child with deafness but no apparent cause.

Introduction of rubella immunisation is an important preventive measure and the change in policy to immunise all children in early childhood should further reduce the incidence of congenital rubella. Mumps immunisation is likely to have a significant effect in reducing the incidence of unilateral deafness. Introduction of the vaccine against *Haemophilus influenzae* will prevent some of the post-meningitis deafness.

Secondary prevention by screening (identifying the condition as early as possible in order to minimise handicap) is well developed for congenital hearing losses. It is important to remain vigilant for late onset hearing losses in order to minimise the effects of these.

SCREENING

Most agree that screening for hearing difficulty is worthwhile. However the ages at which screening is carried out and the type of test used varies considerably. Screening should fulfil the criteria discussed in Chapter 8. Clear local guide-lines should be available as to who should be tested (universal screen or selective screen), at what ages, what test, who is responsible for doing it, and what the subsequent action should be.

Children at risk of deafness

- History of meningitis or encephalitis
- Children with cleft palate
- History of recurrent otitis media
- Significantly delayed or unclear speech
- Children with cerebral palsy
- Parental suspicion of deafness

The two screens used most often are distraction testing at 6–8 months and audiometry at 4–6 years. Other tests are used at other ages for whole population screening or selective screening but their use needs careful evaluation. Most of the tests used are quite difficult to do well, and staff must be trained carefully if the screen is to be performed well. Health visitors and school nurses most commonly do the screening.

Screening test for hearing

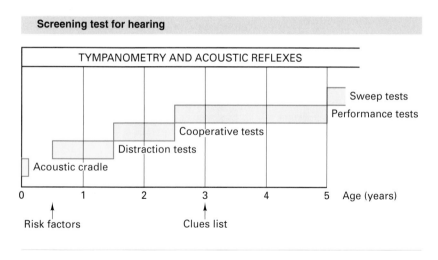

AUDIOLOGICAL ASSESSMENT

Sound intensity is measured in decibels (dB) which is a logarithmic scale of sound pressure. The scale has been arbitrarily set with 0 dB as the quietest sounds that a 'normally' hearing person will hear. Sound frequency (the pitch or tone) is measured in Hertz (Hz) or kilohertz (kHz) and is a measure of sound waves in cycles per second.

Neonatal testing

At present, where this is done, it is normally on a selected high risk group of infants. Probably 50% of the deaf children will be diagnosed by testing the 10% of babies going through Special Care Baby Units. If other risk factors are taken into account then neonatal screening is even more efficient.

Newborn infants at risk of deafness

- Family history of deafness
- Low birth weight
- Significant birth asphyxia
- Severe jaundice
- Congenital rubella or CMV infection
- Neonatal meningitis
- Malformation of the face or external ears

A number of tests have been developed that will test hearing in the newborn. The acoustic cradle measures behavioural responses (e.g. head turning, change in respiratory and heart rates) in relation to sound and compares them with sound free periods. Auditory brain stem evoked responses (BSER) measure electrical activity in the brain in response to sound. Oto-acoustic emissions measure sound reflected from the normally functioning cochlea. All these methods require complex equipment and are time consuming. The best method or combination of methods still has to be established. Any child with normal findings on neonatal testing should be reassessed later in the first year of life because some hearing losses are progressive and may not be apparent in the neonatal period

Parental clues lists

It is often stressed that we should listen to what parents say about their child – they are usually right. This is certainly true of deafness. If this is supplemented by giving parents information on what to look out for, it may be one of the best ways of identifying deafness. This is now well established in many Health Authorities, using *Hints for Parents* given to parents soon after birth with an explanation of how to use it. Parental questionnaires later in the first year of life may give additional information helping to focus screening on high risk children.

Distraction testing

This is commonly used as a screen at 6–8 months and can be used for testing up to about 18 months. Two testers are needed – one to sit in front of the child and hold the child's attention and one to be behind the child and present the sounds at the appropriate time. The child should be able to sit steadily on the parent's knee and be able to turn the head to either side. The tester in front attracts the child's attention to an object, then removes or covers the object; at just the right moment the tester behind will present the test sound sometimes to one side, sometimes to the other. The child should turn towards the sound. The test sound should be presented at 35 dB (very quiet). Warble tones of known frequencies and intensity can be used (e.g. a Meg warbler) or minimal voice ('ooh ooh' or humming for low tone, 'ss ss' for high tone) or a Manchester rattle turned very gently for high tone.

Hints for parents (produced by Dr Barry McCormick, Nottingham Hearing Services Centre)

CAN YOUR BABY HEAR YOU?
Here is a checklist of some of the signs you can look for in your baby's first year:

Tick if
response
present

Shortly after birth
Your baby should be startled by a sudden loud noise and he should blink or open his eyes widely to such sounds.

☐

By 1 month
He should show the additional response of becoming still if you make a sudden prolonged sound.

☐

By 3 months
He should quieten or smile to the sound of your voice even when he cannot see you. He may also turn his head or eyes towards you if you come up from behind and speak to him from the side.

☐

By 6 months
He should turn immediately to your voice across the room or to very quiet noises made on each side.

☐

By 9 months
He should listen attentively to familiar everyday sounds and search for very quiet sounds made out of sight. He should also show pleasure in babbling loudly and tunefully.

☐

By 12 months
He should show some response to his own name and to other familiar words. He may also respond to 'no' and 'bye bye'.

☐

IF YOU SUSPECT THAT YOUR BABY IS NOT HEARING NORMALLY EITHER BECAUSE YOU CANNOT PLACE A DEFINITE TICK AGAINST THE ITEMS ABOVE OR FOR SOME OTHER REASON THEN CONTACT YOUR HEALTH VISITOR FOR ADVICE. SHE WILL PERFORM A SIMPLE HEARING SCREENING TEST ON YOUR BABY BETWEEN SEVEN AND NINE MONTHS OF AGE AND WILL BE ABLE TO HELP AND ADVISE YOU AT ANY TIME IF YOU ARE CONCERNED ABOUT YOUR BABY AND HIS DEVELOPMENT.

Although simple in concept, skill is required in carrying out the tests correctly. Attention to detail is most important.Children with a hearing loss are often very alert to other clues and appear to pass the test. These clues may be auditory (e.g. creaking floorboards, tester's movements) visual (e.g. shadows, tester's hands coming into view) or olfactory (e.g. perfume worn by the tester). Children may wrongly fail the test if their attention is too fixed in front or if not developmentally ready for the test. However if testers are properly trained the distraction test can be very effective.

The age range of the test can be extended by using visual reinforcement – the child receives a visual reward on turning to the correct source of the sound.

Cooperative testing

Testing between 18 and 30 months is perhaps the most difficult. The child will often no longer respond to distraction testing and is not yet mature enough to understand performance testing. From about 18 months of age if the child's language is developing reasonably well, they may respond to cooperative testing. Simple instructions ('Give it to mummy', 'give it to teddy', 'give it to dolly') are used with a quiet voice without the aid of lip-reading. The words must have the same rhythm or the child will guess. It is hard to get a child of this age to concentrate at minimal voice.

Performance tests

These can be carried out from about 24–30 months. The child is conditioned to perform a task (e.g. placing a brick in a box) at the command 'go'. Once the child is conditioned, the tester can reduce the test sound down to threshold level, making sure that there are no visual clues to the sound being made and that the interval between sounds is varied. 'Go' tests low frequency if the 'g' is not stressed too much. Other sounds are then used such as 'ss', warble tones or even pure tones.

Speech discrimination

This test involves the child identifying objects or pictures by name. The words used are chosen so that the sounds may be easily confused, e.g. 'house' and 'cow', 'man' and 'lamb', 'chick' and 'fish'. The words are monosyllabic so that the rhythm of the word does not give a clue. It is necessary to check that the words are within the child's vocabulary. The McCormick Toy Discrimination Test uses objects normally within a young child's vocabulary. It is therefore applicable for use with the younger age group. The Reed test uses sets of pictures and is designed for use in school age children. Children with normal hearing should be able to distinguish between all the test items at a listening level of 40 dB.

Pure tone audiometry

The commonest screening test used at 4–6 years is sweep audiometry. This tests the child's ability to hear sounds at a set level (20, 25 or 30 dB are most commonly used) across the main speech frequencies (generally 500 Hz–4 kHz). More detailed audiometric testing can be used when there is concern about the hearing.

Measurement of hearing

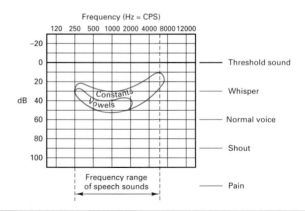

Standard procedures for audiometry have been recommended by the British Society of Audiology and the British Association of Otolaryngology and training is required to carry out the test adequately. Testing should be in a quiet environment; this is often hard to achieve and acoustic cups over the ear pieces helps to cut out background noise. Giving the child a task to do (e.g. putting pegs in a board) when they hear the noise can help with concentration.

Tympanometry

This is a test of middle ear pathology rather than hearing. However since the commonest cause of hearing loss is middle ear disease, this is sometimes used for screening. It is relatively simple to do and requires a minimum of cooperation from the child, so can be used at any age. Unless combined with a test of **hearing**, it will not pick up children with a sensori-neural loss.

Sound is most readily transmitted across the tympanic membrane when it is most compliant which is when the pressure is equal on both sides. A sound is passed into the ear and the amount of sound reflected back is measured. By varying the pressure in the external auditory canal and measuring the reflected sounds at different pressures, the pressure in the middle ear can be inferred from the point at which least sound reflected. In a normal ear, this is at atmospheric pressure. With serous otitis media compliance is reduced at all pressures because of the presence of fluid in the middle ear; this gives rise to a flattened curve. With an obstructed Eustachian tube the pressure in the middle ear is reduced and maximum compliance of the tympanic membrane is at negative pressure.

Tympanometry findings

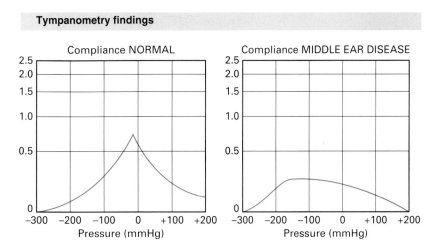

Compliance NORMAL — Pressure (mmHg)

Compliance MIDDLE EAR DISEASE — Pressure (mmHg)

Electrophysiological testing. These are objective methods of testing for an intact auditory system of which brain stem evoked responses (BSER) is the method most frequently used. It is particularly useful in babies and children who are difficult to test by other methods. Some children need to be sedated for the test. Although useful as an objective test it does not give as much information as the subjective tests because they also measure the child's **response** to sound and can be more frequency specific.

ASSESSMENT OF A CHILD WITH SENSORI-NEURAL DEAFNESS

This should be undertaken by a specialist team.

Audiological and otological assessments need to be carried out to determine as far as possible the degree and type of deafness. In a young child this can be difficult; it may be necessary to give provisional estimates and be prepared to revise them later.

General paediatric assessment should be carried out looking for associated problems and any clues as to the cause of the deafness. Overall development should be assessed as this will affect management; many tests of development are heavily weighted towards verbal items thus putting a deaf child at a disadvantage. Assessment of vision is particularly important not only because visual problems are more common, but because the deaf child will rely heavily on their vision for communication and it is particularly important that any of the common visual problems be detected and treated early. There may be indications from the history or examination of a cause of the deafness. This may not affect management of the child significantly, but parents are anxious to know the cause, particularly if it may be inherited. Unless the cause is known the family should be referred for genetic counselling. Investigations, such as viral antibodies, urinanalysis, thyroid antibodies, ECG, CAT scan, are sometimes carried out.

Parents need opportunities to discuss the diagnosis of deafness and its significance. The diagnosis may have come as an unexpected blow, or as a relief that someone finally believed them.

Language and educational assessment. A speech therapist and teacher of the deaf will normally be involved at an early stage. This will provide a useful source of counselling and parents will be anxious to know what they can do to help the child. The educational psychologist will need to see the child at the stage that formal education is first being considered.

HEARING AIDS

It is important to emphasise that hearing aids will not restore the hearing to normal. It is particularly hard to amplify high tones effectively. Where a severe or profound hearing loss is suspected, miniature post aural aids can be fitted from a few months of age. Use of hearing aids from this young age is likely to give the best chance of developing speech and aids may be accepted better.

Post aural aids are most commonly used and there are many different types available. Many severely deaf children require commercially available hearing aids in order to get the power and complexity needed. Tailoring a particular hearing aid to a particular child is a highly specialised field. Radio aids are also used, and are particularly useful in the classroom; the teacher wears a microphone, her voice is picked up by the child's receiver and fed into the hearing aid. This cuts out a lot of the problem with background noise. Radio aids are also useful at home with young children, because the parent can wear the microphone and keep in touch with the child more easily when out of visual contact.

Two hearing aids are normally issued, unless there is only a mild loss or a very marked difference between the two ears. Binaural hearing levels are better and localisation of sound is better. Ear moulds need to fit well so that the volume can be turned up sufficiently without causing whistling from feedback. In infancy this can cause considerable difficulties; the child's ear is growing so fast that unless there is an efficient service, by the time one set of ear moulds are ready the child may have grown out of them.

A few profoundly deaf children gain little benefit from conventional hearing aids. Vibrotactile aids may give some benefit; these are worn on the wrist and cause vibration in response to sound. The information given is limited but does alert the child to look for the source of sound.

The development of cochlear implants has given new hope to the most profoundly deaf children. At present they are being used primarily in children who have become totally deafened after learning to speak (e.g. post meningitis). The indications for use are likely to widen as experience is gained. They can be intracochlear where up to 20 electrodes are inserted into the cochlea through the middle ear, or extracochlear where electrodes are placed on the surface of the cochlea. The electrodes are attached to a receiver placed under the skin behind the pinna. The child wears a microphone which picks up sound and transmits it to the receiver. As with any hearing aid the hearing is not restored to normal, but encouraging results are being obtained.

Management of unilateral loss. This is clearly less of a disability than bilateral loss, but should not be ignored. Overall hearing levels are slightly reduced and localisation of sound is affected. If the better ear develops serous otitis media or is blocked with wax, the child can become significantly disabled. Hearing may be totally lost in one ear (a dead ear). Hearing aids are unlikely to help because the distorted amplification in that ear is so inferior to the quality of hearing in the hearing ear that it provides no benefit. The most important thing is for the child, parents and teachers to be aware of the problem and position themselves accordingly.

COMMUNICATION METHODS

Management of the deaf child has long been divided into the oral and manual schools of thought. Those advocating an oral/aural approach may argue that, however deaf, children can learn to speak and understand speech, that speech is the only way that they will integrate into the hearing world and that learning to sign will inhibit speech development. Those in favour of manual methods consider that deaf people have a right to learn their own language (sign language e.g. British Sign Language or BSL) as their first language and that this will enable them to communicate most fluently and effectively. Many now see a place for both in the education of deaf children depending on the severity of the hearing loss and the progress of the child. Total communication (a combination of speech, signs, lip reading, gesture and body language) is now more often used as a way of maximising communication and enabling a child to learn the value of language and may be a more effective way of teaching speech.

EDUCATIONAL PROVISION

A severe hearing impairment poses particular difficulties in education. Deaf children not only find it hard to learn to speak but also find it hard to learn to read and write because they have not acquired the necessary language. Spoken or written language is fundamental to **most** parts of the curriculum.

A variety of resources may be available for education of the hearing impaired child. More children are now able to be educated in their local mainstream school because of earlier diagnosis, better amplification and more help within the schools. Teachers of the deaf will support some of these children within the ordinary classroom. There may be a unit for hearing impaired children attached to a mainstream school; there is a

Disability associated with various degrees of deafness

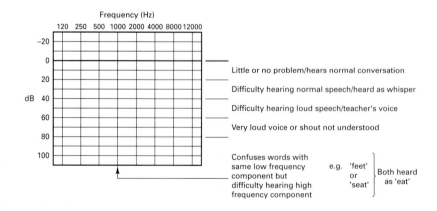

teacher of the deaf in the unit to support the children, but they will spend a variable amount of time in the ordinary classroom. Special schools for hearing impaired children cater for the most severely impaired children, but there should still be encouragement to integrate with hearing children in a local school for some of the time.

It is important that teachers who have a hearing impaired child in their class are aware of the sorts of problems that may arise and how they can be overcome.

A check list for those concerned with teaching deaf children

- the child should sit in a front seat with the better ear directed towards the teacher if there is deafness in one ear only.
- the child should be able to watch the face of the teacher whilst she is talking to the class, and the teacher should try and face the child when important instructions are being given;
- the teacher should try to avoid talking with her back to the class;
- the child should be allowed to turn round to see the faces of other children participating in class discussions;
- it is not necessary for the teacher to shout or use exaggerated lip movements;
- the teacher must be aware of the increased concentration required of the hearing impaired child to understand speech;
- the child must be encouraged to participate in all activities involving language and be a full member of the class;
- the teacher must be aware of the hazards that face the deaf child from teasing from the other children in the class;
- if the child has a hearing aid, it is necessary for it to be checked each day;
- there are some situations where the deaf child is particularly at risk, such as during games and on the road;
- where there is a high tone loss the child may appear to hear but will get things wrong because they do not hear accurately;
- any special attention given to a deaf child should be handled as unobtrusively as possible.

MANAGEMENT OF CONDUCTIVE HEARING LOSS

Many children have brief episodes of conductive hearing loss which may pass unnoticed and not require any treatment. However, persistent mild losses or frequent intermittent losses do cause problems. Nearly all hearing losses from serous otitis media will resolve spontaneously in time, but difficulties may arise while waiting for it to get better.

The most important aspect of management is making the appropriate people aware of the problem. If the parents understand the problem, they can compensate to some extent by getting the child to look at them when they speak, raising their voice a little, checking comprehension. It is also important that teachers are aware when the child's hearing is reduced.

Medical management of serous otitis media appears to have little to offer. Anecdotally some children are said to respond to a variety of medicines, such as decongestants and antihistamines. Some people advocate a prolonged course of an antibiotic because organisms can be cultured from aspirates of middle ear effusions. Co-trimoxazole for six weeks is often used.

Surgical management for serous otitis media is much debated. There is little doubt that many children get temporary improvement in hearing with myringotomy and adenoidectomy with or without grommets. Long term there is little if any improvement in hearing over and above untreated ears, but short term improvement may be of great value in young children. Occasional congenital abnormalities of the middle ear are amenable to surgery.

Hearing aids are better at correcting conductive hearing losses than sensori-neural losses. Congenital abnormalities can often be helped considerably by hearing aids. If there is an abnormal pinna there may be difficulty keeping the aid on and if there is an atretic canal there is nowhere to insert the mould; bone conduction aids can help in this situation. Surgery to the pinna and canal may help and ear prostheses with or without an implanted receiver have developed considerably in recent years.

Hearing loss from serous otitis media can also be helped by a hearing aid, either when repeated surgery has failed, is difficult or inadvisable, or while awaiting surgery. Children with Down's syndrome often have glue ear, but surgery is difficult and they may benefit from hearing aids. Down's syndrome children also may develop a sensori-neural hearing loss.

Glue ear and language

There is uncertainty about the relationship between glue ear in early childhood and the development of language and later school performance. Researchers have felt there must be a link but it has been hard to find. A recent big study from Dunedin, New Zealand has demonstrated an association. It is likely that the multiplicity of factors that go into determining progress in language and at school has confounded much of the research. A likely picture is that: a bright child from a family where a lot of language is used, can get intermittent deafness without their language being affected, because the hearing loss is compensated for; a less bright child, in a family who use limited language, with the same hearing loss, may have difficulty learning language, but with normal hearing would have managed all right. This means that every child with glue ear needs assessment individually and decisions on management should take into account these other factors.

REFERENCES AND FURTHER READING

Chalmers D, Stewart I, Silva P, Milner A 1989 The Dunedin study. Clinics in Developmental Medicine. Mackeith Press, Blackwell Scientific, Oxford
Haggard M P 1990 Hearing screening in children – state of the art(s). Archives of Disease in Childhood 65: 1193
Haggard M P, Pullan C R 1989 Staffing and structure for paediatric audiology services in hospital and community units. British Journal of Audiology 23: 99–116
McCornick B 1988 Paediatric audiology 0–5 years. Taylor & Francis, London
Tweedle J 1987 Children's hearing problems: their significance, detection and management. John Wright, Bristol

22 Language

Associated problems

	Incidence (× expected)
Non-readers	× 12
Poor number work	× 9
Poor design copying	× 8
Behaviour problems	× 4
Clumsiness	× 3
Impaired visual acuity	× 3

Language is probably the most highly developed of all human skills. Large parts of the brain are involved with speech, sound production, understanding speech and coding ideas into language. Language is required as a vehicle for thought and to convey ideas. Inner language enables us to think through, rather than act out, problems and outer language enables expression of feelings.

The table shows just how common severe speech disorders are, as found in the 7 year olds studied in the National Child Development Study. At age 5 at school entry approximately 5% of children were recorded as unintelligible. Children with language problems also had a high incidence of associated educational difficulties. Of those with marked speech defects, 38% had emotional problems. Boys were twice as common as girls, they were more likely to be preterm, younger children of large families and from social classes IV and V.

Epidemiology of speech disorders in 7 year olds (from the National Child Development Study)		
Intelligibility	Difficult to understand (%)	Many or all words unintelligible (%)
Teachers' reports	10.7	2.4
Doctors' reports	13.5	1.4

Children with delays in development of spoken language will also be delayed in acquiring the written form, as children normally read or write with an understanding of those words that they have already acquired in the spoken form. A cycle has been described of children with delayed language leading to delayed reading and writing, cutting the child off from gaining satisfaction in his schooling and leading to truancy in the early secondary school.

Skills required for spoken language

It is quite remarkable how young children learn to distinguish a wide range of sounds in their environment, to imitate them, to attach meaning to them and to put them together into recognised grammatical constructions. We have only to recognise the difficulties that adults have in learning languages with a different vocabulary and grammatical structure. All the skills are dependent upon intact sensory and motor systems, upon the integration of these systems, and upon complex co-ordination of motor activity in speech sound production. The child also must have listening skills and an understanding of gestures and symbols from cues such as toys and pictures. This whole collection of skills needs to be supported by appropriate intellectual development, the will to communicate and an environment in which the necessary opportunities for language acquisition are available.

Skills required for spoken language

- Hearing: to listen to others, to monitor one's own voice
- Auditory discrimination: to recognise (centrally) the difference between sounds
- Phonology: the ability to produce these sounds
- Semantics: the ability to ascribe meaning to patterns of sound that are remembered (vocabulary)
- Grammar: the ability to use words within a framework of knowledge that modifies the ending of the word according to use, e.g. tense (morphology) and constructs sentences according to particular rules, e.g. word order
- Encoding: translating objects, actions, etc, into the words that symbolise them
- Decoding: the ability to relate the spoken word to the object or action for which it is a symbol

---

Normal language development

Some of the major milestones in language development are shown in the accompanying diagram. The diagram is an over-simplification of a complex development of skills.

Development for speech

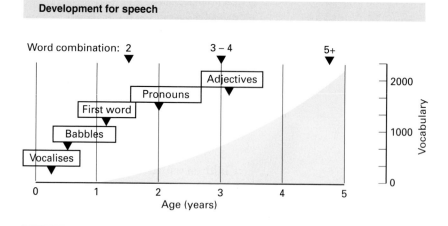

The newborn is not only able to hear but also has some ability to discriminate sound. The baby's cry is not a single uniform ability. Mothers learn very quickly to distinguish the cries of their baby from cries of other babies in the hospital and to know which cries mean anger and frustration. Within the first few weeks a baby will start to 'coo' in response to a parent; 'conversations' take place with alternating parent and baby vocal contribution and parents describe their babies 'talking to them'. The baby rapidly develops a whole range of vocalisations, glugs, grunts, laughs, in response to the appropriate situations.

In the first year the baby learns to discriminate sounds and in his babble practises them. The number of sounds that the child produces rapidly increases but some sounds such as 'th' may not be produced until the child is 5 or older. Vowel sounds develop first, then the back consonants such as 'g' followed by the lip and tongue consonants such as 'b'. In the first year of life comprehension of words must develop before there can be meaningful expressive language. At first the child can only understand the words when there are clues as to the context in which the word is used. The child then proceeds to reflex labelling of the object when the object is in sight. Blind children may have some language delay at this stage because of the importance of seeing the object to relate it to the spoken word.

Later the child acquires the proper meaning of the word in that the word is internalised as a symbol for the object. He may then use the word as a means of acquiring the object, e.g. 'drink', 'biscuit'. At first words have very narrow meanings, for example dog may mean the dog present in the household, though the meaning will gradually widen possibly to include all animals, but then just to include all species of dogs, toy dogs, models of dogs, pictures of dogs. The first meaningful words appear on average at the age of 1 year though with a very wide range of normal.

Between 18 months and 2 years most children will be saying simple two word combinations. These are usually of the noun-pivot type in which a small series of pivot words such as 'bye-bye', can be linked to a wider number of nouns, such as 'daddy bye-bye', 'milk bye-bye'. Sentences gradually increase in length and other parts of speech, adjectives, adverbs, pronouns, are introduced. Word length and intelligibility also increase. The child will want to listen to increasingly complex speech such as nursery rhymes and stories, and develops quite an amazing memory, frequently having verbatim knowledge of fairly long stories. Language is increasingly used in play in which children animate their toys and converse with them. However most of the speaking of young children in play is a monologue rather than an attempt to communicate. Language is increasingly used in the pre-school child to ask questions, initially of the 'what' variety but by 3 years extending to the 'where' and 'who' variety and at 4 the 'why' variety.

TYPES OF ABNORMAL LANGUAGE DEVELOPMENT

Language disorders fall into several categories. The most common is delay in language development with the speech produced resembling that of a younger child. Other children have language development that is deviant and abnormalities of structure and word combination occur which are not typically found in the speech of younger children. In another group, children have problems with the intelligibility of their speech with or without associated abnormality in the content of the speech. All aspects of language must be assessed separately using procedures such as the Reynell Developmental Language Scales and the Edinburgh Articulation Test, for comprehension, expression and articulation may be affected to different degrees.

Stammering is a particular type of speech disorder where there is a lack of fluency. It is a very common finding in pre-school children at the stage when there is a rapid expansion of vocabulary and increase in sentence length. Persistent stammering occurs in about 4% of children. The development of the stammer goes through several well defined stages. Initially there is simply repetition of initial speech sounds, and these increase in frequency with the prolongation of sounds, hesitation and blocking, in which speech completely stops. Associated with blocking there may be grimacing movements of the face. As the stammer develops, hesitation and blocking become more severe and the problem becomes one of absence of speech rather than the initial repetition. Particular words which are apt to set off the stammer are specifically avoided. The stammer becomes an increasing handicap in terms of oral work in the classroom and social relationships outside the classroom. It obstructs any form of employment in which communication with the public is essential. Stammering can be a source of great unhappiness and worry. Other children can be particularly unkind.

Differential diagnosis

Many children have no obvious cause for their language problem and some will simply be at the extreme end of the normal range.

General delay. Late talking is a common presentation of general delay. It is important that a general assessment of ability is carried out because management in a generally delayed child will be directed to overall improvement in skills. However even if there is some general delay, the language may be delayed over and above that of the rest of the development or be deviant, which would warrant specific intervention for this. Children with Fragile X syndrome often have specific language problems in addition to the delayed development.

Hearing loss. A child with a known severe hearing loss will be anticipated to have difficulty with speech. In the past, even severe deafness was often picked up because of failure to speak. We would now hope that these children are identified earlier but still some children slip through. Other children with mild, moderate, intermittent or high tone loss may not be identified at early screening. These children often present with speech problems. Those with a high tone loss are a particularly difficult group because they will hear very quiet sounds and it is hard to convince their parents that there is a hearing problem. But, although they will hear speech, the high tones (elements of the consonants) will be missing and speech will have little meaning to the child. All children with language problems should therefore have a good hearing assessment including high tones.

Environment. It is hard to know how much the lack of a stimulating language environment has on the development of language. There are well documented anecdotes of children growing up totally isolated from speech, and it is not surprising that they develop no speech. However most children growing up in homes with relatively little speech (e.g. profoundly deaf parents) acquire speech satisfactorily, presumably from relatives, friends and neighbours. Most children from socially deprived environments with little conversation also develop adequate speech, though this is a group at risk of having delayed language development. This may be because of lack of input in a child who is linguistically vulnerable, but there could be an element of heredity. Expressive language is often more delayed than comprehension.

CNS damage. In view of its complex nature, it might be expected that language would often be affected by CNS insults but it is rare to have isolated language problems following birth asphyxia, meningitis, or encephalitis. Although speech is normally an activity involving the right side of the brain, the young brain is highly adaptable and can use other areas not normally used for this function if that part is damaged. Acquired aphasia with fits (the Landau Kleffner syndrome) is an example of a specific language problem with what is presumably a CNS disorder. Degenerative disorders in the older child may present with a speech problem.

Specific language disorders. This is a diagnosis made by exclusion of other factors, but there are some special characteristics. Deviant language often falls into this group. There may be associated neurological problems, e.g. clumsiness, epilepsy. Boys are 4 times more affected than girls and there is often a family history of language difficulty. The cause is not known.

Psychiatric disorders. Language disorder is a characteristic presentation of autism. The child may appear to be deaf. Speech may have started to develop but is then lost at the age of 18 months to 2 years.

Elective mutism is a strange disorder that frustrates professionals. The child is reported to have normal language at home and the parents may tape it to prove this. In a social situation the child does not speak at all or if he does it is in a very quiet voice, and maybe via another child rather than an adult.

DISORDERS OF ARTICULATION

The child may develop normal language. Some of these conditions are congenital and some acquired.

Structural defects. Tongue abnormalities either congenital hypoplasia (small immobile tongue) or macroglossia in Hurler's syndrome, Down's syndrome, Beckwith's syndrome can causes problems. Tongue tie is virtually never a cause of speech problems. A cleft palate is often associated with hearing loss, but also causes abnormalities of the speech because of nasal escape of air and immobility of the palate. Palatal disproportion and submucous cleft of the palate are less obvious but can cause similar problems.

Muscular defects such as myotonic dystrophy, fascio-scapulo-humeral dystrophy and myasthenia gravis may present with speech difficulties.

Neurogical defects such as cerebral palsy may be associated with problems in articulation; spasticity of tongue, lips and palate gives rise to slow laborious speech, feeding problems and drooling; involuntary movements and incoordination also affect speech. An isolated bulbar palsy may present as a feeding or speech problem. Articulatory dyspraxia is a familial disorder causing incoordination of speech organs. Nuclear agenesis (failure of development of the cranial nerve nuclei) causes lower motor neurone problems.

ASSESSMENT

There are a number of screening tests or guidelines for identifying children with language disorders. They tend to be complex and quite time consuming. In early life enquiry about the major milestones and talking and listening to the child will usually reassure that language is developing normally. Doctors seeing a child in the clinic or surgery have particular difficulty here, because the command from a parent to 'speak for the doctor' is almost certain to ensure that no speech is heard. Parents' description of their child's language can be misleading; reports of comprehension of speech may in fact be comprehension of gesture or situation; reports of combining two words may be phrases that the child understands as a single word e.g. 'sit down'; parents will understand poor intelligibility because they are used to it. If there is concern about language development, an assessment of all aspects of language (not just speech) is required.

Concentration. Children with language disorders often have very poor concentration. They will flit from one thing to another and it is hard to

Language development

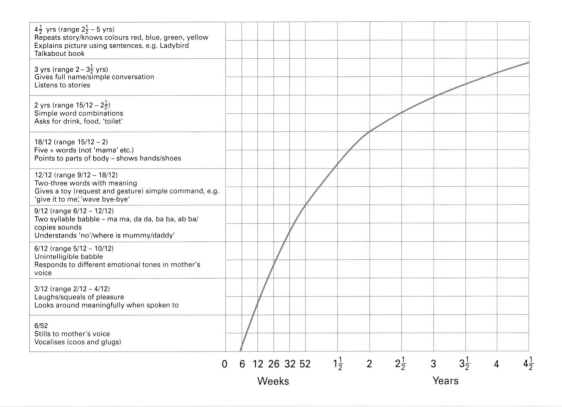

$4\frac{1}{2}$ yrs (range $2\frac{1}{2}$ – 5 yrs)
Repeats story/knows colours red, blue, green, yellow
Explains picture using sentences, e.g. Ladybird
Talkabout book

3 yrs (range 2 – $3\frac{1}{2}$ yrs)
Gives full name/simple conversation
Listens to stories

2 yrs (range 15/12 – $2\frac{1}{2}$)
Simple word combinations
Asks for drink, food, 'toilet'

18/12 (range 15/12 – 2)
Five + words (not 'mama' etc.)
Points to parts of body – shows hands/shoes

12/12 (range 9/12 – 18/12)
Two-three words with meaning
Gives a toy (request and gesture) simple command, e.g.
'give it to me', 'wave bye-bye'

9/12 (range 6/12 – 12/12)
Two syllable babble – ma ma, da da, ba ba, ab ba/
copies sounds
Understands 'no'/where is mummy/daddy'

6/12 (range 5/12 – 10/12)
Unintelligible babble
Responds to different emotional tones in mother's
voice

3/12 (range 2/12 – 4/12)
Laughs/squeals of pleasure
Looks around meaningfully when spoken to

6/52
Stills to mother's voice
Vocalises (coos and glugs)

0   6   12 26 32 52 $1\frac{1}{2}$ 2 $2\frac{1}{2}$ 3 $3\frac{1}{2}$ 4 $4\frac{1}{2}$

Weeks   Years

10% of children below their 'developmental step' require further investigation.

engage them in an activity. If concentration is poor, this area needs addressing before any work can be done on language.

Inner language. The first stage that a child must go through is the understanding of symbols, e.g. that a cup means a drink, that you can pretend to give teddy a drink, that miniature toys and pictures represent real things. This will be delayed in general delayed development, but not deafness.

Comprehension. Understanding of speech must come before you can use it effectively. Initially this is of names of objects 'where's the *cup*?', then linking two objects 'put the *spoon* in the *cup*', then three or four words together 'put the *spoon under* the *cup*', 'put the *spoon behind* the *blue cup*'. Only the words in italics are being tested (spoons normally go in cups, so comprehension of the word 'in' is not being tested). You also need a choice for the spoon and for the cup (if you give a child a cup and a spoon, there is a high chance he will put the spoon in the cup whatever you say).

Expression. Initially this will be naming objects, then pictures. Getting an older child to look at a book or play a game may produce more complex language, but you need to be alert to listening in on conversations between child and parent. Beware the child who has a wide range of 'cocktail party' conversation – they have learnt a lot of set phrases, but when you probe more deeply, the comprehension of language is poor. This occurs typically with hydrocephalus.

Articulation. Some sounds are naturally acquired later than others e.g. 'r', 'th', and particularly consonant clusters e.g. 'str' spl'. With most delayed but normally progressing articulation, reassurance can be given. Deviant articulation needs addressing.

Semantic and pragmatic areas. This covers the use of language in a more complex way i.e. grammar (word endings etc.), word order ('John hit Mary' has a different meaning from 'Mary hit John'), conversational arts (turn taking, empathy). These may be lacking in children with specific language disorders.

Any more complex assessment of the language itself should be done by a speech therapist. There are a number of tests that they can use to assess different aspects. The Reynell Development Language Scale is one commonly used and covers children from 6 months to 6 years. It gives a score for comprehension and expression which can be recorded as an age equivalent score. If the child's first language is not English, it is important that an assessment in the first language is done if possible.

An important part of the paediatric assessment is establishing any associated problems and possible causes (as much to reassure the parents of a lack of association with, say, a forceps delivery, as to find a cause). This means taking a history looking particularly at birth history, feeding difficulties, serious illnesses, otitis media. Family history may reveal family members with similar problems; family history of learning difficulties or hearing problems may also be relevant. Assessment of general development is important in looking for possible causes of the language problem as well as considering management. A general examination of the child should reveal any associated handicaps of which clumsiness is the most common. It should include a search for dysmorphic features which may suggest a particular syndrome. Examination of the mouth is particularly important if there is an articulation problem. Investigation should include a hearing test, but other investigations only when specifically indicated (e.g. chromosome analysis for Fragile X).

MANAGEMENT

For many young children where language is delayed rather than deviant, a period of observation to establish normal progress is all that is required. Parents can be encouraged to talk naturally with the child rather than trying to teach the child words.

Speech therapy is the mainstay of management for language disorders. Some have changed their name to 'language therapists', to indicate that they do more than teach children to speak. Parents sometimes get frustrated that the speech therapist is not 'teaching their child to speak', but helping attention control and understanding of language are vital first steps for many children. Speech therapists are investigating a variety of different ways to help children other than individual therapy. Language groups and short bursts of intensive (daily) therapy are methods being used that may be more effective as well as more efficient ways of using speech therapy time.

Many children with language disorders get into Day Nurseries, particularly those with socially deprived backgrounds; nursery nurse training includes language development through play and many of these children may benefit simply by being in a linguistically rich environment. Nurseries may have a speech therapist visiting to see individual children or to work out language programmes for nursery nurses to use with specific children or to advise generally on helping children with language problems.

For children with severe articulation problems there are devices to help with visual feedback on speech sounds produced. These can be helpful with the older child.

With fluency problems below the age of 8 years treatment is not required and parents should be recommended to avoid correcting the child. Drawing the child's attention to the stutter is likely to exacerbate it rather than improve it. Older children may benefit from intensive courses using the technique of the syllable timed speech in which a regular unaltering rhythm is imposed. Cutting out auditory feedback of the child's own voice also helps stuttering.

Education

For many children their problems will have largely resolved by school age or soon after. However some of the children will go on to have reading and writing problems. The language problems may continue to be sufficiently severe to interfere with normal education. These children will need additional help within school, which may be provided by a unit specifically for language disordered children. Specialist teachers and speech therapists will work with the children in school, but there will be opportunities for integration into mainstream classes. There are a small number of special schools for children with the most severe problems. Many of the children will have improved sufficiently by secondary school age to integrate into mainstream school though they may need continuing support. A very small but significant number of children have such severe problems that they fail to learn even socially useful speech.

Alternative communication methods. Those with severe language problems, mental retardation or severe motor problems affecting speech may need to rely on alternative methods of communication. For those with isolated severe language problems, Paget Gorman is a signing system designed to help with English language development, because it is structured like English and builds up ideas and words in the same way. The problem with Paget Gorman is that very few people use it, so in those where spoken language does not develop adequately, opportunities for communication are limited. Some language disordered people learn British Sign Language, so that they can communicate within the deaf community.

Makaton is the signing system used with children with severe learning difficulties and some with physical disabilities. This is a signing system based on the signs in British Sign Language, but has limited vocabulary.

Bliss symbolics is an alternative communication system, particularly useful for people with severe physical disabilities.

Computer assisted communication is a developing area and has great potential for helping children with severe speech problems, though the system must be carefully chosen to help with a particular child's needs.

Voluntary agencies

The main national organisation in the UK involved with language disorders is the Association for all Speech Impaired Children (AFASIC). They have a regular newsletter, advice centre and some local branches. They are also involved in providing courses for parents and professionals and helping research. There may be other local groups set up to support families of a child with a language disability. Failure to communicate adequately is such a pervasive and frustrating disability that parents welcome the opportunity to link up with others in a similar situation.

REFERENCES AND FURTHER READING

Bath D 1982 Developing the speech therapy service in day nurseries: a progress report. British Journal of Disorders in Communication 16: 159–173
Bishop D, Mogford K 1988 Language development in exceptional circumstances. Churchill Livingstone, Edinburgh
Butler N R, Peckham C, Sheridan M 1973 Speech defects in children aged 7: a national study. British Medical Journal 1: 253–257
Cooper J, Moodley M, Reynell J 1978 Helping language development. Edward Arnold, London
Gilham W 1978 First words language programme. Allen and Unwin, London
Jeffree D, McCorkey R 1976 Let me speak. Souvenir Press, London
Reynell J 1980 Language development and assessment. MTP Press, London
Rutter M, Martin A 1972 The child with delayed speech. Clinics in Developmental Medicine no. 43. Heinemann Medical, London

23 Learning and Health

Educational medicine is concerned with the different ways that health and education interact. In its crudest sense, it involves the general fitness of children to receive education and in its more sophisticated sense, it is concerned with the ways particular health problems or disabilities produce learning difficulties. Achievement or failure to achieve, results from a complex mix of individual, medical, social and educational factors. No one professional group has the monopoly of knowledge and no one group can function effectively without an understanding of these multidisciplinary aspects. Paediatricians, teachers and social workers are all experts on children, but see childhood from different perspectives. It is important to understand these differing professional views, but also to resist straying too far into areas where we lack training and authority.

The presence of learning difficulties and their implications also have large emotional overlays for parents and children. The involvement of the community paediatrician may raise expectations from parents, children and teachers that we may be unable to meet. Parents may look for a medical cause and also a medical cure; teachers may be looking for practical medical advice; children may just want to feel better about themselves as they become conscious of their learning difficulties. Involvement of the paediatrician should, therefore, start with a discussion of the 'problem' as perceived by parents, children and teachers, their expectations of the paediatrician (and of the child) and of their feelings about the learning difficulties.

This chapter will discuss three aspects of educational medicine:
(1) general factors affecting learning
(2) the effects of illness on learning
(3) specific learning disorders

FACTORS AFFECTING LEARNING

The school

Children spend at least ten years of their life at school and it would be surprising if the quality and content of this experience did not have some, if not a major effect upon their behaviour, academic attainment and success in adult life. Rutter (1979) in '15 000 hours', studied the intake of 12 London comprehensive schools in 1970, comparing assessments at age 10 in primary school with those at age 14 and examination results at age 16. They showed that children did much better in some schools than in others, and that these differences could not be explained by differences in their intake. For example, the intake of one school contained 31% of children with behaviour problems, which was reduced to 10% by the age of 14. In another school the intake contained 34% of children with behaviour problems, which had risen to 48% by the age of 14. The type of school which produced best results largely followed the model of firm and consistent discipline, high academic standards, homework, school uniform and a wide range of extra-curricular activities in which children could engage and take responsibility. Other characteristics such as modern buildings and facilities were not shown to be important factors.

The pastoral side of education in both primary and secondary schools can do much to compensate for adverse social circumstances and to supplement the positive influences of family life. Indeed the hallmark of many successful schools is that they not only influence their children, but that they also influence parents and the surrounding community. In return, parents and community can make a great contribution towards the life of the school. The strength of such feeling becomes very evident when the school is deprived of resources or threatened with closure.

Social life

Although the quality of education has an important influence upon educational attainment, social inequality has a very large effect as shown by data from the National Child Development Study (Wedge & Essen 1982, Wedge et al 1973). The reasons for this are diverse and complex, but include such elements as material resources (housing, nutrition), pre-school opportunities for learning, parental and teacher expectations, and parental interest and involvement in their child's education. Among the parents of 11 year olds followed in the National Child Development Study (Wedge et al 1973), neither mother nor father had visited the school of three in every five children in the previous 12 months in the disadvantaged group, compared to only one in three of the other children.

The consequences of early sensory, social and emotional deprivation have been extensively studied. Children brought up in institutions which provided material care, but where emotional needs and stimulation were not provided were found to have poor language development, poor school attainment and an impaired ability to form emotional attachments. The newborn infant fixes on a human face, and, under normal circumstances, this will be reinforced by the mother and thus the child is encouraged to take greater and greater interest. The neglected child becomes apathetic and does not learn the joy of taking an interest in his surroundings. Others will find the world a hostile place and learn to react negatively to contact. Lack of early linguistic stimulation will impair the development of language. Restricted language in turn delays the development of basic reading and writing skills. Such children often

The roots of educational failure

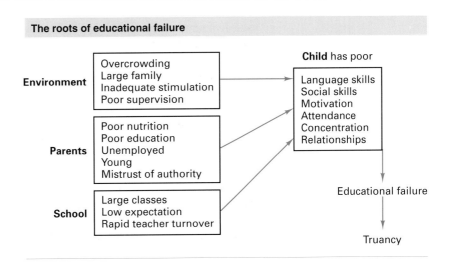

become more aggressive and impulsive and are less able to rationalise and think through conflicts because of lack of inner language. Knowledge of shape, colour, size, texture is needed as a basis for early education and this need may not be met if the child is reared in dull surroundings. Neglected, suppressed children may, at school entry, have little understanding about the sea, mountains, farms, animals which is assumed in some teaching materials designed for children of this age.

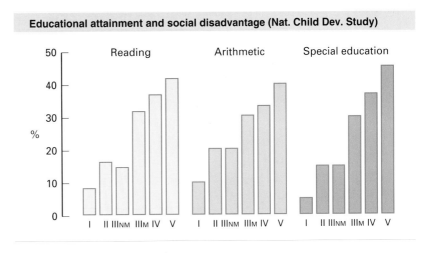

Educational attainment and social disadvantage (Nat. Child Dev. Study)

The ability of a child to succeed in school is determined by a mixture of inhibitory and facilitating factors. They may compensate one another and include such factors as opportunity to receive education, intelligence, temperament, health, disability, social disadvantage or advantage, and quality of teaching. These factors are also not independent of one another so that, for example, social disadvantage may have a negative effect upon health.

Health and well-being   For some children with obvious physical, mental or sensory disability, their learning problems can be explained by a medical diagnosis. However, using the framework of impairment (the medical 'lesion'), disability (the functional consequence of the impairment), and handicap (the limitations in lifestyle and activity that stem from the disability), we can see that like impairments do not produce like disabilities and handicaps. Two children may have identical levels of visual impairment or hearing loss and similar intelligence, yet one may be functioning at the top end of a mainstream school and another may be lacking in basic skills. The importance of the medical diagnosis must not be allowed to hide other factors which have led to a much greater disability arising from a similar level of impairment. Other social and environmental factors may act to prevent, minimise, or increase the disability.

For most children with learning problems in mainstream schools or children with moderate learning difficulties in special schools, there is no spot medical diagnosis, but up to 50% may be found to have a medical condition or risk factors which have contributed towards the learning problem (Lamont & Dennis 1988). For some this may be a single problem such as fragile X, or a conductive hearing loss; for others it may relate to past medical history which led to a prolonged period of ill health and poor school attendance; and for others, it is a combination of problems that might be minor individually, but which collectively are important.

Risk factors in children with moderate learning difficulties (after Lamont & Dennis 1988)

No medical risk factors	58%
Definite medical risk factors:	42%
• prenatal	13%
• perinatal	24%
• postnatal	5%
Possible risk factors	37%
Family history of learning problems (both parents)	51%

POOR SCHOOL PROGRESS

The following scheme is offered as a framework for the medical assessment of children who have been referred because of poor progress in class.

Limited intellect?
(see also Chapter 24)

Poor educational achievement does not always indicate poor educational potential. However, where teachers' and educational psychologists' assessments indicate that one basis is limited intelligence rather than limited opportunity, the paediatrician has a role in its investigation. Errors, of course, can be made and the danger of a medical label that lowers expectations and changes expectations into self-fulfilling predictions must always be borne in mind. Parents may have differing views to those of teachers and psychologists and may have information on their child's strengths and areas of achievement that have not been observed in school, for example in elective mutism. The following questions should be asked.

Is there a specific condition or syndrome associated with mental handicap?

Fragile X would be an important example, affecting 1:10 of boys and 1:22 of girls with moderate learning difficulties. Diagnosis of specific conditions may be helped by the careful recording of a family tree and physical examination for dysmorphic features. Positive identification of a named condition will help in establishing a prognosis, alerts one to look for known associated impairments, provides an explanation for parents and teachers, gives access to medical literature on management and should indicate the often neglected need for genetic counselling. It is easy with such a diagnosis for the child to 'become the syndrome'. The child is *an individual with the syndrome* and we need to remember the large range of individuality in appearance, personality and attainment.

Are there any events in the past medical history which may be the cause of mental handicap?

Some events may be relatively straight forward in providing an explanation, for example a history of congenital infection or head injury. In other cases, it may be much more difficult: for example birth asphyxia may be cited as a cause of cerebral palsy, whereas antenatal and genetic factors are much more likely, perinatal factors accounting for only 8% of cases (Hall 1989).

Perceptual difficulties
(see also Chapters 20–21)

Problems with hearing and vision need to be considered in every child with learning difficulties. In the past, they were sometimes missed (hopefully now a very rare event), particularly where testing is difficult.

VISION? What is the near and distant visual acuity? Are the visual fields full? Assessment of visual fields is not routinely required, though it is important in children with neurological defects, for example cerebral palsy, where a hemiplegia may be associated with a homonymous hemianopia. The hemianopia, if unrecognised, may inhibit the development of reading and writing skills. In any report written for teachers, it is important to remember that their training does not include the ability to understand medical shorthand, so telling a teacher that a child's visual acuity is 6/12 is usually not helpful. The teacher in a special school for visually handicapped children will understand this, but most children with impaired vision will be in ordinary school. What the teachers really want to know is a practical application of the child's visual ability, that is the size of print that the child can read easily in a book or on the board. Information in this form is a good starting point for sorting out a child's individual needs.

HEARING? Hearing losses of as little as 20 db or common fluctuating hearing losses can impair school work and lead to behaviour problems in individual children. Children should never be labelled as uncooperative in hearing tests, as this avoids making a diagnosis of either deafness, a behaviour problem, or a degree of mental handicap which renders the child unable to perform that particular test which is appropriate to his chronological age. The effect of any level of hearing loss depends upon a range of factors including concentration, intellect, level of stimulation at home and the need to learn a second language on starting school. Teachers need practical advice on the level and frequencies of hearing loss, the effects of that hearing loss in the classroom and playground and how they can help, for example by appropriate position of the child's seat in the classroom.

Language
(see also Chapter 22)

A child's language development is the most reliable predictor of educational progress. Time and skill are therefore required to make a proper assessment of language and the child's linguistic background. Assessment of expression, comprehension and articulation is important using information obtained from parents and teachers as well as personal observations. Minor problems of articulation are of little significance, but other concerns, particularly about comprehension, may indicate the need for assessment by a speech therapist. Specific language difficulties, in the absence of other developmental problems, are uncommon. Diagnosis may be difficult and incorrect labels such as mental handicap or behaviour problems made instead of expressive or receptive language problems.

It may, on the surface, seem easy to identify children who are non-English speakers. However, unless we ourselves are also fluent in Hindi, Urdu or any other language that the child may speak, we will fail to identify the child who may have considerable delay in his own language. The parents are also likely to speak little English, adding to our difficulties in making a proper assessment. This challenge is one which needs to be taken up earlier rather than latter in the child's school career and, hopefully, long before school entry. Investments in time, patience, an interpreter or, better still, a multilingual speech therapist are essential.

More commonly children enter school who speak English as a second language, but whose skills in English are not as well developed as those of the language in use at home. Most young children will rapidly expand their English vocabulary with appropriate help in school, for example by 'English as a second language' teachers in primary schools or through special units for children of secondary school age. However, a superficial examination may fail to reveal the depth of individual children's difficulty in English and their comprehension may be inadequate for educational purposes. Combinations of factors should be recognised such as a minor hearing loss which may assume much greater significance in a non-English speaking child.

A second language should not be regarded as a problem, but as a potential asset in the international community. The child who is bilingual requires to have this advantage valued rather than ignored. Language is an important part of cultural identity as well as simply a means of communication.

Dialect problems such as a strong regional accent may produce temporary difficulties in understanding. Learning difficulties that in the past have been ascribed to this cause, for example in children of West Indian origin, are more likely to be due to other factors such as preschool experience or differences in the cultural setting between home and school.

Other perceptual difficulties including disorders of visual perception, body image and coordination can be associated with learning difficulties. It is estimated that 5–15% of children may fit into this category of the 'clumsy child'.

Long-standing illness

About 10% of children have some form of long-standing illness that may affect school progress through a variety of mechanisms.

Absence from school. This may be because the child is ill at home or requires frequent hospital out-patient or in-patient attendances. There are obvious conflicts between the demands of treatment and education, though clearly they are inter-dependent. School doctors may be asked by education authorities for their opinions as to whether a certain degree of nonattendance is reasonable on medical grounds. These are difficult issues. It is important that the doctor is not seen by the child and parents as an inquisitor whose job it is to establish innocence or guilt. The doctor's task is to see how a particular child's medical management might be structured so that his educational needs can be more adequately met. Examples might relate to the scheduling of appointments in relation to school holidays and timetables or by the school health team taking a greater role in day to day medical management.

Non-treatment absences. These may be common in children with chronic illnesses where school absence is greater than can be explained by the child's illness or disability. Important factors may be parental anxiety, combined with a desire to protect against actual or potential adverse factors, for example bad weather or a minimal upper respiratory infection. Parents may also be trying to make some sort of compensation for the loss of quality of life caused by the illness or simply, and understandably, are adopting a softer approach. The child may, through anxiety or intent, exaggerate the effects of symptoms. There may also be a degree of collusion between parents and children. The doctor's role is to understand the underlying factors, to provide reassurance and support and to explain the importance for the child's future in keeping up with school work.

Other children may be withheld from school, whilst in very good health, under the pretext of illness, but with the intention of helping mother look after the house, a younger child or an elderly relative. There are often very real difficulties at home and a sympathetic and helpful attitude mobilising services through the general practitioner and health visitor may be more successful than a critical approach.

Present but ill. In some cases the child is present at school, but is receiving treatment that does not adequately control their symptoms. Examples would include children whose activity is limited due to asthma, who are distracted by itching from their eczema or whose attention span is interrupted by petit mal attacks. The underlying problem may be inadequate treatment being prescribed (unfortunately a fairly common occurrence), poor compliance or real difficulties in providing an effective therapeutic regime. Compliance may be poor because parents do not understand the treatment or the techniques of administration, for example of inhalers. On other occasions, families may not be sufficiently well organised to ensure that they have a continuous supply of medicine, although they might recognise the need. Occasionally, parents may deny the existence of a specific diagnosis and therefore withhold treatment. The child may be reluctant to accept the discipline of regular medication, even when it is successful in controlling symptoms. This is often a problem among adolescents, for example those with diabetes, who may attempt to manipulate or sabotage the effects of treatment.

A thorough review of treatment and compliance is often needed in order to optimise control of symptoms. School health services can have an important role in the day to day monitoring of medication and its effectiveness. For a few children, treatment results in some improvement, but, in spite of an optimal regime, there is still significant disability. In this instance, awareness and understanding of the disability and the provision of additional educational resources can serve to minimise the child's educational difficulties.

Treatment is interfering with the ability to learn. Learning difficulties as a side effect of drug treatment are rare, but do need to be considered in children with learning problems who are on long term medication. Medicines that may cause drowsiness such as some of the older antihistamines and anticonvulsants should be considered in this context.

The child's reaction to his illness. Some children in response to chronic ill health will adopt a 'sick role' in which their conception of disability is generalised into many other fields of activity in which it does not apply. Fortunately, most children will rise to the challenges faced by ill health, but a few use it to shield themselves from other demands, such as education. Parents and teachers may, to some extent, collude with this, by regarding the child as 'delicate' and decrease pressure and expectations of him. In the real world, children with a disability will need more education and not less if they are to compete for jobs when they leave school. Children should therefore be encouraged to take a positive attitude to their health problems and may sometimes require a fairly firm approach to their school work. Parents and teachers will need support in this as they often find it difficult to apply pressure and standards to children with disabilities. Occasionally, the sick role is part of a much deeper and more generalised depression. In these circumstances, discussion with the Child and Family Therapy Team may be needed.

The reaction of other children. Successful integration of a child with special needs requires careful consideration of the possible attitudes or reactions of other children. Minor features that draw attention to a child as being different, for example wearing glasses, may provoke comments from class members that might add to the misery of a child who is already feeling sensitive about his altered appearance. Peer group reactions or pressure may have an adverse effect upon the use of glasses, other aids or appliances or the use of medication in school. Children may be amused by the abnormal gait of a child with cerebral palsy or the language difficulties of a child with a stammer. Children may also be frightened of a child with a disfigurement. It is easy to see how a child with a disability can become isolated and unhappy and, as a consequence, work poorly in school.

Managing these problems in the classroom may prove to be extremely difficult. They first of all need to be recognised. Many children will choose to suffer in silence as peer group pressure dictates that you do not tell the teacher. Other children have personalities that do not succumb to this type of treatment and will not fit into the role of victim. It is certainly a valuable experience for a class of children to gain understanding about disability and learn to overcome the fear and prejudice that can be a common reaction. One should not under-estimate the skills required of a teacher to do this and too often the solution is to remove the victim to more secure surroundings. To some extent, problems can be prevented through promotion of self-esteem from an early age and by providing support and an open channel for communication of hurt feelings. Education also has the challenge of reversing the attitudes to disability that children too often acquire from their families and the local community.

On occasions, the opposite problem is seen in which classmates become overprotective and provide too much assistance, inhibiting the development of self help skills.

Unnecessary restrictions. Teachers in mainstream education have probably received little or no instruction about childhood illnesses, but will inevitably have to deal with the common health problems that will affect the children in their charge. Without proper information, teachers are unlikely to wish to take responsibility for activities which they may regard as involving extra risk. Thus a child may be excluded for incorrect reasons from lessons such as PE, chemistry or metalwork and might be sent to the medical room or indeed home as a strategy for dealing with all medical concerns. The loss in education may be very significant. It is the role of the school medical team, with parental permission, to explain to the teacher the nature and consequences of the child's problems. Usually, there would be no limitations: a negative statement about lack of limitations is as important as a positive statement imposing restrictions. The school medical team must be willing to accept responsibility for the advice that they have given the school. The 1981 Education Act, with its emphasis on the integration of children with special needs, broadens the role of teachers in the care of children with disabilities.

Physical well being

Lack of sleep. Children who are tired, for whatever reason, are likely to perform poorly at school. Lack of sleep may be caused by the failure to apply an appropriate (or in some cases any) bedtime. Noise and overcrowding may also be contributing factors. It is accepted that the amount of sleep that children require in order to not feel tired the next morning varies very widely. A survey of television programmes that children claim to watch often provides a good indication of bedtime, provided that the paediatrician is also suitably informed or has a copy of the *Radio Times*. Many children who cannot tell the time appear to have a built in clock which tells them precisely when a particular programme is on. Older children may be tired because they are out late at night. Children who are tired often present with behaviour problems which include short attention span and general argumentative behaviour; they are frequently not obviously tired. Paediatricians may need both to advise on bedtimes and on methods of implementation. (The management of sleep problems is discussed in the chapter on behaviour).

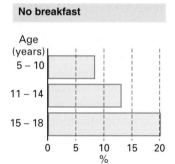

No breakfast

Age (years) — 5–10, 11–14, 15–18; % axis 0, 5, 10, 15, 20

Lack of food. Not all children will want or eat breakfast; however, among 15 000 ten year olds studied from the 1970 birth cohort, 2.6% never ate breakfast and 18.9% had breakfast 'sometimes', this being a more common occurrence in manual social classes (Haslam et al 1984). There appears to be a 'no breakfast syndrome' in which the child often appears tired and unwell at school. They may be seen by the school doctor or nurse because they have fainted or referred with abdominal pain. A noticeable improvement is seen after a mid-morning snack or dinner at midday. They are, in practice, often going 18 hours without a meal, so these symptoms are not surprising. This is a sensitive area and needs to be taken up with some tact, promoting better eating patterns, without being openly critical.

The role of poor diet as a cause of developmental delay is discussed in Chapter 15. There is a strong association between failure to thrive, iron deficiency and learning problems and convincing evidence that nutritional supplementation results in improvement (Granthan-McGregor et al 1991). Careful assessment of nutritional status is therefore an important part of the medical examination. Long-term learning problems may result from prolonged poor nutrition over the first two years of life when brain growth is rapid. There is little evidence to support the case for additional vitamins and minerals in children who are not clinically deficient.

Overworked? The situation of a child being tired and unable to benefit from schooling because of excessive hours of work outside of school is largely historical as the hours and ages and suitability of paid work undertaken by children is strictly regulated. A paper round or a Saturday job may be regarded as good work experience. However, there are instances where children are given excessive burdens in housework, in a family business or are set by their parents unreasonable amounts of extra school type work at home with the aim of improving their attainments. These situations are fortunately rare, but can usually be identified by asking the child to take you through what they do in a typical day. Advice to parents or the help of the Education Welfare Service, one of whose roles is to regulate employment of children, may be needed.

The most common problem in this category is impaired development due to a lack of early childhood experience, which may be coupled with lack of parental support for child and teachers resulting in limited contact between parents and school and little encouragement to do well. Neither the parents nor the child expect success. This area is discussed in detail in Chapter 15. Although prevention is the best strategy, improvements at any stage can come about through changes in opportunity, experience and home life (Rutter 1979).

Problems at home

Many children are able to dissociate themselves in school from disruption and turmoil at home, and find there a 'haven' in which they can thrive. More commonly, family disharmony may present in school life as aggressive behaviour, lack of work coupled with poor attainment, excessive anxiety or depression and withdrawal. Children in the first category cannot fail to come to the attention of teachers, but children in the latter categories may be relatively hidden. Violence at home, lack of continuity of parenting and rules, episodes of reception into care, many moves of house and school provide an unstable and unpredictable background from which it is difficult to make educational progress. Anxiety and aggressive feelings arising from the home situation are displayed in the school setting.

General approaches must include obtaining a full social history, seeing the child and family over a period of time, discussions with teachers with pastoral care responsibility, the primary health care team, clinical psychologists, child and family therapy services, education welfare officers and social workers. Notes often record the families as 'difficult to engage' which usually means they do not come to appointments and have a profound mistrust of the services, keeping us at arm's length.

Behavioural problems
(see also Chapter 26)

School refusal. This is a fairly frequent problem encountered by the school health services. It is discussed more fully in the chapter on behaviour. A wide range of contributory factors need to be explored including anxiety about separation from parents, relationships with other children, particular lessons, changing for PE or use of school toilets. An early return to school is essential before a pattern of non-attendance becomes too firmly established and before the continuity of school work and relationships is severely disrupted.

Conduct disorders. Truancy from school and/or the presentation of behaviour problems within the classroom are a frequent cause for consultation between teachers and the school health team. The outcome may often be poor in terms of educational attainment and adjustment in adult life. The keys to management in school are a warm caring attitude, firm consistent discipline, counselling, stimulating lessons and improvements in self image. Quality teaching and continuity of adult-child relationships are essential components. The school health team may become involved in a counselling role or because of wider associated health or family problems.

Depression. Depression is commonly seen in the upper age groups in the secondary school. It is often described as 'boredom' with general withdrawal and inactivity. The child may be very easily upset or cry for reasons that cannot be explained. Although this may be transient, it often coincides with times when there is increased pressure from examinations and the need to formulate plans for the future. Counselling is needed for some and a few suffer serious depression with suicidal thoughts. Exploration of the depth as well as possible causes always needs to be made.

Poor attention control. Whether or not this is a psychiatric entity, it is certainly a problem in an educational setting. Children with a limited attention span, poor concentration and who fidget, are going to do badly whatever the subject matter taught. They also tend to be punished for their inattention. Underlying problems may be hearing difficulties, tiredness, effects of medicines, solvent abuse, mental handicap or neurological disorders, for example petit mal.

Solvent abuse. Solvent abuse often goes unrecognised. However, up to 14% of children admit to knowing someone who misuses drugs of some kind. Teachers may notice impairment of concentration, deterioration in behaviour with swings in mood. Solvent abuse may be suspected from the smell of the breath, spilt solvent on the clothes or a perioral rash. Management involves control of access, explanation of risk and exploration of underlying factors. Abuse of other substances should be considered in all children with unexplained behaviour problems.

Child abuse. Deterioration in school work may present as a feature of child abuse. Children with learning difficulties, particularly those from deprived backgrounds, are much more vulnerable to sexual abuse than other children (McCormack 1991).

Psychotic disorders. These are extremely uncommon, and perhaps as a consequence of their rarity are not correctly diagnosed for some time. For example, a secondary school girl's written work was described as 'lively and imaginative' without the recognition that her essay revealed elements of delusion and thought disorder. She fatally stabbed a teacher the following week.

Differences in culture

Cultural differences in outlook, behaviour and social norms as well as in clothing and language may cause difficulties in adjustment to the school environment. Children may 'adapt' by staying within their racial group or schools may recognise the diversity of their catchment population and modify their own institution to reflect the needs of the community. Conflicts can, however, develop between standards and patterns of behaviour expected at home and at school. Pupils may find that many of their peer group have different freedoms at home. In order to appreciate the importance of these issues, the teachers and school medical team need to acquire information about the cultural backgrounds of the families whose children attend the school. Useful sources of information are *Asian patients in hospital and at home* (Henley 1979) and *Child health in a multicultural society* (Black 1990).

FORMAT OF ASSESSMENT AND REPORTS

A paediatric assessment may be carried out formally under the 1981 Education Act, as part of a full assessment in the Child Development Centre or within a consultation or series of consultations in a paediatric clinic or at school. The consultation is dissimilar to most in paediatrics in that the results are intended for use by the Education Authority as well as for the parents and child. There should not usually be any conflict of interest here, but the paediatrician must be aware of the different nuances in a consultation where a child is seen at the request of the Education Authority rather than the parents. The parents must not feel side-lined in this situation and the philosophy should be to address the consultation and its findings to the parents first and to regard the transfer of information to the Education Authority as a secondary activity following full discussion with the parents and child. The child is the subject of this assessment and, like his parents, must feel in control and informed. Children are anxious about changes in their school, teacher or content of lessons, as these activities take up the major part of their waking life. They are aware of their successes and failures and of their achievements relative to their peers. The consultation must, therefore, focus on the child's strengths as well as his weaknesses. The approach, too often seen in the past, of listing 'defects' only serves to reinforce poor self esteem. Lack of self esteem is often an important factor in maintaining low levels of attainment. Until a child can feel good about himself, it is difficult for him to face school tasks with confidence.

Report

The report should be written in plain English as it is intended to be understood by parents and teachers. If medical terms are used, then they should be explained. The report starts with a description of the child. This must include strengths as well as weaknesses and relevant past medical history. The description of a medical condition must include an interpretation of the effects of that condition upon the child's daily life and activities at school, for example with regard to mobility, self help, hearing in the classroom or ability to read normal size print. The need for medical management and follow up at home and at school should be described in terms of medication, therapy (eg physiotherapy, speech therapy), aids, appliances and adaptations or special transportation to school. Advice from others, eg speech therapist or child psychiatrist, may be required to incorporate into the report or to be sent separately. Negative, as well as positive findings, must be included, for example normal vision and hearing. The report should be comprehensive, covering physical health, development, mobility, hearing, language, vision, behaviour, feelings, social skills, interests and accomplishments.

BRIGHT CHILDREN

Very intelligent children can make poor school progress if their special needs are unrecognised or unmet (Lobascher & Cavanagh 1977). In some instances, this may result from boredom because the educational programme is not sufficiently challenging. Others may present with psychosomatic symptoms, behaviour problems or feelings of isolation from their peer group. Some may have high levels of anxiety about failure and this may impair their ability to concentrate. Parental expectations may also be high and children may be put under great pressure resulting in a lifestyle that lacks a reasonable balance between utilising obvious talents and enjoying leisure pursuits. Children may derive from this situation high self expectations in which it is not permissible to fail or be anything but best or top all the time. Management involves encouragement of relaxation and honest communication, and an acceptance of the child as a person unqualified by demands for success. Failure should explicitly be allowed so that the child does not have to convert such fears into physical symptoms or open revolt. A sense of humour is an asset to be treasured in an intelligent and serious mind, and can become an essential survival aid.

CLUMSY CHILDREN

Clumsy children are those showing difficulties in motor coordination which is more poorly developed than their other abilities (Gordon & McKinlay 1980). Various estimates from 5 to 15% of schoolchildren have been made. Boys are affected more often than girls. The clumsiness may be associated with learning problems or with emotional problems. The latter may well be as much a reaction to how adults respond to their difficulties as to their own frustration. The label has become a popular one and should not hide children with specific neurological disorders such as cerebral palsy, cerebellar ataxia or lower motor neurone disorders. For this reason, a careful neurological examination should always be carried out. 'Clumsiness' is sometimes quite a difficult term for the paediatrician to understand as it represents the rare use of an ordinary English word to describe a medical 'condition'. In the Oxford Dictionary it means 'awkward in movement'; in medical literature, it becomes ennobled to 'a deficit in the acquisition of skills requiring fluent coordinated movement, not explicable by general retardation or demonstrable neurological disease'. Management has been described, perhaps unfairly, as finding out what the child cannot do, and then making him practice it over and over again.

Aetiology

Much of what is said about the aetiology of clumsiness is speculative. The children probably form the lower part of the normal distribution of gross and fine motor skills rather than having a discrete disorder (Hall 1988). Genetic factors may also be important. It is, however, difficult to separate these out from environmental factors, in that parents with high degrees of fine and gross motor skills tend to provide opportunities and encouragement of their children to develop these skills from an early age. Some children go through a transient stage of clumsiness during periods of rapid growth such as in adolescence, when their perception of body image does not keep pace with changes in body size. Organic factors which are insufficient to cause gross neurological impairment, may contribute towards later clumsiness, but it is difficult to provide convincing evidence for this in individual children.

Although clumsy children are frequently slow to develop laterality, the suggested association of handedness with neurological or perceptual deficits cannot be supported. Those 'left handers' who do have difficulties are usually those who have some dysfunction of the preferred side and hence transfer to the non-preferred side (Bishop 1983). Likewise, a number of 'right handers' have difficulty with functioning on the left and have hence transferred to the right. As the right handed group is much larger than the left handed group, incorrect conclusions can be drawn about the significance of left handedness unless the function of the non-preferred hand is examined. Further examination of the phenomenon of crossed laterality (differences in the side of dominance of eye and hand), has established that this too is unimportant as a reason for poor gross motor or fine motor functioning.

Natural history

Anecdotal evidence suggests that clumsiness improves with maturation either during the first two years of schooling between five and seven years of age or at adolescence. However, Losse et al (1991) in a follow up study of children at age fifteen to seventeen years, who were first seen when they were six, found that the majority of children still had motor difficulties, poor self concept and poor academic attainment.

Presentation

Clumsiness may present with difficulties or delays in developing self help skills such as dressing. The child may have difficulty with fastening buttons or shoes, assembling a zip and some children may almost strangle themselves whilst attempting to put on or take off a jumper. The child may be very poor or untidy at feeding himself, either missing the target area of the mouth or being unable to capture the food on the plate with a spoon or transfer it to the mouth without spillage. In play, the child may have trouble with such material as jigsaws, building blocks or with drawing. Climbing through a hoop may turn out to be an impossible task where the child is unable to work out the correct sequence of movements. Some children may present with the problem of frequent falls. Older children may be referred because of associated learning difficulties, particularly poor handwriting. Others will come to attention because of extremely poor performance in PE. Such skills are important within their peer group and a noticeable lack of skill may result in social isolation. It is not unusual for emotional problems to be the main cause for referral. Improper understanding by teachers or parents may result in a child's difficulties being attributed to laziness or naughtiness, thus adding to the child's feeling of frustration.

Examination

There are standardised tests of motor performance, using scores based on activities such as pencil control, cutting with scissors, catching in one hand or balancing on a board, eg TOMI (Test of Motor Impairment, Stott et al 1984). However, for most clinical purposes, simple observation of appropriate tasks is usually adequate, followed by a detailed assessment by an occupational therapist and physiotherapist where there is a significant disability.

Fine motor skills. The clumsy child may have difficulty in building a tower of bricks, in repetitive fast tapping, pronation and supination movements or finger-thumb opposition sequences. The movements are jerky and imprecise. Drawing may be difficult and such exercises as tracing or colouring within lines may demonstrate the child's difficulties in classroom activities. Threading beads, a discipline which involves accurate eye-hand coordination is a useful test. It should be remembered that repeated activities that focus on the child's difficulties may be a distressing experience and the child may 'refuse to cooperate'. Observation of the emotional reaction or interaction with parents is often as important as the motor difficulties themselves.

Simple tests for school entrants to identify clumsiness

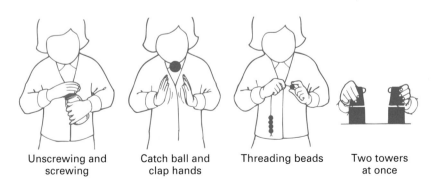

Unscrewing and screwing   Catch ball and clap hands   Threading beads   Two towers at once

Gross motor skills. The child usually has problems with such exercises as standing on one leg, hopping, skipping, kicking a ball or heel-toe walking. Most five year olds should be proficient in these skills. In the older primary school child, the clap-catch test, in which the child is required to throw a ball into the air, clap the hands and then catch the ball, may be quite impossible. Walking on the lateral aspects of the feet is another useful test. Associated movements of the upper limbs is seen normally in younger children, but persists after the age of ten in clumsy children.

Mouth coordination. The difficulties with motor coordination may sometimes be demonstrated in the muscles of the face. There may be difficulty with exercises such as blowing, whistling, tongue protrusion, licking, clenching the teeth or rapid in and out or side to side movements of the tongue.

Management

Management involves the practice of appropriate tasks in order to improve skills in those areas which the child finds difficult. These tasks start within their own level of ability so that confidence can be boosted and success ensured. Specific measures aimed at relieving tension or anxiety within the child or family may be needed. Remedial teaching at school and sympathetic encouragement may be required to help the child overcome associated learning difficulties. A detailed assessment by an occupational therapist, physiotherapist and educational psychologist will determine the level and nature of difficulty. Without this, a blind attempt at improving motor function may involve the child in attempting tasks which are quite impossible for him and where success, even if obtained, will not generalise into other areas such as writing.

Activities may be centred around awareness of body image, eg drawing around the whole body, identifying parts, or in singing games which involve imitation of posture or gesture. Other activities can introduce awareness of rhythm such as dance. Swimming may be useful to develop coordination, though confidence in the water is a prerequisite. Eye-hand coordination can be developed through such activities as drawing, tracing and work with scissors. Practical training in self-help skills in eating and dressing is often useful. The development of skills often results in improvements in confidence and self-esteem. Sometimes the emotional problems need to be tackled in a more direct way when they block progress in other programmes or in school work.

PROBLEMS WITH READING AND WRITING

In general, problems with reading and writing are the professional concern of teachers rather than doctors. However, medical, developmental or behavioural problems may be associated with learning difficulties and, in practice, it is important to identify or exclude these. It is also desirable for two professions who work exclusively with children to share some understanding of their work.

General reading difficulties

It is estimated that approximately two million adults in the UK, comprising 6% of the adult population are illiterate. 25% of children leaving the infant school at age 7 have significant reading difficulties and 10% of those tranferring to the secondary school at age 11 have persisting problems. In many, the problem is part of a general learning difficulty which depresses achievement and understanding in all areas of the curriculum. In others, there is a specific difficulty confined to reading, with much better results in other areas. However, educational opinion is quite divided on the issue of whether within the spectrum of children with difficulty learning to read, there is a special group called specific reading difficulties or dyslexia, which is quite distinct from the rest. Reading difficulties are likely to give rise to parental anxiety and in the child, loss of confidence, a sense of failure and emotional problems. Reading is an essential skill in most school subjects and many jobs in adult life. A third of children with conduct disorders are described as having reading difficulties. Which is cause and which is effect may not always be clear; however the strong association is well recognised. It has been proposed that early identification of children with potential reading problems, coupled with appropriate teaching, will do much to prevent the establishment of these difficulties (Lansdown 1978).

Skills required for reading

- The ability to understand and use spoken language. A delay in speech and language development is often found in the history of children who are later found to have reading problems and may alert teachers to the need for careful early assessment of any difficulties.

- The ability to recognise visual symbols. Visuomotor problems are regarded as much less significant than language in the causation of reading difficulties. However, the task of sorting out similar letters such as p's, b's, d's and q's, differentiating the m from the w and correctly orientating letters such as s may give rise to difficulties in writing as well as in reading. Children with visuo-spatial problems may also have sequencing difficulties. They may be unable to remember a telephone number or the order of the months of the year. They may have important spelling problems, having difficulty with the order of letters.

- They must have normal sound perception and discrimination. Children who have difficulties in reliably classifying speech sounds and in producing rhymes often go on to have reading problems (Bryant & Bradley 1985).

- They must be able to relate written symbols to oral sounds and to relate words and spaces in print to words and phrases in speech.

- They require a well established lateral preference. This does not mean that left handedness or crossed laterality causes problems in reading or writing, but confusion over laterality does. Children require a 'directional' approach to print in order to be able to read.

- Normal emotional development is needed. Defects in concentration, and impulsive behaviour are found more commonly among children who have difficulty in reading.

- They require normal memory.

Reading, writing and spelling problems are often related, but not rigidly so. Some children are able to read words which they cannot spell and others can spell words which they are unable to read. Reading difficulties are more common in manual social classes and with ascending birth order. They are increased in schools with a high rate of teacher and pupil turnover. Unfortunately, these educational disadvantages often go together.

Assessment

Some reading tests eg the Schonell test scores the ability to read individual words graded by difficulty. They are not tests of 'real' reading in that the words are presented as lists out of context. Speed in reading is obtained by scanning the text rather than by the recognition and interpretation of individual letters. The Neale reading test involves recording errors accumulated whilst reading a particular passage.

Remedial help

Systems have been devised which concentrate upon the analysis of presumed basic problems, such as visuomotor difficulties and the introduction of programmes designed to improve these skills. However, they often improve these 'underlying skills' but not reading. Early identification and individualised help are important, before secondary emotional and other problems become established. The teacher must gain the child's confidence and interest and the programme should be designed to achieve early success which is recognised and rewarded by parents and teachers.

SPECIFIC READING DIFFICULTIES

Specific reading retardation (sometimes called dyslexia), occurs in some 4 to 10% of junior school children. This term defines those children whose reading problems cannot be explained by low intellect. The term 'dyslexia' is a descriptive term for children with specific reading difficulty: it is not a 'disease' for which one can imply a common aetiology and regarding it in the framework of a medical model is generally regarded as unhelpful. It is more commonly seen in boys (ratio of 3 or 4 to 1) and there are frequently others in the family with reading problems. Language difficulty is frequently found at earlier stages of development. The children may also have trouble with writing and sometimes arithmetic. Many features of their writing simply resemble those of younger children, such as reversal of pqbd, but others are quite different as shown in bizarre spelling or mirror writing. Left/right confusion (which is distinct from crossed laterality) is common and the children show difficulty in sequencing from left to right, this being a necessary skill for reading and writing in English. The sequencing difficulties affect order as well as direction, producing difficulties in memorising tables or other sequences such as the days of the week. Handwriting is often very poor and becomes even more untidy through alterations and indecision. Misuse of grammar is also seen.

Secondary problems may arise if the child's intrinsic reading difficulties are not appreciated. Pressure, criticism or even punishment may be applied when an obviously intelligent child is failing to progress as expected. The child's reaction may set up emotional barriers, which may themselves present formidable barriers to progress.

Aetiology

A large amount of educational and psychological research has been carried out on the complex skill of reading and on children with reading difficulties. The result has been a series of associations, the most important of which is with language problems, but it has not been possible to isolate factors that can be successfully harnessed into a remedial programme. For example, visual problems were thought to be important and children were treated with tinted lenses or monocular occlusion, however the claims of benefit from this form of management have not been substantiated (Hall 1988).

There may be coding/decoding difficulties, but this perhaps represents a description of the problem rather than a formulation of a cause. Neurological causes have been proposed particularly with regard to left or right cerebral hemisphere location of function. Visuo-perceptual problems have been proposed because of the incorrect orientation of the letters p,b,q,d, though this is a normal feature of younger children. The ability to retrieve visual or auditory information from the short term memory may be lacking. Others have stressed the importance of integration of senses, vision, fine touch and spatial awareness.

Management

Management of complex problems of reading difficulties is clearly the role of the teacher and advice given by the paediatrician through ignorance is not likely to be warmly received. All approaches depend upon analysis of the child's individual ability and difficulties. They build upon the child's strengths and begin with tasks that he can be expected to achieve. This is important as many children have lost confidence by the time that they start to receive extra help. They need to find again the pleasure that reading and writing can give. Detection and intervention at the earliest stages of learning to read may prevent greater problems developing. This model of secondary prevention certainly fits with the professional strategies of community paediatrics.

REFERENCES AND FURTHER READING

Bishop D V M 1983 How sinister is sinistrality? Journal of the Royal College of Physicians 17: 161–71

Black J 1990 Child health in a multicultural society. British Medical Journal Books, London

Bryant P E, Bradley L 1985 Children's reading problems. Blackwell Scientific, Oxford

Gordon N, McKinlay I 1980 Helping clumsy children. Churchill Livingstone, Edinburgh

Grantham-McGregor S M, Powell C A, Walker S P, Himes J H 1991 Nutritional supplementation and mental development of stunted children: the Jamaican study. Lancet 338: 1–5

Hall D M B 1988 Clumsy children. British Medical Journal 296: 375–6

Hall D M B 1989 Birth asphyxia and cerebral palsy. British Medical Journal 299: 279–82

Hall M 1988 Dyslexia. Not one condition but many. British Medical Journal 297: 501–2

Haslam M, Morris A, Golding J 1984 What do our ten year old children eat? Health Visitor 57: 178–9

Henley A 1979 Asian patients at home and at hospital. The King's Fund, London

Idjradinta P, Pollitt E 1993 Reversal of developmental delays in iron-deficient anaemic infants treated with iron. Lancet 341: 1–4

Lamont M A, Dennis N R 1988 Aetiology of mild mental retardation. Archives of Disease in Childhood 63: 1032–8

Lansdown R 1978 The learning-disabled child: early detection and prevention. Developmental Medicine and Child Neurology 20: 496–7

Lobascher M E, Cavanagh N P C 1977 The other handicap: brightness. British Medical Journal 2: 1269–71

Losse A, Henderson S, Elliman D, Hall D, Knight E, Jongmans M 1991 Clumsiness in children – do they grow out of it? A 10 year follow-up study. Developmental Medicine and Child Neurology 33: 55–68

McCormack B 1991 Sexual abuse and learning difficulties. British Medical Journal 303: 143–4

National Dairy Council 1981 Nothing for breakfast. Taylor Nelson

Rutter M 1979 The long-term effects of early experience. Developmental Medicine and Child Neurology 22: 800–15

Stott D H, Moyess F A, Henderson S E 1984 The Henderson revision of the test of motor impairment. Psychological Corporation, San Antonio, Texas

Wedge P, Prosser J 1973 Born to fail? Arrow Books, London

Wedge P, Essen J 1982 Children in adversity. Pan Books, London

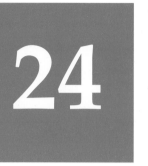

24 Learning Disability

'They're people like us, but they've got this extra little bit in their cells, its called a chromosome ...'

[Quote from 12 year old girl asked what she knew about children with Down's syndrome]

How do we describe the problems of people who have a mental handicap, and how, apart from the physical basis of their handicap, are they different from us? One of the difficulties is that the term 'mental handicap' does not match current terminology and we should rather speak of intellectual impairment, and of learning disability, using the term handicap only to describe the ways in which children are unable to fulfil their normal roles. The baby who has Down's syndrome may not be handicapped in any way during its early weeks, but by the age of 5 years will have special needs for help in coping with the intellectual and the social demands of a primary school class. However, habit dies hard and the terms will be interspersed throughout this chapter!

Measured IQ has for many years formed the basis of categorisation of people with mental handicap. The terminology used differs between different professional groups, and changes periodically as each new term is seen as a derogatory expression. The word clever has been used in its present sense since 1716 and genius since 1749 but terms used to describe people who are mentally handicapped change quite frequently illustrating society's current attitude to people who have a disability.

Terms used in health and education

IQ	Prevalence/1000 pop.	WHO (1968–1971)	Education (1981)
0–20 20–35	0.5	Profound Severe	ESN(S) Severe learning difficulties
35–50	3.0	Moderate	ESN(M) Moderate learning difficulties
50–70	20–30	Mild	

IQ figures are no longer quoted by educational psychologists when assessing a child's educational needs: instead they prefer to describe a child's current abilities and to indicate ways in which they can best be taught. It has therefore become progressively more difficult to define the child with severe and with moderate learning difficulties.

In the past children with profound, severe or moderate mental handicap as defined by WHO, were considered 'unsuitable for education in school'. Following the 1971 Education Act those children were classified as Educationally Subnormal (Severe) and the special schools who were pioneers in setting and achieving educational goals appropriate to their abilities were known as ESN(S) schools. Children with mild mental handicap, who had previously been called feeble minded, were labelled Educationally Subnormal (Moderate) and the schools they attended, which had previously been called schools for mentally defective children, were now known as ESN(M) schools.

Following the 1981 Education Act, the terms SLD (Severe learning difficulties) and MLD (Moderate learning difficulties) came into use. Until recently one could still talk about a child who would benefit from education in a school for children with severe learning difficulties. Now that such children are being accepted into mainstream schools we describe their need for special help without attaching a label. However the two groups, those with severe and those with moderate learning difficulties have distinct characteristics and it is convenient also to consider separately their needs for health care.

Severe learning difficulties

Most children who have severe learning difficulties have a recognised impairment which accounts for their disability and many of them have multiple disabilities. Parents and siblings are usually of normal ability. There is an excess of males, partly due to sex-linked recessively inherited conditions, such as that associated with the Fragile X. The social class distribution of severe learning difficulties is similar to that of the general population; family size is average but may be affected by parents' decision to limit their family following the birth of a handicapped child.

Conditions causing severe learning difficulties. The Oxford mental handicap register (Elliot et al 1981)

Diagnosis	%
Down's syndrome or other chromosomal abnormality	26.5
Other abnormality of CNS	9.0
Cerebral palsy	6.5
Birth injury	2.0
Infective, post-infective, or immunological	2.0
Metabolic or nutritional	2.0
Psychiatric syndromes	4.0
Cerebral anoxia	1.5
Cultural/familial causes	1.0
Degenerative diseases of CNS	1.5
Epilepsy	1.0
Recognised syndromes of unknown aetiology	1.5
Other conditions	3.0
Subnormality (not otherwise classified)	4.0
No known cause	34.5

Moderate learning difficulties

Most children who have moderate learning difficulties have abilities in the lower range of normal variation, and have no single recognised impairment. Parents and siblings are often found to have learning difficulties. More boys end up in special schools, but this reflects the prevalence of difficult behaviour, not of moderate learning difficulties. Social class distribution shows a gradient with many more children belonging to more disadvantaged families. Family size is above average.

Diagnosis is important both to parents and to professionals looking after the child who has a mental handicap. Once the possibility of learning difficulties is suspected, the twin threads of intervention are diagnosis and assessment. For the parent struggling to come to grips with their child's disabilities, a diagnostic label helps them to see the reality of the impairment, and gives them something to hang on to, a group to which, however unwillingly, they belong. To the professional, a diagnosis is also a tool for understanding the child's present condition, for recommending interventions, and for sharing an understanding of prognosis with parents. However, assessment of the child's present skills and deficits in order to organise appropriate teaching and therapies must take place whether or not a medical diagnosis has been made.

GROUPS OF CHILDREN WHO SHARE COMMON NEEDS FOR HEALTH BASED SERVICES

Disorders diagnosed at or soon after birth

In any group of children who have severe learning difficulties between a third and a quarter will be children who have Down's syndrome. This is a diagnosis which is usually obvious at birth and parents faced with this diagnosis deserve a coherent, continuous service. Cunningham's work with a cohort of children in Manchester did not show that intensive programmes improved long term developmental outcomes, but indicated that early intervention is highly valued by parents. A community based early intervention service is described later in this chapter.

Children with multiple handicaps

Children with multiple handicaps may have a motor or sensory impairment as well as other disabilities; many also have epilepsy. Some of these children are unable to move without help, and need total nursing care, others are able to crawl, roll, or walk with difficulty and need a great deal of safe space to do so. All need help with dressing, washing, feeding and toilet. Many need night care. Communication varies from eye contact only to short phrases. A survey carried out for Mencap by Hogg and Sebba found that parents of children with profound and multiple disabilities spent 1–2 hours a day feeding their child, and another 2–3 hours dressing, washing, and toileting. In addition to this time was spent in play activities and therapy. Parents who care for a child with multiple disabilities need an easily accessible multidisciplinary service, one-stop shopping for medical, nursing and therapy advice and treatment in a child development centre, local specialist clinic, or school. They also need readily available respite care.

Degenerating CNS

This group contains a large number of rare conditions with different symptomatology, associated handicaps, and rates of progression. What they have in common is very often the period of uncertainty before diagnosis, and always the more or less gradual loss of the normal child, and the inexorable progression of the disease. The distress this causes to the child's family is often echoed by the sorrow felt by others involved in helping the child and family in the home, school, and hospital clinic.

Families who have a child with a degenerating condition need help matched to their own changing needs and those of their child. At the time when their child first shows signs of regression, they need expert assessment, appropriate referral, and accurate diagnosis. Their need then is for sensitive counselling and introduction to the services they will soon come to need. At this time counselling should also be offered to the extended family, and to the staff of the school or nursery which the child may attend. As the disease progresses families may need to accept shared care of their child in the form of respite care and of help at home. The doctor must also talk to the family about their child's approaching death, helping them through timely decisions about where they would like this to take place, and about the stage at which the child might be allowed to die without intrusive heroic resuscitation.

Handicap and poorly controlled fits

A high proportion of people with severe learning difficulties develop epilepsy, either during childhood or early adult life. Their fits are often difficult to control and they may need a combination of anticonvulsants. A few children have consistently difficult epilepsy, where control can only be achieved with frequent changes of medication and at the expense of unwanted sedation. The aetiology of their handicap may be unclear, as in the Lennox-Gastaut syndrome, or fits may be associated with tuberose sclerosis, or follow a severe brain illness or injury. In any case, not only are the fits themselves disabling to the child and his family, but they may be associated with intellectual deterioration. Frustratingly, when the fits are under control the child makes progress, only to regress when once again they return. The families of these children need open access both to outpatient assessment of medication, and inpatient treatment when needed. School and nursery staff, as well as parents, need an understanding of first aid treatment of fits, of the use of rectal diazepam and clear guidelines as to when urgent hospital admission is needed.

Challenging behaviour

Rutter (1970) found that 50 per cent of children with mental handicap had some behaviour problems. Many of these problems relate to the mismatch between the developmental stage the child has reached and their chronological age. Behaviour which can be tolerated in a 2 year old, such as terrible tantrums in the supermarket, and inability to recognise danger, is more unacceptable in the 10 year old with learning difficulties. The family may be one which functions well despite problems, functioning may be adversely affected by their child's behaviour, or the family may be thought to be one which would have had problems even without a handicapped child.

Problem behaviours

- may occur in all situations, or at home and in one other situation (eg school) or only at home
- may be pervasive, or may involve only one field of behaviour (sleep, eating, elimination)
- may cause the child's ability to be severely or moderately impaired

Other factors affecting the nature of behaviour problems are the choice of school, the age and the size of the child. However, a much smaller group of children with mental handicap, possibly 5 per cent, have severe repetitive apparently causeless often destructive behaviour. The difficulties caused to their families and to all services by these children is out of all proportion to their numbers. These children are at an extremely early developmental stage, but are fully mobile with restless and often destructive behaviour. They are the children it is difficult to engage in any planned activity, and who often find it hard to relate either to adults or other children. Some of them have obsessional behaviour, and irrational fears. These children need one-to-one attention for all their waking hours. They and their families need a carefully planned service involving expert psychiatric and psychological help. Well planned and freely available respite care is essential.

Other genetically important syndromes

A large number of the syndromes causing learning disabilities have genetic implications for the child concerned, for parents, siblings and for the wider family. This subject is dealt with more fully in another chapter. It is most important for the paediatrician to be alive to the possibility of a new diagnosis at all stages in the care of the child and of the family and to have access to a clinical genetics service. Sometimes, for instance when siblings may be planning their own families, it is important to be able to point out the absence of a genetic element in aetiology.

Severe learning difficulties of unknown aetiology

Parents whose child appears normal and well grown, but who has severe learning difficulties of no known cause face an added set of problems. Firstly in themselves, understanding the basis of their child's difficulties: 'What is it? What do we say when people ask? Was it our fault?' and then in the accusing looks from bystanders, when their child displays behaviour consistent with his developmental stage. It is most helpful to them if a diagnosis can eventually be established to explain their child's problem even though this may have no genetic or therapeutic implications.

CARE FOR CHILDREN WITH SEVERE LEARNING DIFFICULTIES

Relief care

This is any period of respite offered to families caring for a child with chronic illness or a handicapping condition, and may be for a few hours, a few days, or for a longer period while a family takes a holiday. Most relief care is provided informally by extended families and by friends, but may be provided by health or by social services, in a hospital, hostel, or foster home. Parents and their children often need relief from one another during school holidays, and holiday playschemes specialised or integrated, make an important contribution.

Parents of 'normal' children use informal sources of relief care constantly. If a child is handicapped, these informal arrangements may still work, sometimes for a variety of reasons they do not. This is where formal arrangements for relief care can make the difference between coping and exhaustion, and between a loving family and an abusing one. Possibilities for relief care should be discussed with parents at regular reviews from an early age.

Preschool child who has a handicapping condition

An account was given in an earlier chapter of some of the processes involved in recognition, assessment and management of the preschool child who may have special needs. In particular the evolution of the hospital based child development centre was described, together with developments both in education and social services. The service described below was set up to meet the needs of a group of children and their families already identified from the time of birth as having special needs for intervention from health, education, and social services.

A community based service for preschool children and their families

The Nottingham Down's Syndrome Children's service began in 1985 as an attempt to coordinate and give a direction to already-existing health and education services in the community. Prior to this medical follow-up had been through the ordinary hospital paediatric clinics, and usually families were seen at six monthly intervals, sometimes by the consultant, but more often by changing junior staff. Child health doctors in the community were likely to see the children only when their names were brought forward from a central observation register at around two and a half years of age, and a doctor was sent to consider whether the child should be referred to the education authority so that a teacher counsellor could be involved.

A medical student's project (Rhodes 1984) showed that only about half the families were referred for speech therapy, less than a third to the physiotherapist, and although all families eventually met a pre-school teacher, the ages at which children were referred varied widely. Each family had a health visitor who could call on the expert knowledge of her specialist health visitor colleague but often family health visitors felt unsure of their role with families who had a child with a disability. Referral to a parents' organisation (both MENCAP and the Down's Syndrome Association have local branches) did not routinely take place.

The idea of a specialised, community based clinic developed during meetings with therapists, teachers, and specialist health visitors and with parents who felt the current state of affairs to be unsatisfactory. This was to be a regular meeting place where parents could meet all those professionals who felt they could help children with Down's Syndrome, in an informal atmosphere. The local Down's syndrome Association were interested in this idea, and promised support. Plans for the service were discussed with service managers for each profession, and with the paediatric committee. The monthly clinic was to be a focal point for the service.

The venue needed to be near the city centre, accessible by public transport, and with enough space for people to sit and chat informally, as well as rooms in which one-to-one work could take place. A church hall which had been newly renovated, and whose owners were looking for a community project turned out to be ideal. The hall itself was a large room with a coffee bar, there were several smaller rooms, available storage space, and modern toilets with changing space for children. The facilities made a remarkable contrast with many well remembered church hall clinics.

When the service began children were referred by health visitors, by the speech therapist, by hospital and community paediatricians, and by word of mouth through the parents themselves. From the start, an informal atmosphere prevailed. Coffee making was an important part of the proceedings. Specialist health visitors took on the very important role of hosts to the clinic, introducing parents to one another, and to the professionals. Parents from the local Down's Syndrome Association came to each session to meet and support the parents of the younger children.

The service runs on a supermarket principal, parents are put into a position where they are able to choose the services they will use, but the mainstay of the service is parent to parent support. At the clinic sessions paediatrician, health visitors, speech therapist, and teacher counsellors circulate among the parents chatting informally, and explaining their services. Few formal appointments are sent out; when they are, it is usually because there has been a request for health advice for a statement of educational need. People who would like to see the paediatrician or the physiotherapist book in as they come. The physiotherapist uses an adjacent room, to give herself space to demonstrate exercises. The team from the Children's Hearing Assessment Clinic visit every other month making regular, and opportunist tests of children's hearing. A social worker from the local Community Mental Handicap Team visits the clinic regularly, as does a welfare rights worker.

The clinic is quite unstructured, most of the real work goes on elsewhere. Since the clinic began, hospital paediatricians have come to refer all babies who have Down's syndrome born in the Nottingham hospitals to the community paediatrician at the time of the diagnosis; this gives an opportunity to visit the family in hospital, to counsel and to provide an introduction to the community based services. All parents are given the opportunity to meet another parent at this early stage. Although some people are ready to take this up at once, others find it easier to meet informally at the clinic, where they can choose their contact. They can also hear from service providers what they have to offer, and choose whether and when they are ready to take this up. The second visit is made at home together with the family health visitor, to establish working relationships with the primary health care services, and to emphasise that children with a disability are entitled to, and should take advantage of, all the normal services available to children and families. Where follow up in hospital is also needed excellent communication has been established.

The speech therapist provides a home visiting service for the youngest children, and runs makaton groups for children over 18 months. The teacher counsellors also visit at home and workers are involved in negotiating common policies, with the idea of using a key preschool worker where the services overlap.

Not all parents of children who have Down's syndrome choose to attend the clinic, but the service covers all preschool children in the district who have Down's syndrome, and regular checks are made with health visitors and other workers to ensure all children are receiving appropriate services. By means of this service, every family in the district who has a child with Down's syndrome has the opportunity of appropriate services from the time of the child's birth. Although some families wish to have time to adjust before accepting specialist services, we have found that no child has reached his first birthday without the family accepting some form of intervention.

LOOKING AFTER CHILDREN WITH SEVERE LEARNING DIFFICULTIES IN SCHOOL

The special school for children with severe learning difficulties is likely to be a day school for between 50 and 150 pupils, depending on the size of the catchment area. The children's ages may range from 3½ to 19 years, and their range of ability is quite as wide as that met in a comprehensive school. Teachers in such a school will not only have expertise in special education, but will have experience and understanding of a range of medical conditions and their educational implications. The role of the school doctor in a special school is to work as a team with nurses and therapists based in school who together provide health care to individual children, and support to their families. Working in mainstream schools it may not be easy to draw together the team involved in the care of the child with severe learning difficulties; however multidisciplinary review is even more important in those situations. Whereas in a special school teaching and other staff acquire a wide understanding of the health problems of children with severe learning difficulties, of the needs of their families, and of the service networks involved, in the mainstream school no such background knowledge can be assumed. Health care reviews within school provide an opportunity not only for parents to discuss their child's health and progress, but also for relating children's health care to their educational needs both in special and in mainstream schools.

An important part of the work lies in understanding the anxieties of staff about the children they teach, and demands the ability to think of a child's medical condition in terms of how it affects his life in school, and to interpret this to his teachers both on an individual basis and by taking part in the provision of formal in-service training for teachers and other education staff. The paediatrician must be ready to provide support and counselling both to health care and to education staff who work with children with disabilities.

Care of the child and family

The first school based review should take place during the term before the child starts at the school. This is an opportunity for parents and the health care team to meet and to exchange information, and to agree on communication issues. Summaries of medical assessments made in the community, hospital and Child Development Centre need to be available, but discussion must take advantage of the parents' unique knowledge of their child's abilities and disabilities, strengths and needs and reactions when unwell or uncomfortable. This last is especially important if the child has difficulty in communicating. It is useful to cover points, such as self help skills, mobility, language development, as well as up to date information on vision and hearing. A description by the parents of a day with the child gives insight not only into skills but also into the gaps to be tackled by therapy intervention. Any current medication must be discussed, and agreement reached as to who will give it, as must the use of rectal diazepam, and the procedure to be followed should the child need admission to hospital. It is rarely appropriate to examine the child at this review, especially if he is shy and nervous; by the time the next review takes place both he and his parents will be more confident in school.

Wider issues include any problems at home with the child's physical care or behaviour, or with parents' or siblings' health. Does the family use any respite care facility? This is an opportunity to outline local facilities which are available to families when they wish to take advantage of them. Does anyone visit the family at home? Community nurse, specialist health visitor, social worker? Is the family aware of their welfare rights?

Finally, the doctor should outline the health care available in the school, and negotiate communication between health care team and teaching staff as well as with the family doctor and the hospital paediatrician. Both in special and in mainstream school there should be a discussion with the head teacher, and with the class teacher about how this child's health is likely to affect his schooling.

A second review should take place when the child has been at the school for a few weeks to discuss any unforeseen problems which have arisen, and to make plans for the child's future medical care. This care is always shared with the family's general practitioner and good communication is essential. It is difficult but necessary to give children and their families a specialist service and at the same time keep them in touch with the family doctor who has continuing responsibility for the health care of the whole family. It may also be useful to share care with a colleague in hospital paediatrics if a child needs frequent access to inpatient treatment, but the practice of subjecting families to long waits in hospital out-patient departments in order to spend three to five minutes with a doctor (often a different one at each visit) is one which has little to recommend it.

Further medical reviews can be tailored to the needs of each child and family. The advantage of working in a school and visiting it regularly is that the paediatrician can see children when problems arise. Parents, teachers, the school nurse, the therapists, and sometimes the child himself can ask for a review. This allows for prompt medical advice and intervention when the need arises.

It remains useful to have regular periodic reviews in order to meet parents, to update records, and check surveillance.

Annual hearing testing is recommended for children who have Down's syndrome, and for those with fragile X. For other children testing should be undertaken if there are concerns. Vision should be checked in school if possible. If the child does not attend an ophthalmology clinic, vision should be tested as regularly as that of other children.

Specific questions should be asked to elicit any behavioural or emotional problems. Sometimes unacceptable behaviour is condoned from children with severe learning difficulties, particularly when the child is in a mainstream school, and this needs careful counselling.

Receipt of benefits, relief care and home intervention should also be reviewed. Examination should be carried out as clinically relevant. All reviews include discussion with school staff as appropriate.

LOOKING AFTER CHILDREN WITH MODERATE LEARNING DIFFICULTIES IN SCHOOL

Who and where are the children with moderate learning difficulties? The majority of children identified as having special educational needs have mild to moderate learning difficulties which, when combined with their problems of socialisation, make them difficult to teach. These children may attend a special school or be catered for in their local school. Papers written about the aetiology of moderate learning difficulties generally refer to those children attending special schools or receiving special services. Lamont et al (1988) and Lamont & Dennis (1988) point out that, in the schools they studied, a substantial proportion of children had measured IQs within the normal range. Children who have reached MLD schools are those who have been difficult to teach in mainstream school often because of behaviour problems. Where such schools still exist the children in them are likely to come from among the most disadvantaged families.

In a school for children with moderate learning difficulties in Nottingham in 1990 there were 114 pupils, age range 5–16 years.

A total of 22 children had brothers or sisters in the same MLD school

4 families have two brothers in the school
2 families have a brother and a sister
1 family has four children in the school
6 children have sibs who previously attended the school

Many parents gave a history of problems with their own schooling, and had difficulties with literacy.

> **In the school of 114 pupils, 20 were on the child protection register**
>
> 7 for physical abuse
> 7 because of sexual abuse
> 3 were thought to be at risk
> Another three were on the register for neglect

In the ordinary comprehensive school serving the same area 7 children out of 700 were on the child protection register.

Recent studies, such as those of Lamont & Dennis (1988) have drawn attention to the need for careful medical evaluation of these children. The paediatrician caring for children in this group is not only aware of the need for diagnosis of possible handicapping conditions but also of the need to look for undiagnosed or undertreated ill-health and secondarily handicapping conditions, since these may be further inhibiting the child's ability to benefit from and enjoy his education. Once these unmet needs are identified, the paediatrician can work towards the provision of appropriate remedial services. If medical factors are found which may contribute to the aetiology of the child's learning difficulties, these must be explained fully to parents. They have the right to understand any genetic implications, and to have access to voluntary organisations and parents groups.

An account of the medical investigation required for the child who fails in school is given in Chapters 18 and 23. Provision of appropriate health services for these children in their schools may reduce their vulnerability and need for services in adult life. We need to be quite clear about the role of medical assessment, in helping children with moderate learning difficulties and their families. It is not for health workers to take over the leading role from education or from social services. The role of the doctor is to look for medical factors in the aetiology of moderate learning difficulties, to assess whether health problems are contributing to the child's difficulties in school, and if possible, to arrange treatment of those problems with the least possible disruption to the child's education.

The school doctor and nurse, working as a team in school, should review the health of all children with special needs annually. This may be done as a notes review undertaken with teaching staff. Special attention should be paid to the areas of growth, and to hearing and vision testing. Parents should be asked if they have any concerns about their child's health.

There is a general impression that families of children with moderate learning difficulties find it difficult to use the available health services, or that they simply do not care. In our own health district, doctors working in MLD schools complained that parents did not come to annual medicals. When a group of doctors sat down to consider the reasons for this, it was discovered that there was no real rationale for routine annual examinations. Sensory deficits should be discovered by surveillance programmes, and health problems do not arise at convenient annual intervals. It is not surprising that parents will not travel long distances on awkward and often expensive bus journeys, to see a doctor who does not help them because their problem is not a health one!

Children are now selected for medical examination on the basis of:

- Parental request
- Past medical history
- School concern re health or behaviour
- School nurse's observation

Safeguards

All children are examined fully on school entry and at 13+. Health appraisal by the school nurse takes place at ages 5, 7, 11, 14 (hearing, vision, scoliosis, height and weight, general health). The school should be aware of non-protective parents who do not recognise or react to their child's health needs.

If health problems are contributing to the child's learning difficulties, it is the school doctor's job not only to arrange treatment, but (with parent's consent) to interpret those problems to school staff, and to facilitate adaptation of the school environment to the child's disabilities. This may include involvement with health service managers in planning for better provision of health care services within the school, and advising education authorities on the adaptation of the school environment to children's needs. Educational medicine is concerned not only with the health of the child, but with the effects of the child's health on his schooling and with making the school a place where each child can reach his/her maximum potential.

The 13+ review

This is a built-in opportunity for the paediatrician to take extra time to look at each child. The first look is towards the past to review the ascribed cause of the child's handicap. If a likely cause was found during earlier assessments, does it still seem as likely? Sometimes medical understanding has progressed since a tentative diagnosis was made, or dysmorphic features have become more obvious as a child grows up. It may be appropriate to repeat chromosome analysis or other tests, or to refer the family to a dysmorphologist for further appraisal. If a cause is already known, do the parents understand its implications for their child as an adult and are the family fully aware of any genetic implications?

Looking at the present involves a thorough look at all aspects of caring for the child as in previous reviews, paying special attention to testing of hearing, vision and to the development of self help skills.

Looking towards the future involves the paediatrician beginning with the family the difficult adjustment towards perceiving their disabled child as an adult. One of the reasons that this is difficult is that while the young person is becoming physically mature and going through the emotional changes of puberty, he remains dependent and immature in other ways. It is very difficult to grasp just what being an adult means for young people with severe learning difficulties and they and their parents need to be given a chance to start talking this through. Parents of children with moderate learning difficulties also have often justified concerns about how their child will cope with life after school.

The school staff and their colleagues in careers and social service departments will at this time be beginning to talk about prospects for training and employment, or about structured day care. Health care staff need to talk about appropriate adult services.

OTHER ISSUES

Support of staff in school

The work of the school doctor also includes providing day to day support for both health care and school staff. Staff who work full time with children with disabilities have particular needs for support. Working with children with profound handicaps who make desperately slow progress, can make staff uncertain of their own abilities and worth. They need to be able to talk through the goals of their work and its benefits to both child and family. The illness and death of a child arouses feelings of grief, not only for the child's death but also for her life. The paediatrician has a part to play in the support of the bereaved in school as well as the child's family.

A seriously ill child

The child who has a degenerating condition may still be able to enjoy the experience of attending school, and the company of his friends and teachers. The presence of a child who may become seriously unwell in school naturally causes anxiety to school staff. Both staff and parents should feel free to talk about their concern that a child may die in school. The school nurse and doctor will be the natural people to consult. It is the school doctor's responsibility (in consultation with the GP and hospital consultant) to talk to parents about the possibility that their child might be taken seriously ill, or even die, in school. When such a discussion has been held, the doctor should talk to the head teacher and class teacher and anyone else who may be concerned to ensure that everyone knows what the parent wants done in the event of their child being taken ill (eg to be called to the school, rather than to meet the child at hospital). The doctor should also write this clearly in the notes to be held in school with a clear signature, the parent should NOT be asked to sign this. The doctor should also agree to provide 'cover' to come and give advice if necessary, and to provide counselling for any staff involved if and when it is wanted.

Planning health care

Helping to plan health care provision in schools involves identifying unmet needs in order to bring appropriate health services to children with learning difficulties. Effective planning demands a knowledge of the changing prevalence of handicap within the community, and an understanding of the burden of disability, as well as the changing pattern of educational provision. A present issue is the rise in prevalence of children with severe multiple disabilities. In common with all children they are receiving better medical care and living for longer. The numbers of multiply handicapped children in schools have risen gradually. Many such children had previously been cared for at home or in institutions. It is important to measure the health care needs of this very dependent population, and to plan how to recruit and train staff to meet their needs within schools.

The young adult

When the child reaches school leaving age, the school doctor will be involved in providing health information for the assessment carried out for the Disabled Persons Act. An outline of the provisions of this Act, and of the information required is contained in the chapter on special needs.

A great deal of the responsibility for the health care of the adult with a handicap will remain with their family doctor. Where paediatric handicap services are holistic, those for adults are specialised. Psychiatrists in mental handicap provide a specialist service for people who have behaviour problems or mental illness in addition to their learning difficulties. There is no equivalent of the school health service in day centres for adults, so that the family doctor may have to resume care for a young person with whom he has had little to do in the past 16 or more years. In many areas community nurses, and community mental handicap teams help to bridge the gap between paediatric and adult services.

Community MH nurses

Community mental handicap nurses are registered nurses of the mentally handicapped (RNMH) and who are experienced in caring for people in residential as well as community settings. They work individually and as members of multidisciplinary health care teams, and are core members of community mental handicap teams. They provide an invaluable practical home based service to families with a member who is learning disabled across the age range. As well as offering practical nursing skills, they are trained in the management of behaviour problems, and in counselling skills.

Community MH teams

This is a team of workers whose aim is to meet the specialised needs of people with learning difficulties. The team varies in structure according to the personnel available and the local philosophy of the service; generally it consists of a community nurse, social worker, clinical psychologist and occupational therapist. Each team usually serves a population of about 100 000.

Functions of the community mental handicap teams

- to provide a service to people with mental handicap, wherever they live
- to facilitate access to health care and to housing and social services
- to support families and other caring groups
- to ensure adequate liaison between health care and other caring agencies involved, including the child health services, when the child passes from paediatric to adult services

HEALTH EDUCATION FOR CHILDREN WITH LEARNING DISABILITIES

Children with moderate learning difficulties have a wide range of educational needs, abilities and personal and social characteristics, many of which have a bearing on school health education and on the service offered by school nurses and doctors.

The 1981 Education Act says that a child could be defined as having a learning difficulty if he has *'significantly greater difficulty in learning than the majority of children of his age'*. While this is a useful working definition pointing up differences, it is important also to recognise that children with learning difficulties have a great many similarities with other children of their age and gender.

Children with or without learning disability are alike in:

- the way they grow and develop
- their emotional need for affection and for caring relationships
- their physical needs for rest, exercise, warmth, shelter
- their nutritional needs
- their hobbies, interests and leisure pursuits
- the pressures they face as children growing up in the 1990s.

But they also differ. It is also important to remember the backgrounds of children with learning disabilities when planning health education programmes. Studies indicate that the population of children attending MLD schools are not representative of the school population as a whole and this has implications for health behaviour, health beliefs and health education (Combes & Craft 1987a).

Social background

Occupation. Pupils in MLD schools come almost exclusively from working class families. In the 1981 Census, 43 per cent of the population in Britain were in social classes III, IV and V (manual occupations). This contrasts with 100 per cent of pupils in the ESN (M) (now MLD) schools in the study by Gillies (1978), and 89 per cent in the study by Pappenheim (1982). Social Class V is greatly over-represented. In the 1981 Census 4.1 per cent of the general population were in social class V in contrast to 43 per cent of pupils in ESN(M) schools in the study by Gillies.

Income. Unskilled or semi-skilled jobs tend to be particularly vulnerable to the down-swings of economic recession. Hence in Stoke, 30 per cent of the fathers and 66 per cent of the mothers of the ESN(M) pupils were unemployed (Combes 1984). The Inner London Education Authority survey found that 35 per cent of parents of ESN(M) pupils were unemployed (ILEA 1984).

Family size and structure. Many children with moderate learning difficulties come from relatively large families. In Stoke the average number of siblings for ESN(M) pupils was 2.8, ranging from 0–9 (Combes 1984).

In London 21 per cent of children at MLD schools had 3 or more siblings under the age of 16 (ILEA 1984). Large family size and low income combine to make overcrowding more likely. Combes (1984) found 10 times the local rate of overcrowding for families with a child at an ESN(M) school. Traditional family patterns may be less common among children in MLD schools, with higher than average numbers of one-parent families, divorce, re-marriage and Local Authority care (Combes 1984, ILEA 1984).

Patterns of disadvantage. Many pupils with moderate learning difficulties experience a combination of these social factors which amount to significant social and material disadvantage. Combes (1984) calculated an index of disadvantage (comprising one point each for factors such as social class V; no parental income; free school meals; family disruption; 3 or more siblings; overcrowding). Thirty five per cent of the ESN(M) pupils scored 3 or more points and 10 per cent scored 5 points. The ILEA Survey (1984) used a similar index and found that 88 per cent of the children in MLD schools scored at least one point (as compared with 70 per cent in ordinary schools) and 35 per cent scored 3 or more points (23 per cent in ordinary schools).

Ethnic background. In the past West Indian children were over-represented in ESN(M) schools. In 1972 (the last year in which the DES collected statistics on ethnic background), West Indian pupils amounted to 0.85 per cent of the total school population, but 3.26 per cent of the ESN(M) school population. However the ILEA report of 1984 found very little difference between the percentages of West Indian pupils in ordinary and special schools (although there was still an over-representation in units for language impairment and in schools for children with emotional and behavioural difficulties).

Asian pupils were under-represented in ILEA ESN(M) schools – 5.6 per cent as opposed to approximately 10 per cent in ordinary schools. But these figures are not replicated in areas such as Birmingham and Sandwell where the proportions are commensurate with the general population (Jervis 1987).

A profile of the slow learner: teachers recognise slow learners as the pupils who:

95%	need clear, step by step, repeated instructions
93%	need extra explanations of subject matter
88%	need constant extra help
87%	have reading difficulties
87%	lack concentration
87%	have difficulty in comprehension
84%	do not absorb information
82%	have writing difficulties
82%	are easily distracted
81%	lack basic knowledge or skills
81%	do work of poor quality
80%	are slow learners and slow to respond
80%	are easily confused

From: Bell & Kerry 1982

Characteristics of the children

Bell & Kerry (1982) asked over one hundred teachers to list the main classroom cues which indicated to them that a pupil might have learning difficulties. These cues were circulated to a further two hundred teachers and the percentage figures in the table refer to the proportion of these teachers who concurred with those cues.

Implications for chool health education

Taken by itself the table offers a model of cognitive deficit, indeed the very phrase 'learning difficulties' encourages a focus on deficit, but the picture for each individual child is far more than a sum of that child's scholastic difficulties. However, the list does offer two pointers when we consider health education. Firstly, it forces us to carefully consider the pace, the clarity and the manner in which the subject is approached. Secondly, the way in which help is institutionalised and delivered to children identified as having learning difficulties, can have unintended consequences because of the attached stigma of going to a special school in a society which places emphasis on examination success. Self-esteem and feelings of self-worth have enormous significance when it comes to personal health choices and health related behaviour. School health education has an important part to play in fostering children's sense of themselves as valued individuals who can make decisions and influence the world around them.

Similarly the social background of children with moderate learning difficulties requires equally sensitive attention. Much of the thrust of health education tends to focus on individual responsibility – whether or not to smoke, whether or not to eat junk food, whether or not to exercise. However, as the well-researched National Child Development studies (Kellmer Pringle et al 1966, Fogelman 1976) and the Black Report (Townsend & Davidson 1982) have shown, within this society life chances are closely linked to social class. As we have seen, pupils with moderate learning difficulties are more likely to come from families in social classes IV and V, which links to decreased disposable income, increased risk of disease, illness and accident, decreased available choice about where to live and what to eat. Children's health can be adversely affected by damp housing and limited diet and a school health education programme and a school medical service which focuses on individual choice where only very circumscribed personal choice exists runs the risk of doing more harm than good. However, where the programme is planned in consideration of how and what choices can be made, no matter how small, then successes can be achieved.

'It is therefore essential that teachers use the process of listening to what pupils have to say about their lives outside school, providing an opportunity for them to express their health-related interests and of using both these to inform their teaching ..... this listening is particularly important where there is a big difference between pupils and teachers in their health-related experiences. It can be all too easy to teach health education unthinkingly in a way which reflects the teacher's experiences and values rather than those of the pupils, because health education is so much about personal experiences. Many teachers are from middle-class backgrounds and have lifestyles which are in sharp contrast to those of their working class pupils. This makes the process of listening to children and involving them in a dialogue about health, essential.'

(Combes & Craft 1987a)

Teaching approaches

The characteristics of children with learning difficulties have to be taken into account when planning health education. For example, forcing pupils with poor literacy skills to spend a large part of a lesson reading and writing only reinforces their difficulties in those skills, whereas a lively and well-structured discussion of a topic with a short group summary for each pupil's file can make learning enjoyable and fun. Short attention spans suggest that we use a variety of approaches within a session – perhaps a brief talk, a few slides, then some drama or art work. The 'Special Health' programme has a unit on learning approaches, prompting teachers to extend their range of methods (Combes & Craft 1989). The pace at which new topics are introduced and old ones consolidated depends upon the particular pupils in a class. Again, a range of teaching methods and resources can allow the same topic to be revisited in new ways.

Language is an important consideration, particularly for those who might be invited into a class to teach for specific lessons only and who are not trained teachers. Difficulties may be compounded because of the 'technical', biological terms which may be involved and with which pupils are unfamiliar. It may also be that personal embarrassment caused by talking about usually private and intimate matters makes us use convoluted phrases and incomprehensible euphemisms. Pupils are far more likely to know the common or slang names for parts of the body. Useful rules are to keep sentences short, establish mutually understood vocabulary as you go along, give frequent summaries of the ground covered up to that point and check out that pupils *are* understanding, not just nodding politely.

With regard to available teaching resources, teachers have always had to adapt material to meet the needs of their pupils with learning difficulties. In 1988 the Health Education Authority published a free, comprehensive, annotated list of health education resources, reviewed by teachers of pupils with mild and moderate learning difficulties (HEA 1988).

Influences on children's health-related behaviour

The list of factors which influence the health-related behaviour of children with moderate learning difficulties will be very similar to the list for any child.

Factors influencing health-related behaviour

- Family (parents, siblings, the wider family circle)
- Family circumstances (income, housing, etc)
- Child's ethnic and religious background
- The media
- Pop stars
- Peers
- Teachers and school environment

However, a child might be perceived to be unduly influenced by neighbourhood mainstream friends because she/he does not want to run the risk of being excluded from the group and its activities.

As with all school health education programmes the primary task is to offer children information in a way they can understand it so that they can make informed choices.

THE FUTURE SERVICES FOR CHILDREN AND ADULTS

Enormous changes have taken place in services for people with a mental handicap in recent times and especially over the past twenty years. From being regarded as people with a condition to be managed by doctors and nurses, often within hospitals, learning disabled people are gradually being integrated into their local communities. Many of the changes have begun in the children's services, and have been cumulative. For example, inclusion of children with a mental handicap within the education system, has led to provision of health care services in schools, which has led to a demand for appropriate services for adults.

The closure of large mental handicap hospitals has led to a demand for suitable sheltered accommodation within communities, which has never been fully met. Integration of children with learning difficulties into the mainstream of education is likely to lead to dissatisfaction with large adult day centres. The effect of 'Caring for People' on these demands has yet to be seen; responsibility has been placed firmly with social service departments, with encouragement to cooperate fully with voluntary bodies and private agencies in the provision of services.

In the meantime health services are enjoined to cooperate with social service departments, and to provide help when requested. Much work remains to be done before the respective roles of all agencies under the provisions of the 1989 Children Act, the 1986 Disabled Persons Act, and the Health and Social Services Act are fully understood.

REFERENCES AND FURTHER READING

Bell P, Kerry T 1982 Teaching slow learners in mixed ability classes. DES Teacher Education Project Focus Books. Macmillan Education

Combes G 1984 Drinking patterns and beliefs among ESN(M) schoolchildren and their implications for health education. PhD. Thesis, University of Keele

Combes G, Craft A 1987a Health education for children with special needs. In: David K, Williams T (eds) Health education in schools. Harper Education Series

Combes G, Craft A 1987b Parents, schools and community: Working together in health education. Health Education Council (available from CEDC)

Combes G, Craft A 1989 Special health: A professional development programme in health education for teachers or pupils with mild or moderate learning difficulties. Health Education Authority, London

Craft G, Cromby J 1991 Parental involvement in the sex education of students with severe learning difficulties. A handbook. Department of Mental Handicap, University of Nottingham Medical School

Craft A and Members of Nottinghamshire Sex Education for Students with Severe Learning Difficulties Project 1991 Living your life: a sex education and personal development programme for students with severe learning difficulties. LDA

Department of Education and Science 1987 Sex education in schools. Circular 11/87. HMSO, London

Elliot D, Jackson J M, Graves J P 1981 Oxfordshire mental handicap register. British Medical Journal 282: 789

Fogelman K R 1976 Britain's sixteen year-olds. National Children's Bureau

Gillies P 1978 A study of mildly subnormal adolescents in Nottingham: Their characteristics and health knowledge, accompanied by a survey of parental and teacher attitudes towards health education. MSc Thesis, University of Nottingham

Health Education Authority 1988 Health education resources for pupils with mild and moderate learning difficulties. HEA, London

Inner London Education Authority 1984 Characteristics of pupils in special schools. RS 962/84. ILEA Research and Statistics, London

Jervis M 1987 Across the cultural divide. Special Children 9: 20–22

Kellmer Pringle M, Butler N R, Davie R 1966 11,000 seven year olds. National Children's Bureau, London

Lamont M A, Dennis N R 1988 Aetiology of mild mental handicap. Archives of Disease in Childhood 63: 1032-8

Lamont M A et al 1986 Chromosome abnormalities in pupils attending ESN(M) schools. Archives of Disease in Childhood 61: 223-6

Lamont M A et al 1988 The socio familial background and prevalence of medical aetiological factors in children attending ESN(M) schools. Journal of Mental Deficiency Research 32: 221–32

Pappenheim J 1982 Special school leavers: The value of further education in their transition to the adult world. Greater London Association for the Diabled

Rhodes K 1984 Parent's views on the services for preschool Down syndrome children in Nottinghamshire. BMSc Dissertation

Townsend P, Davidson N (eds) 1982 Inequalities in health: The Black Report. Penguin, Harmondsworth

25 Emotional and Behavioural Problems

The range of emotional and behavioural problems presented by children is endless, therefore only the general issues and the most significant points will be discussed here. Each problem, however simple it may seem, occurs as the end result of complex interaction of numerous aetiological factors. An appraisal of any particular behaviour or emotion must take into account these factors and also consider what other influences are at work in maintaining the disorder. It is often the case that a self-perpetuating cycle develops with a strong tendency to continue. The concept of a vicious circle is useful when discussing behaviour problems with parents and it may be helpful to actually draw up a list of the various contributing factors. Some of these will be difficult, if not impossible to influence. It is therefore important to focus therapeutic efforts on those parts of the cycle that are most likely to change in response to interventions. It may be helpful to use several different therapeutic approaches at the same time; for example supporting the parents whilst working directly with the child and at the same time attending to any problems that have occurred at school.

Some 7 per cent of 3 year old children have moderate or severe behaviour problems, as defined by their parents. At 5 years of age approximately 10 per cent of children are reported to be often disobedient and 'quick to fly off the handle'. By 7 years old some 20 per cent of children showed some form of antisocial behaviour such as destructiveness or disobedience, with or without hyperactivity. This steady increase of problems may be due to parent's changing perception of what is unacceptable at different ages and the fact that larger children make more of an impact, rather than to a true increase in bad behaviour. Generally, behaviour problems have been found to be more than twice as common at home than at school and boys are noted to show more difficult behaviour than girls.

Serious disturbance

The majority of difficult behaviour is non-specific and does not necessarily indicate a serious disturbance. For example, children who steal may be doing this simply because they can get away with it. On the other hand, it may be the outward manifestation of profound disturbance. Even something as serious as fire-setting could be seen as normal experimentation by an inquisitive child. Nevertheless this explanation can only be used once and further attempts at fire-setting would imply pathology in family function. A few symptoms are almost invariably indicative of significant abnormality. Generally, the more symptoms present, the greater the risk to the child.

Childhood behaviours indicative of serious disturbance	
Symptom	Disturbance
Deliberately destructive	Hostile relationships, low self esteem
Deliberate messing	Lack of self worth, inadequte care
Wandering off	Poor supervision
Running off	Lack of affectionate and/or intolerable distress
Deliberate self harm	Low self esteem or intolerable distress
Age inappropriate sexual behaviour	Sexual abuse

HABIT TRAINING

Basic training in the habits of every day life is an important developmental task that parents seem to find increasingly difficult because of the extensive demands on their time and energy. Most children go through a developmental sequence for establishing routines in the different areas of everyday life.

The development sequence of everyday habits
1 Feeding
2 Sleeping
3 Eating
4 Going to the toilet
5 Going to bed and getting up
6 Dressing and undressing
7 Washing and cleaning teeth

There is no doubt that some children have more difficulty getting into a daily routine than others, especially those with a difficult temperament. Nevertheless, it should be possible to achieve a regular habit with even the most trying child, provided that the parents insist on keeping to a routine and a time schedule. Once the routine is established, things can then be relaxed a bit to allow family life to be more flexible and adaptable. The relevance of training a child in the routines of everyday life may seem obvious, but it is surprising how many parents find this difficult, and how many clinicians underestimate its importance. Failure to achieve an acceptable routine in everyday life will result in daily hassle and distress for the family.

Pervasive habit training disorder

Some children present with a wide range of problems relating to the routines of everyday life. There will be problems getting the child to sleep at night, arguments over dressing, unsettled meal times and sometimes associated toileting problems. In such instances it is best to start by tackling the problem that comes earliest in the developmental sequence, before attempting to improve some of the others. The management of pervasive habit training disorder involves agreeing a strict routine with the parents. It helps to write this down so that the parents can be reminded to keep to the strict time sequence, if necessary using timers or alarm clocks to keep everybody to schedule. Close supervision will be needed to ensure that the agreed routine is maintained.

Young children enjoy and benefit from routine and regularity in their life. It helps them to feel secure and makes argument and discussion over daily routines much less likely to occur. The benefits of establishing these routines at an early stage are all too obvious and parents need to understand that it is best to get in first and establish a routine which suits the family, rather than to follow the routine set by each child.

Unwanted habits

Nail-biting and thumb-sucking. Large scale surveys of children show that habits such as nail-biting and thumb-sucking occur quite frequently. Approximately 30 per cent of five-year-old children bite their nails, suck their thumbs or both and about the same number have eating or sleeping habit problems. These habit disorders are rather more likely to occur in girls than in boys. In addition, roughly one in four children experience twitches and tics at some time in their development.

Most of these habits are strongly age dependent. Finger and thumb sucking under the age of three years is quite normal, but there is evidence that after the age of four it may cause problems.

The adverse effects of finger and thumb-sucking

- Malformation of the mouth and face
- Difficulty in responding to questions
- Interference with spontaneous speech
- Restricted use of play material
- Negative interactions with parents
- Perceived by others as being immature

Nail-biting and thumb-sucking are particularly difficult habits to influence. Both require a cooperative effort between the parent and the child. Reassurance may not be sufficient in itself, since many parents find it difficult to ignore these behaviours. A recent approach to this problem involves identifying the times and circumstances when the child is most likely to thumb suck. Then the child is taught to make a clenched fist with the thumb inside the fist and to hold it in that position for a count of 20. The child has to repeat this whenever the circumstances arise where thumb-sucking may occur. If the child is actually found thumb-sucking at any time, then the fist clenching exercise is repeated at least once. A similar approach can be used for other simple habits where first a behaviour is identified that makes the habit impossible to perform, then the child's cooperation is gained and most important of all, the approach is kept playful and good-humoured.

Masturbation. Although masturbation in young children provokes a range of strong feelings in parents and other adults, it is really just like any other habit. It occurs more frequently when children are bored, emotionally upset or excited. The principles of disrupting the habit are also the same. Hands need to be kept occupied and any satisfaction from the behaviour should be kept to the minimum by withdrawing attention or by dressing in clothes that make access more difficult.

TICS

Tics are simple, repeated and unwanted movements that have no purpose and can only be controlled by will-power over a period of minutes. They are made worse by emotional stress, but also by boredom and excitement. Tics are not present during sleep. The usual onset of childhood tics is between two and fifteen years, with one peak around the age of seven years old and another in early adolescence. Only a very small number continue into adulthood.

Features associated with tics

- Overactive behaviour
- Family history of tics (about 15%)
- Other habits
- Speech disorder
- Obsessional behaviour
- Emotional problems (more common in males)

It seems likely that all tics are based on the neuro-physiology of the startle response. The most common tic is eye-blinking and the next is the facial tic and then a head-twitch, and so on in the same progression as would occur when a person is startled. The most extreme form of tic known as Gilles de la Tourette Syndrome involves multiple and complex tics including vocal expletives. There is evidence that neuro-transmitter imbalance is an important factor in the production of tics and that environmental and psychological factors are also important in maintaining the movements.

A simple explanation of the nature of tics may reassure some parents, but many will want some more specific instructions. The primary goal is to deal with any stress and achieve optimal arousal levels. Any comments or actions that draw attention to the tic must be stopped, both at home and school, since they will have a major influence in maintaining the symptom. Other approaches such as deliberately practising the tic or keeping a detailed diary of tic frequency may sometimes be helpful.

Treatment with drugs such as Haloperidol that influence neuro-transmitters can be effective in controlling severe tics. Unfortunately, they all have potentially serious side effects and should only be used by clinicians with specialist experience and only then, if a tic is causing a severe handicap to the child's development.

EATING PROBLEMS

The close relationship between food and feelings is the cause of considerable concern for parents. Most of the worry about children's eating is unnecessary, because the majority of childhood eating problems resolve spontaneously. But at the same time most of the eating problems of adult life can be traced back to childhood. Significant feeding problems occur in 10–15 per cent of very young children and are likely to be associated with having a young mother and being an only child with a low birth weight. By the time that the children start at school about 1 in 4 children are described as being faddy and are more likely to come from smaller and better off families. Children with feeding problems are more likely to have stomach aches, vomiting, and headaches, but there is no way of telling if this is due to a common factor such as food allergy. There is no difference between boys and girls in the overall rate of eating difficulties.

Obesity

Childhood obesity appears to be increasing in frequency in western countries. Some 10–15 per cent of pre-school children are overweight The follow-up of these fat children shows that there is a strong tendency for the obesity to continue. The onset of obesity after the age of 4 years seems to have a much worse prognosis than an onset in infancy. Weight reduction is notoriously difficult and requires major changes in parental attitudes and dietary behaviour patterns. Parents need to understand that whatever they think may have caused the obesity, weight can only be lost by eating less than the child actually needs. Parents must take full responsibility for their child's weight, since it is the parents who have bought, prepared and served the food that the child has grown fat on. It should be made clear to parents that if a child is slimming, hunger is a positive sign that should be rewarded with praise and cuddles rather than more calories.

Food fads

Various factors such as parental attitude to food, family dietary and eating habits have been implicated in children's abnormal eating patterns. More severe eating problems are likely to be associated with problems in the parent-child relationship and by emotional stress affecting the child or parent. Most fussy children seem to do extremely well in other respects. Physical growth, haematology and biochemistry are usually well within the normal. It is essential to find ways of banishing emotions from meal times and to take a long term view, gradually introducing new foods over a period of years. At the same time it is important for parents to avoid becoming a slave to the child's fads by allowing the fussy child to control family meals with demands for separate food.

Some children seem to develop a 'phobia' of particular foods. Forcing a child to eat the feared food may make things worse, but avoiding it will only maintain the problem.

It is not unusual for toddlers to use food refusal as one way of asserting their independence or to find out how far they can push their parents. This type of negativism is best dealt with by a 'take it or leave it approach'. The hunger drive can be used to good effect and it is quite acceptable for children to miss two or three meals, provided that their weight is satisfactory and fluid intake (without calorific value) is kept within the normal range.

Anorexia

More extreme forms of food refusal can occur in a range of conditions, most of which are fuelled by emotional distress. Symptoms that are similar to anorexia nervosa can occur in prepubertal children, in which case they are almost invariably the result of obvious stress factors at home or at school. Occasionally the food refusal may be part of a more general despairing state where the child seems to give up completely. This condition may occur after an illness and can be seen as a failure to convalesce; intensive rehabilitation will then be required. The typical features of anorexia nervosa occur more frequently in adolescent girls than in boys.

Characteristic features of anorexia nervosa

- Loss of more than 20% of expected body weight in relation to height
- Preoccupation with food and body weight
- Concern about being too fat in spite of being underweight
- Persistent refusal to maintain an appropriate weight
- A tendency to set high standards and to be obsessional
- A feeling of being out of control and difficulty in communicating feelings

---

Mild or undeveloped forms of anorexia nervosa are quite common and are best dealt with before lack of food intake leads to the many secondary symptoms of starvation, such as lowered mood and amenorrhoea. Recent treatment approaches for anorexia have been aimed at encouraging the child to take responsibility for their weight and eating, using 'eating and feeling' diaries. Young people with anorexia nervosa seem to find communication at an emotional level especially difficult. They are therefore encouraged to examine their feelings in relation to eating and it may help them to carefully record the details of what they have eaten and how they felt about it. At the same time a reasonable target weight range should be agreed and progress closely supervised. Younger children may benefit from their parents taking more active control of their eating and being prepared to be quite tough and determined that their child will eat appropriate amounts of food.

Food and behaviour

Undernutrition in the weeks just before and after birth can have an adverse effect on brain function which may be lasting and result in poor school performance and an increased rate of behaviour problems. The brain uses about two thirds of the sugar available in the body. It has been claimed that sugar causes difficult and aggressive behaviour in school children and that it interferes with learning. There is some evidence that sugar might increase movement in children, but there is no convincing evidence that sugar affects other aspects of behaviour. Caffeine in coffee and tea does have a general alerting effect, but is unlikely to change children's behaviour.

Food allergies are quite common in young children during the first few years of life, but become less frequent as they grow older so that by the age of five years most of the problems have resolved. The chief symptoms are diarrhoea, abdominal pain, and skin rashes. There are theoretical reasons why salicylates, occurring naturally in food, might have an effect on behaviour through their influence on the production of prostaglandins in the brain. Removing salicylates as well as artificial colourings and preservatives from the food of hyperactive children has been claimed to result in an improvement within a few days in at least 50 per cent of cases. Unfortunately, in most cases this is likely to be due to the 'halo' effect of a special diet. Properly controlled research suggests that only a very small number of children are affected by food additives and an even smaller number improve on an exclusion diet (some estimates suggest 25 per 100 000 children). If parents are keen to try an exclusion diet to improve their child's behaviour it is as well to be supportive, rather than undermining of their efforts. Better behaviour often results, although in most cases this is more likely to be due to the child's experience of more consistent and firm management than to removal of allergens or toxic substances.

CHILDHOOD SLEEP PROBLEMS

It is reported that one in three infants and children up to five years old have disturbed sleep and, of these, about 30 per cent could be regarded as having a serious problem. Fortunately, children sleep better as they grow older and, by eight years old, the frequency of sleep problems is down to one in 10. The newborn infant spends most of the day and night asleep, but has a short sleep cycle of about 20 minutes. By three months old children spend more time awake during the day than during the night, but there are still four to five periods of nocturnal wakefulness. Around the age of six months, most children spend up to 15 hours asleep during the night and a clear day/night sleep pattern is normally established. Therefore, it is better to wait until at least six months of age before taking any action to deal with a child's disturbed sleep pattern.

Why worry

There is evidence that sleep deprivation adversely affects children and, indeed, their parents. Lack of sleep leads to poor concentration and irritability after 24 hours of wakefulness, followed by anxiety and feelings of depression after 48 hours. These symptoms are shared by both children and adults. But paradoxically, as children become more tired, they tend to speed up, becoming restless and apparently energetic; whereas most adults slow down and run out of energy. Parents also need time for themselves, time to communicate and to enjoy being together. A sleepless child can make this very difficult.

Since parents cannot force sleep on their child, they should concentrate on making sure that they are providing the right conditions for sleep: that the child is lying in bed with the light turned off and the bedroom door closed. Resting in bed at night is almost as restorative as sleep itself. Sleep is therefore not the absolute goal for parents to aim for, rather they should aim to get their child to bed in good time and ensure that the child stays there.

The management

Children are quick to realise that by playing up at bed time, they can control their parents and obtain extra attention and cuddles. It often seems that children are better at training their parents into a night time routine than the other way round. Hypnotic drugs are contraindicated because they have side effects and are ineffective in the long run. Complying with the child's wishes may seem an easy way out, but this too has side effects and is no long term solution.

Establishing a good sleep habit. At six months, most children have settled into a reasonably stable sleep/waking cycle, but by two years this has often broken down, especially if a regular sleep routine has not been firmly established. Sleep, just like eating, toileting and dressing is a daily habit that requires regular training over a long period before it becomes properly established. How parents organise a good sleep habit will indicate how parents will cope with other developmental tasks where the child's demands have to be given second priority. It is therefore important to focus on sorting out sleep problems before dealing with any other management problems.

There is more to night time than merely sleeping – rest is also important, whether the child is asleep or not. Less obviously, night time is when children begin to learn to feel confident on their own. This is one of the very few times when children are completely alone for any length of time and, therefore, able to develop self-reliance. Children have to grow up relatively quickly in order to cope with our present day society. It is therefore helpful to achieve a reasonable level of self confidence and independence before starting at school. Sleeping in the parent's bed may seem like an easy solution to night time problems, but it is difficult to mature while still dependent in this way. In addition, sleeping together exposes the child to a much more intimate experience of the parent's emotions than is healthy. Children gain a sense of security from parents who are confident and predictable in their childcare. Confusion about what is expected at night is likely to lead to feelings of insecurity and unsettled behaviour during the day. One of the main reasons why children do not settle quickly at night is because insufficient effort is put into getting the bed time routine well established.

The following approach is recommended:

1 Take time to go through the routine carefully with parents
2 It may help to write it all down
3 Agree a bed time that can be kept to rigidly
4 Start the routine one hour before bed time
5 Gradually wind things down
6 Always do the same things in the same order
7 Once in bed, spend no more than five minutes with the child
8 Always say exactly the same words when saying good night
9 Turn the light out and shut the bedroom door

This routine needs some explanation. It is important that the bed time is not fixed too late. The longer a parent stays in the bedroom the more the child is likely to complain when the parent leaves. A few quiet words together is all that is needed before saying the usual good night phrase and leaving the room. The same 'sleep phrase' can also be used at other times during the night if, for example, a child is woken by a nightmare. If the light is left on it gives the wrong message to the child: *that darkness is dangerous*. If the door is left open wide enough for the child to walk through, the message is: *come out anytime you like*.

Ensuring a successful outcome. Most parents can manage to get their children to bed. Any difficulty with this would suggest a disciplinary problem. The child has to be taught to stay in bed – or at least, in the bedroom. Of course, if the child is still in a cot, there is no problem. When children graduate to a bed it is best to aim for a 'psychological lock' on the bedroom door so that the child knows not to come out of the bedroom after having been put to bed, except to go to the toilet or in an emergency.

The quickest way of achieving a 'psychological lock' on the bedroom door is to catch the child at the earliest possible moment after getting out of bed and then return the child immediately – with a tone of voice and facial expression and a manner that is so impressive that the child remains in bed. The child's reaction to this will let the parents know if the performance was good enough, or if they will have to practise a bit more. Parents who are unable to control their children enough to keep them in bed at night are also likely to have similar problems in other more dangerous situations. Children should be considered to be at risk until parents have achieved this first stage of discipline. If the child stays in bed, but calls out, cries or screams, it is important, *provided the child is safe and well*, that the parents do not respond in any way. This 'in at the deep end' approach is effective in a few days if parents can keep to it.

Parents often say they have done it all before and it has not worked, but on checking carefully it is usual to find that they have not really carried it through. Either the child has been allowed out of the bedroom or the parents have eventually responded to the crying which shows the child that it is worth carrying on crying because someone will respond in the end.

Reasons for failing to establish a good sleep routine and possible solutions

The problem	Possible solutions
The child creeps out without parents knowing	Fit an alarm to the door or a movement detector
The child might suffer some harm	The bedroom must be totally safe
The room must be entered to check that the child is all right	Look through the keyhole or use a mirror or a baby alarm
The neighbours complain about the crying	Warn them first. They will normally be supportive
One parent gives in	Both parents must agree. The tougher parent should look after the one that gives in
The crying is too distressing	Try a personal stereo or ear plugs
The child will not stay in bed, but stays in the room	Dress in a warm all-in-one suit
The child vomits with screaming	Clear it up with the minimum of fuss, avoiding any eye contact

This rather tough approach can only be justified if it is clear that the child is not ill or in discomfort, but is just crying to get his own way. It is best to carry it out any time between the age of 6 months old and starting at school. The difficulty of keeping to this sleep programme should not be underestimated, and parents will often need intensive support on a daily basis to help them persevere. It is always best to see both parents together before they tackle sleep problems. Any slight disagreement is likely to be magnified using this tough and demanding approach.

An alternative approach

Some parents lack the confidence and motivation to carry out the demanding approach described above. There is an alternative approach where the parent spends progressively less time in the child's bedroom each night, following a carefully worked out schedule. This can be effective, but many children soon grasp what is happening, and return to their previous ways.

There will always be a few who are against causing a child any distress at all, fearing that it must inevitably lead to long-term psychological harm. There is no evidence to support this view which makes the unrealistic assumption that distress can somehow be avoided in life. In fact, children cannot have all their wishes met, so denying their unreasonable demands in the context of a loving family, can have a positive and protective effect on children. Success in establishing a good night time routine leads to increased confidence and happiness all round, making all the hard work well worth the effort.

ENURESIS AND ENCOPRESIS

Many of the issues related to enuresis and encopresis are similar. The one major difference being that soiling provokes much stronger negative reactions than wetting. Enuresis is much more common than encopresis and will therefore be dealt with in more detail. The 1946 British National Survey found that most parents started to sit their children on the pot well before the end of the first year and there is no evidence that early training has any adverse influence on the achievement of continence in any way. It may well be that delayed toilet training makes it more difficult for some children to gain continence.

Most of the usual explanations that parents use to help them understand enuresis have been shown to be mistaken. Deep sleep has not been found to play any part. Sleep EEGs have shown that enuresis can occur at any stage of sleep although wetting is more frequent in the stage just before waking and occurs less frequently during REM sleep. The notion that incontinent children have a smaller bladder capacity than normal has a certain logic to it, but the issue is far from straight forward. The average urine volume voided is about 80 ml at two years of age, increasing to around 225 ml between seven and eight years old. The ability of the bladder wall (detrusor) muscles to relax as they become stretched keeps the pressure around 15 cm water until micturition occurs when the pressure increases to about 50 cm water. In young children the detrusor muscle contracts at relatively low volumes leading to a rise in pressure and an urge to micturate which has to be inhibited by contraction of the external urethral sphincter.

Urine volume per voiding has been found to be significantly less in enuretic children. However, under light anaesthesia bladder capacity is the same for continent and enuretic children at 40 cm water pressure. The total output per 24 hours is also the same. These findings suggest that it is the functional immaturity of bladder function that leads to small amounts of urine being voided, rather than small structural capacity.

The observation that wetting is frequently worse when a child is emotionally distressed has led to the commonly held view that it must be the emotion that actually causes the enuresis. However, enuresis presents in much the same way as other conditions, such as asthma, nail biting, or tooth ache – they all get worse if a child is distressed for any reason. There are very few aspects of development that improve with emotional stress and regression under the influence of threatening or stressful influences is part of normal functioning.

Children who have experienced stressful life events do have an increased rate of incontinence, but there is also an increase in a whole range of maladaptive behaviour. What does seem to be important is the timing of the stress. For example, children admitted to hospital between the ages of 2–5 years are more likely to continue wetting than children who have not been admitted.

The relationship between stressful life events, emotional states and enuresis is highly complex. If enuresis is primarily a symptom of emotional disorder, one might expect more girls than boys to be affected or at least for the sex ratio to be equal, since the frequency of adverse life events is much the same for boys and girls. Enuresis in school age children is at least twice as common in boys than in girls, although if girls do wet they tend to be more emotionally disturbed than boys.

Enuresis

Enuresis is a specific developmental delay and this implies that one or more aspects of maturation are significantly delayed by 20 per cent or more in relation to the rest of the child's general development. The commonly recognised specific delays in development involve speech and language, reading and arithmetic, fine and gross motor skills, bowel and bladder development. It is likely that hyperactivity and some forms of impulsiveness also occur as specific delays in development.

Specific developmental delays share the same characteristics

- A higher incidence in boys
- A tendency to be more serious in girls
- Normal progression through maturational stages
- Evidence of heritability
- Good response to specific training and little response to other treatments
- Early regression under stress
- A tendency to be associated with other specific delays
- Increased vulnerability to psychosocial stress
- Associated with secondary emotional distress, frustration and low self esteem
- Normal development in most other areas
- A strong tendency to improve spontaneously

There is a 68 per cent concordance rate for enuresis in monozygotic twins compared with 36 per cent concordance for dizygotic twins. The steady improvement of enuresis with age is well documented as is the superiority of treatments involving training over other therapies. These findings all support the view that enuresis is primarily a specific developmental disorder as defined above.

The implications of enuresis. The developmental model described below is essentially an interactive one that takes account of a range of different factors and at the same time is capable of integrating a wide range of different theories. The outlook for a specific developmental delay is good in the sense that it improves with time, but ineffective training or stressful experiences will delay the attainment of skill competence. According to this model the delayed skill will remain vulnerable and is likely to be the first skill to be lost as a result of regression under stress.

Secondary enuresis may not at first appear to fit the model, since it characteristically follows a stressful event after a period of continence. However, the concept of children being either continent or incontinent is unhelpful because continence is only gradually achieved and is always dependant on the relationship between bladder maturity and adverse emotional or physical stress factors that affect bladder control. This is why the main features of primary and secondary enuresis are the same, the treatment is the same and the outcome is much the same as well.

Day wetting is more common in girls and they in turn are also more likely to have bacteruria. Diurnal wetting is also linked to a higher rate of psychiatric disturbance, but none of these findings is contrary to enuresis being primarily a specific developmental delay.

Deliberate urination that causes wetting of the bed or elsewhere is very different from accidental incontinence and should be seen as a provocative antisocial act. Clinical impression suggests that children who indulge in this unusual behaviour are disturbed and are using it to

An explanatory developmental model of enuresis. Any explanatory model of enuresis has to be able to integrate all the research findings and provide a satisfactory explanation for the complex relationship between enuresis and psychosocial stress too.

This illustrates the typical relationship between the rate of skill acquisition and age, with a high rate of development early on eventually reaching a plateau. The normal course of development is not a smooth one, rather it is characterised by advances and regressions under the dual influences of training and stress

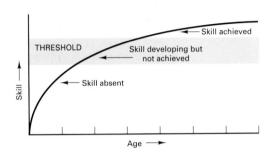

Specific training speeds up the rate of development of skill competence and stress of any kind (physical and emotional) may slow down development or lead to regression and loss of skills

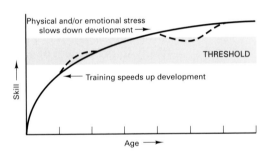

This illustrates the developmental curve of a typical example of specific developmental delay

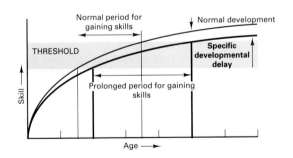

In a child with a specific developmental delay, a prolonged period is spent passing through the threshold and the plateau is established nearer the threshold than normal. In the event of a stressful experience, the specifically delayed skill is likely to be lost before other abilities

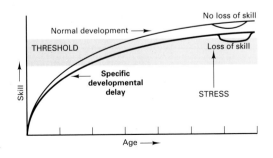

signal their distress about their care within the family.

The feeling of failure and the development of a low self-esteem resulting from the many negative experiences associated with enuresis is likely to become apparent around the age of 6–9 years of age, when children start to have a more clearly developed concept of self-image. It is also difficult for children to feel grown up and mature while they are still wetting the bed. Treatment should, therefore, not be postponed in the hope that the child will grow out of it.

Toilet training

Less than 1 in 10 children with enuresis have some physical cause for the wetting, most commonly a urinary infection. This needs to be excluded before any continence training programme is put into effect. Toilet training in one form or another is the most effective way of managing enuresis. However, it is important that toilet training is undertaken at the appropriate age. Most parents start potting their children between the ages of 5 and 9 months, an age at which most children can sit unsupported. Another accepted sign of readiness of toilet training is the ability to indicate a wish to pass urine and showing signs of distress when wet. There is some evidence that if training is delayed beyond 20 months the likelihood of persisting incontinence is significantly increased.

The first step in the treatment of day or night time wetting is to record the frequency of accidents, while at the same time giving high praise for being dry. Simple explanation of the significance of wetting and its developmental nature should also be given. If this fails to produce improvement after two weeks, daytime wetting is then best dealt with by visits to the toilet at intervals that are frequent enough to ensure that the child remains dry and then gradually increasing the gap between the visits. The use of individually designed reward charts with stars or smiley faces indicating success are generally helpful, but take a lot of organisation to do properly.

Increasing a child's involvement in the clearing up process after accidents is also helpful. Cleanliness training helps to increase children's awareness of the inconvenience of wetting. When wetting occurs, the child has to remove the wet clothes or sheets and put them to soak or in the laundry. They are then replaced with dry items. The more the child takes responsibility for this cleaning up process the better. Parents must understand that this is a training technique and not a punishment. They will also need to supervise the cleaning up and provide assistance at an age appropriate level. This training approach helps children to become more aware of the wetting and less inclined to pretend that it does not exist. It also makes any success more noticeable for the child.

Moisture sensitive electric buzzers that sound the alarm on micturition are available in many different forms, although they all make use of urine to complete an electric circuit. These gadgets can be used for day or night time wetting and if used according to the instructions, should result in an 80 per cent improvement rate. However, social and motivational factors are crucially important in determining the outcome of these training interventions.

The so called Dry-Bed Technique seeks to maximise motivation and raise social rewards for dryness. On the first night the child is woken up every hour, given a drink and guided to the toilet. If urine is passed in the toilet the child is praised and appropriately rewarded. The dry-bed training programme also includes a buzzer apparatus that is used to identify a wetting incident. If wet, the child has to do the '20 times routine'. This involves going to the toilet 20 times, counting up to 20 on each occasion. For the first week the child has to perform the 20 times routine every night before going to sleep even if the bed was dry the night before. But after that, it is only performed after wetting. There are several variations of this approach, but they all have in common an emphasis on overlearning, ie repeating something more times than might seem necessary. This rather extreme approach is remarkably successful if carried out properly, but is best reserved for the highly motivated families.

Lifting or waking children at night to go to the toilet may be quite successful, but it fails to train the child and the improvement is purely symptomatic. Bladder training techniques are occasionally helpful, but are not worth spending too much time and effort on. Bladder training includes voluntarily prolonging the intervals between voiding or stopping and starting the flow during micturition.

Medication. Desmopressin (Desamino-D-arginine vasopressin), a vasopressin analogue is currently more favoured than imipramine as the drug of choice for symptomatic treatment of enuresis. Desmopressin has been found to be effective for short term symptom suppression. It is administered as a single intranasal dose of 20 to 40 μg before bed time. This recommended dose is independent of age and body weight and can be expected to produce improvement in 80 per cent of children, half of whom will stop wetting altogether. The efficacy of Desmopressin seems to be related to its ability to concentrate urine and thus decrease the output of urine during the night. Desmopressin is relatively free of side effects in comparison with other drugs such as tricyclics. In view of this, they are no longer considered appropriate in the routine treatment of enuresis. Excessive drinking with desmopressin can lead to hyponatraemia.

Encopresis

The term encopresis implies that formed faeces are deposited in abnormal places. This distinguishes it from overflow related to constipation and accidental soiling due to diarrhoea. It is best conceived of as a specific delay in the development of bowel control, having all the characteristic features already outlined. A simple explanation of these issues is usually very reassuring for parents. The management of encopresis is relatively straight forward unless there are secondary emotional or physical factors that may perpetuate the symptom.

The programme outlined in the table may seem rather basic, but it is usually very effective if it is applied to the letter. It is the strong emotions generated by the soiling that undermine treatment by making parents feel angry and children feel unlikable failures. Successful treatment

Main steps in the treatment of encopresis

1 Train the child to sit on the toilet for up to 5 minutes at regular times. The use of charts and timers may be helpful
2 Plan for the child to sit on the toilet frequently enough to avoid soiling. Four or more times a day may be necessary
3 First reward regular sitting and when this is well established, reward passing a stool in the toilet
4 Use diet, laxatives or enemas to keep the lower bowel as empty as possible. Soiling will be less likely to occur
5 The child should take some responsibility for clearing up the mess with help and supervision as appropriate
6 If dirty pants are hidden, the parent should take control of all pants and only provide clean ones for old ones returned

normally reverses these negative processes, but where symptoms continue in spite of treatment interventions, the underlying, disturbed emotions will need attention.

HYPERACTIVITY

Main characteristics

• Short attention span
• Distractibility
• Poor impulse control
• Marked overactivity

Hyperactivity is a symptom that causes considerable confusion amongst parents and professionals. Each of the symptoms are developmentally normal in younger children aged 2–6 years. This makes assessment difficult because there are no generally accepted measures of hyperactivity and the diagnosis is therefore a subjective one. Parents are often quick to diagnose hyperactivity if they find their child difficult to manage. Nevertheless, about 2 per cent of children are noticeably restless and inattentive, many of whom go on to have learning problems at school and pervasive behaviour problems as a result of their symptoms.

A number of different factors have been identified as possible aetiological factors. It seems likely that the condition will eventually be seen as the final common pathway of a number of different causes including genetic, neurochemical and adverse psychosocial factors. The effect of diet on overactive behaviour remains less than certain. What is more certain is that at least 30 per cent of hyperactive children seem to do particularly badly on a range of measures when followed up into adult life. It seems likely that a cycle of adverse relationships, low self esteem and negative experiences is set up at an early age leading to progressively more antisocial behaviour.

The treatment of hyperactivity should be focused on encouraging impulse control and the training of appropriate behaviour. No one method has been shown to be better than another and it is reasonable to create individually tailored programmes that address the most obvious problems at school and at home. Hyperactive children benefit from routine and regularity in everyday life, with firm boundaries set for their behaviour. Concentration exercises can also help: the child is asked to concentrate on a task for a few seconds, timed by the clock, and the time is gradually increased over several weeks, always ensuring that each concentration session gives an experience of success. Stimulants derived from amphetamine have a paradoxical calming effect in children and have been shown to be effective in the symptomatic treatment of hyperactivity, but not to influence the long term outcome when used alone. The use of such drugs should be restricted to clinicians with special experience in this field.

DIFFICULT AND DISOBEDIENT BEHAVIOUR

It is obviously important to focus on prevention as the primary aim of any therapeutic work with childhood behaviour problems. Ultimately it is good parenting that provides the most help for children in the long run. The risk of developing antisocial behaviour is reduced if the child is provided with the high quality care.

Parental qualities that reduce the risk of behaviour problems

- Routine and regularity in everyday life
- Clear limit setting
- Unconditional love and affection
- A high level of supervision
- Consistent care and protection
- Age appropriate discipline and rewards
- High levels of supervision

Difficult behaviour occurs so frequently in children and is so often due to the parent's perception of their behaviour or their mishandling of the child that it is all too easy to reassure parents that there is really nothing wrong with their child or that 'the child will soon grow out of it'. Unfortunately there is good evidence that many behaviour problems have a strong tendency to continue. Indeed, aggressive behaviour is a very stable characteristic and is almost as unchanging as IQ.

Coping with problems

It is not difficult to see that many children's problems are actually caused or at least maintained by their parents. Sometimes parents actually provide examples of the unwanted behaviour and model it for their children. For example, argumentative children have frequently gained experience and been tutored in this style of interaction by their argumentative parents. Similarly, children who are aggressive have frequently experienced at first hand their parents own aggression. It is important to identify this mechanism where it occurs and to be prepared to point it out to parents in a supportive and factual way. This is a delicate task because any approach that is seen as critical of parent's actions is unlikely to produce positive results. The task of parenting is difficult enough as it is and impossible to get right all the time. The consequent feeling of guilt that parents experience much of the time, is the main driving force for the majority of inappropriate and potentially harmful responses that occur between parent and child. Great effort, therefore, needs to be devoted to helping parents feel less guilty while at the same time encouraging and supporting parents in the use of more effective methods of child care.

Antisocial behaviour in children is closely associated with aggressive behaviour in their parents. This leads to a predictable sequence of events called 'the coercive system' as follows:

1. Badly behaved children make it difficult for their parents to use the more subtle forms of management of deviant behaviour and to encourage good behaviour.

2. The naughty child frequently produces an aggressive response from the parent, which then serves as a model or example for the child to follow. Alternatively the parent may give in 'for a quiet life', in which case the child will learn that it pays to be bad.

3. The level of disturbance and aggression in the family rises and anarchy follows, leading to a further breakdown of caring and positive, helping behaviours in family interactions.

4. As a result, the parents tend to become fed up and irritable. They lose their confidence and self-esteem and their children also become frustrated and fed up.

5. Family members disengage from each other, the parents become disunited and the control of antisocial behaviour breaks down, resulting in still further problems and so the cycle continues.

Helping with discipline

Standards of parental discipline vary a great deal from one family to another. What seems to be the crucial issue is for each family to agree and set standards of acceptable behaviour. It is inconsistent discipline that causes far more problems for children than discipline that is consistently too lax or too strict. The word discipline comes from the Latin 'disciplina' meaning teaching or training which gives an indication of how behaviour problems are best dealt with.

One of the most typical ineffectual parent-child interactions that occurs in everyday family life is where a parent asks their child to do something. When nothing happens they ask again and again and again and again. On each occasion the demand becomes more hostile until eventually the parent is driving to screaming pitch. At this point the child wonders what all the fuss is about. After all, it was only a relatively minor thing that was being asked in the first place. Unfortunately this type of interaction actually trains children to take little or no notice of their parents until they become furious. Nagging is tiring and can lead to fraught and hostile relationships within the family. It is therefore best to have a rule that in general instructions are only given once. If it is unimportant, there is no need to repeat it again. If, however, it is important then a warning should be given about the consequences of not doing what has been asked. Most parents are very successful in using this training approach to protect their child from potentially dangerous situations such as playing with fire, running into the street and sticking fingers into electric sockets. Clearly until parents are able to gain this level of control, their children are at risk of accidental death.

Assuming that parents have been able to gain compliance from children faced with danger, the same training approach can then be extended to other areas that the parents feel are important. If parents feel uncertain or uncomfortable about being quite firm with and controlling their children, it may help to point out that if their ultimate aim is for their child to gain self-control then it can only be achieved by the parents giving this control in the first instance. Children are not born with self-control and it does not develop spontaneously without it being provided externally first.

ATTENTION-SEEKING BEHAVIOUR

Disruptive behaviour is often labelled attention seeking as a way of identifying the aetiology. Unfortunately this explanation is not a particularly helpful one. In fact, any behaviour could be called attention seeking. Even total conformity or doing nothing at all could be described in this way. An additional problem is that identifying a behaviour as attention seeking does not provide any helpful insight as to what might be done about it. Giving the behaviour more attention is likely to make it worse. Alternatively, removing attention and ignoring the behaviour is also likely to lead to an exacerbation of the behaviour until the child does eventually get noticed. Assuming the child does actually need extra attention, it is important to get in first and provide this in an appropriate caring way, rather than waiting for the child to demand it. One effective way of doing this is by providing 'quality time' where the child is given undivided and undisturbed attention for a period of 5–10 minutes on a regular basis.

SCHOOL BASED PROBLEMS

Boys are more likely to be excluded from school than girls, with aggressive behaviour being the most common reason for suspension from school. Once excluded, few will return to normal schooling. Boys are also more at risk for specific reading problems which are associated with a higher rate of behaviour problems when compared with children who have no difficulty with reading. There is a highly complex relationship between the bad behaviour and the reading problem, with both having some causative factors in common.

The school itself may have characteristics which encourage or at least allow the development of antisocial behaviour. Even if school intake factors are controlled for, there remain consistent differences between schools in the rate of children's antisocial behaviour. The most likely explanation for these differences is that they have been caused by factors within the school itself.

School factors which are associated with a high rate of antisocial behaviour

- Low staff morale
- High teacher turnover
- Unclear standards of behaviour
- Inconsistent methods of discipline
- Poor organisation
- Lack of knowledge of the children as individuals
- Undervaluing children's work

From school age onwards, antisocial behaviour has a strong tendency to continue as a very stable characteristic. About 50 per cent of the children with bad behaviour continue to cause problems over long periods.

Factors associated with a poor outcome for antisocial behaviour

- High frequency and wide range of antisocial acts, especially aggressive, argumentative and disruptive behaviour
- Truancy and lying
- Fire setting or running off
- Mixing with other antisocial children
- Growing up in extreme poverty
- Misuse of drugs
- Early onset of problems
- Family members with antisocial behaviour or alcohol problems

Assessment

When considering problems that arise within a school setting, it is important to distinguish the five main areas where problems can arise.

School based sources of disturbed behaviour

- The child's own problems, eg separation anxiety
- Difficulties with peers, eg bullying
- Problems with academic work, eg too easy, too difficult
- Problems with teachers, eg poor discipline
- Problems outside of school, eg family breakdown
  (Any combination of the above)

It is all too easy for schools to believe that any problems at school must be due to difficulties at home but children spend a considerable amount of their daily life at school (approximately 15 000 hours in all). It would therefore be surprising if factors within school did not play a considerable part in the aetiology of childhood emotional and behavioural problems.

Teasing and bullying. The majority of all bullying takes place in school or near the school. There are marked differences in the rate of bullying between schools, probably because some schools have an ethos that makes bullying unacceptable. Overall about 10 per cent of children report being bullied at least once a week, and approximately seven per cent of children are identified as bullies. Bullying is more common in primary than secondary school and becomes more subtle and verbal as children grow older. Girls use less physical means of bullying, but are almost as aggressive as boys. Roughly 20 per cent of the victims are also bullies and this group of children tends to be particularly disturbed. The typical bully, on the other hand, tends to have high self esteem and is generally aggressive and dismissive of authority. At least 75 per cent of bullying goes undetected by parents or teachers, and it should be considered as a possible cause for any child whose symptoms of distress do not seem to have a sufficient explanation.

Bullying occurs where there is an unequal power relationship and where any form of aggression is deliberately used to humiliate someone and cause them distress. It should never be tolerated and should always be directly confronted and dealt with immediately. A whole school policy on bullying that includes a commitment from children, parents and teachers to identify and stop bullying has been shown to be the most effective approach. Close supervision of bullies and victims is also helpful.

Non attendance at school. The causes of school non attendance are multiple and complex. Leaving aside those children who are kept at home by their parents, there are three main reasons for not attending school. It is most important to immediately exclude a genuine and acceptable reason for avoiding school such as being bullied or being unable to cope with the work. The other two causes are the neurotic disorders of school refusal due to separation anxiety (worse on leaving the parent) or school phobia (worse on arrival at school) and the conduct disorder of truancy.

Main differences between school refusal and truancy

School refusal	Truancy
Well behaved at school	Antisocial behaviour in and out of school
No academic problems	Poor academic achievement
Associated neurotic behaviour	Associated antisocial behaviour
More frequent at primary school	More frequent towards the end of secondary schooling
More often youngest or only child	More often in children from large families
Stable home background	Unsettled family background
Child remains at home – over involved relationships	Child's whereabouts unknown – poor supervision
Prognosis generally good	Poor prognosis

Management

Because the reasons why children do not attend school are multitudinous, it is important that the problem is not tackled in a piecemeal way. Close collaboration is required between parents, teachers and other professionals, and after a detailed assessment of the problem, a comprehensive treatment package should be drawn up involving all the relevant people. In most cases of school refusal, except where there are genuine reasons for fear of school, the child should be returned as quickly as possible in a firm and determined way. At the same time that the child is returned to school, the underlying causes need to be dealt with, but it is often true to say that 'the treatment of school refusal is to return to school'. This is because once back at school most children usually settle into the routine quite quickly, almost as if nothing had ever happened. The advantage of returning a child to school rapidly is that if it does not work, the underlying causes can be expected to become clear for all to see. Truancy also requires a total treatment package involving all the relevant professionals. The most effective approach here is to construct a programme of education that is appropriate for the needs of the child, while at the same time monitoring and supervising the young person throughout the school day. Any learning problems must also be addressed.

EMOTIONAL DISORDERS

Anxiety states of one kind or another are the most common emotional disorders. The normal stages of anxiety development are described in Chapter 14. Each of these stages can develop into a pathological state and become a disorder if the symptoms are severe, prolonged, handicapping and developmentally inappropriate.

Simple anxiety states

Extreme shyness and separation problems become more significant as children grow older and at school age they can be a serious handicap to a child. In addition some children have a very high level of general anxiety that relates to a wide range of situations. These children usually have a 'sensitive' or 'highly strung' temperament that makes them highly reactive to stress of any kind, including exciting events. The management of generalised anxiety has some important elements.

1. Facing the anxiety. This involves helping the child to learn how to manage the anxiety provoking situation by facing up to it rather than by avoidance. There are two main approaches:

(a) The 'in at the shallow end' approach. The child is gradually exposed to the feared situation, step by step. Anxiety must always be kept to a manageable level. Perseverance over a long period is essential and the process may fail if any of the steps are too large. It is then necessary to go back a stage and start again from there.

(b) The 'in at the deep end' approach. The child is exposed directly to the feared situation and remains with it until the anxiety has reduced to a tolerable level. This approach carries a higher risk if it is not carried through to completion. In addition, everyone concerned must agree that this is a reasonable way to deal with the problem. The advantage of this potentially distressing approach is that it can be rapidly effective, especially in younger children. However, the supervising adults must feel confident in what they are doing.

2. Anxiety is catching. It helps to be aware of the powerfully infectious nature of anxiety. This is seen in the way parents cling to their child who has separation anxiety or where the light is kept on because the child is afraid of the dark. Such anxious responses only confirm that there is indeed something to be frightened about.

3. Linking behaviour and thinking. There is a strong connection between thinking and behaviour. For example, a child who has been helped to think through all the positive things about attending school for the first time is likely to cope better than a child who has heard about all the things that might go wrong. A child who has been taught to behave in a confident way at school is less likely to be picked on by other children. Most children respond well to role play exercises where they practice coping with the feared situation.

4. Thought control. Anxiety is primarily due to the anticipation of feared situations before anything has happened. Thoughts are therefore an important trigger for anxiety. In fact, children are surprisingly good at controlling their thoughts, but they will need encouragement and practice to do this. This cognitive approach requires creative solutions that are tailor made for the child. For example, the child with a fear of spiders could be encouraged to name spiders after a close relative in order to change the perception of spiders to something friendly.

5. Relaxation. There are many types of relaxation, any of which may help a child cope with anxiety. Again, it is best to use a method of relaxation that makes sense to the child and is enjoyable. The relaxation technique can then be used to counter anxiety as it arises in the real world, or in the imagination.

6. Keeping a sense of humour. It is difficult if not impossible to laugh and be anxious at the same time. Laughing and joking is a common strategy used to combat anxiety and all anxious children can be helped if the adults around them avoid becoming too serious with them. For example, the child who is anxious about monsters is not helped by the parent who looks under the bed and checks the wardrobe in order to demonstrate that they are monster free.

Phobias

A phobia is an overwhelming irrational fear of an object or a situation which is then avoided as far as possible. Simple phobias of animals and insects are very common and occur in more than 5 per cent of children. It is the avoidance behaviour that tends to maintain the phobia because the child never has a chance to find out that there is nothing to fear. Most phobias can be traced back to an occasion when there was a genuine reason to be frightened or where the child has witnessed another person reacting in a fearful way. Phobic children may therefore have parents with similar fears. Phobias are best tackled along the same lines that have been outlined above for dealing with anxiety.

Obsessional compulsive disorders (OCD)

There is a particularly strong association between phobias and obsessions, so it is possible to describe one in terms of the other. For example, a dirt phobia can be seen as an obsession with cleanliness or obsessional thoughts about harming someone can be viewed as a phobia of death. There is some evidence that OCD is associated with other problems of repetition and impulse control such as tics and other habits, suggesting a neurophysiological basis for the condition. There is also evidence for an inherited genetic contribution to both OCD and phobias. Although drugs that inhibit 5-HT uptake have been claimed to be effective, behavioural approaches are usually more effective. The aim is to find some way of disrupting or time limiting the obsessional thoughts or behaviour, sometimes called 'response prevention'. Thus, the child who insists on compulsively checking is prevented from doing this more than once.

Post traumatic stress disorder (PTSD)

It is now clear that children experience PTSD in the much the same way as adults, following exceptionally severe stress, outside the normal range of experience. Sexual abuse and near-death ordeals are typical of such events. The three characteristic features are vivid memories and avoidance reactions to the event, together with symptoms of hyperarousal. The symptoms may not be present immediately after the stressful event, but develop within a few days. They would normally be expected to gradually reduce after six weeks, but can persist for many months and be complicated by other psychiatric disorder.

Symptoms of post traumatic stress disorder

Re-experiencing	Avoidance	Hyperarousal
Nightmares	Denial of event	Insomnia
Flashbacks	Social withdrawal	Irritability
Preoccupation with the event	Avoidance of memory triggers	Vigilant and over-reactive
Panic attacks	Regression	Easily started

It is helpful to understand PTSD as the equivalent to an emotional wound. It may seem awful at the time but it can be expected to heal eventually. There will always be an emotional scar, but if the healing process is satisfactory the scar need not seriously interfere with function. The emotional wound must be cared for, but not covered up or it could become infected. Thus, exposing the wound to the fresh air is helpful, ie talking about the stressful event. On the other hand, scratching around in the wound is not, ie forced and unwanted counselling.

ANGER AND AGGRESSION

Much of our everyday understanding of anger stems from the work of the psychoanalysts. Freud, Jung, Klein and others highlighted the importance of anger as a normal, and sometimes unconscious, motivating force. Unfortunately these ideas underestimate the importance of learning and life experiences in shaping behaviour. A better understanding of children's moods and tempers has come from surveys, mostly using parental questionnaires, though some also use reports from teachers and/or direct observation of the children.

Tempers occur more often at bedtime, at the end of the morning and the end of the afternoon, that is, when children are hungry or tired. After the age of two years tempers gradually become shorter and less violent, but whining and sulking increase. Overall, the main cause for tempers is attempts to get the children to conform to accepted standards of social behaviour and relationships. Tempers are generally more frequent in children aged from two to five years with a peak around two to three years old.

Tempers and difficult behaviour are more common in boys than in girls and problem behaviour tends to persist. In fact, about 70 per cent of the children who have significant behaviour problems at three years of age still have them a year later. Children with temper tantrums and their families have been shown to have a wide range of associated characteristics.

Associated features of temper tantrums

Child characteristics	Family and social factors
Speech and language problems	Young or elderly mothers
Wetting and soiling	Single or step parent present
Feeding and sleeping problems	Poor social conditions
Hyperactive and difficult	4 or more children in family
Miserable and tearful	Mothers smoke heavily
Frequent aches and pains	Poverty and unemployment
Frequent minor illnesses	Inner city areas

The table lists statistically significant associations, but they must be interpreted with some care. For example, the link between tempers and mothers who smoke may have an affect heavily may be a direct one: the inhaled cigarette smoke may have an effect on the child or it may be the effect of a difficult child causing the mother to smoke more. Alternatively the link might be an indirect one, such as poor living conditions, which could cause stress reactions in the child leading to tempers and, in the mother, leading to heavy smoking.

About 10 per cent of five-year old boys have temper tantrums at least once a week, but the same frequency of tempers was only reported in 2 per cent of 15 year olds. However, irritability and other forms of angry behaviour tend to continue. It would seem that, although tempers usually decrease with age, there is no evidence that children's experience of anger diminishes over time – it just changes in the way it manifests itself. Thus while anger becomes less obvious, depression becomes more apparent.

Three main approaches to the management of childhood tempers

The approach	The metnods
Prevention	Avoid high risk situations (eg tired or hungry) Plan in advance Divert if possible
Training children to express anger in a more acceptable way	Teaching by example Rewarding self control Training anger management
Ignoring the behaviour	Remove any audience Time out Leave until calm

CHILDHOOD DEPRESSION AND DELIBERATE SELF HARM

Epidemiological studies of depression have noted a gradual increase in the incidence of depression in children from about 8 years of age, with a rapid increase of frequency during adolescence. The emergence of depressive disorder in the middle childhood years coincides with the development of clear concepts of 'self image', 'time' and 'death' around the age of 7–9 years. Thus, younger children may experience misery and distress, but the essential ingredients of depressive disorder, namely hopelessness (concept of time required) and worthlessness (concept of self image required) are not yet fully developed at that age. Puberty seems to be an important trigger for psychotic symptoms of bipolar depression, such as delusions and hallucinations, to become a feature of depression. The classification of the different types of depression is still being worked out. At present it is sufficient to understand that depression presents in a number of different forms, all of which need to be taken seriously.

The distinction between distress, depression and despair is an important one. Distressed children are reacting as expected to adverse circumstances or events. Depressed children, on the other hand, experience symptoms that have grown out of proportion to the situation to such an extent that they have a significant adverse effect on the child, interfering with everyday life. Those who reach the point of despair as a result of extreme stress are very much at risk. They have become overwhelmed by their emotions and often present as unusually withdrawn children who fail to thrive. Depressive symptoms frequently accompany other psychiatric disorders, especially conduct disorder and anxiety states. Thus the presence of lowered mood is a relatively non-specific symptom.

Diagnosing depression

Many of the biological concomitants of depression found in adults have also been reported in children, including a failure of dexamethasone to inhibit cortisol secretion, lower nocturnal and 24-hr plasma melatonin levels and a reduced rapid eye movement latency on the sleep EEG in depressed children. Unfortunately the use of psychobiological markers in clinical practice is of limited value since they fail to distinguish between distress, despair and depressive disorder. Diagnosis will depend on identifying the typical pattern of associated features.

Diagnostic features of depression

1 Lowered mood, misery, tearfulness
2 Persisting for more than 2 weeks
3 Severe enough to interfere with everyday life
4 Associated with two or more of the following symptoms:
   – Feelings of worthlessness
   – Sense of hopelessness
   – Disturbed sleep
   – Altered appetite
   – Irritability
   – Anxiety or phobic behaviour
   – Pessimistic and morbid thoughts
   – Suicidal ideas or acts

Children of depressed parents are more likely to suffer from depression themselves and at an earlier age than the children of non-depressed parents. The same group is also at risk of a wide range of health and behaviour problems. This link between depression in children and their parents is a strong one, but complex and interactive in nature. An interesting and frequent finding is that parent's and children's rating of the child's depression correlate poorly. Parent's ratings are almost always lower than their children's own ratings of depression, confirming the general tendency for adults to underestimate the strength of children's distress.

Suicide

Suicidal thoughts occur in a third of depressed children. The frequency increases with age, (particularly in girls), but suicide attempts are rare before the age of 11 years. There is some evidence that attempted suicide is increasing in frequency in young people and that ever younger children are deliberately harming themselves in response to adverse factors within the home or school. Suicidal children appear to have particular difficulty thinking through the consequences of their actions and in coping with their feelings of anger and depression. The factors associated with suicide are so frequent in the general population that it makes the prediction of suicide virtually impossible.

Main associated features of attempted suicide

Disturbed or disrupted home life
Poor functioning at school
Low self-esteem
Antisocial and aggressive behaviour
Poor impulse control
High levels of dysphoria and depression
Substance misuse (especially alcohol)
High frequency of stressful life events in the last year
Family history of affective disorder
A friend or relative who has attempted suicide.

The management

A diagnosis of depressive disorder during childhood suggests a high level of stress and/or vulnerability. The first step must therefore be to identify all the sources of stress in the child's life and to deal with them as far as possible. Various forms of counselling, supportive psychotherapy and cognitive therapy may be used to help the individual to become more resilient and where appropriate family therapy may also be useful. Parents need to understand that their child is 'ill' in the sense that they should make special allowances for any uncooperative behaviour and at the same time provide additional care and affection. Parents and teachers can play a key role by helping to improve the child's self-esteem.

Treatment with antidepressant medication should be reserved for clinicians with specialised knowledge of child psychiatric disorders. Likewise, the assistance of the Child Psychiatry Service should be sought if childhood depression fails to respond to simple treatment or where there is evidence of suicidal or psychotic thoughts.

TREATMENT APPROACHES

Psychological treatments

This section summarises the main psychological treatment approaches that can be used for childhood psychiatric disorder. A number of treatment strategies for particular disorders have already been outlined. There is a wide range of psychological treatments for emotional and behavioural problems of childhood and there is also a considerable variation in the way in which they are applied, which probably has more to do with the personality and style of the therapist than anything else. What evidence there is suggests that all the main types of psychological treatments can be effective. What is less clear is how much more successful one approach is over another. The powerful positive effects of kindness and empathic care should not be underestimated. Sympathetic support and understanding is often more appreciated and just as effective as high powered 'technical' therapeutic procedures.

Family therapy

Family therapy developed as the result of two major impulses. On the one hand psychoanalytic theory was found lacking in its ability to explain many aspects of child behaviour in a social context and practical treatment approaches did not result from the theory of the unconscious mind. On the other hand, the application of social systems theory to groups of people developed new ways of understanding how organisations worked. In particular, how one part of a social system that malfunctions will affect every other part. It is this basic idea that underpins most family therapy, together with the notion that the family also has an unconscious life of its own.

There are many different forms of family therapy, but all methods share the belief that the family can be treated as a single entity and that many of the symptoms of individual members are actually the manifestation of a dysfunctional family. Therefore the family as a whole has to take responsibility for the malfunction of one of its members. This notion does not appeal to some parents and compliance with treatment can be poor. Family therapy is a specialised therapeutic technique that should only be used by experienced therapists in circumstances where there is clear evidence of primary family dysfunction. The use of family therapy for treating individuals in front of the family audience is unhelpful and should not be regarded as family therapy.

Behaviour management

Identifying the factors that have contributed to the behaviour should be the first step in any management programme. Taking a detailed history of the behaviour and gaining relevant background information can be therapeutic in itself. Parents may sometimes gain insight simply from the experience of being able to step back a bit and look objectively at what has been happening. In every case it is helpful to carefully identify the *Antecedents* of the behaviour, details of the *Behaviour* itself and the *Consequences* of that behaviour – the so-called **ABC** approach.

It is also important to know about the social context in which the behaviour occurs. This means collecting details of family relationships and functioning as well as details about how the child is in school.

Knowledge of these complex interactions is important, but at the same time it should be recognised that the full significance of each aetiological factor can only be guessed at. In every case the diagnostic assessment should arrive at a hypothesis to be tested by the outcome of the treatment.

Keeping a record of the behaviour using the ABC method of analysis can be helpful to all concerned. The diary of behaviour not only helps parents to be more objective about their child's behaviour and their own reaction to it, but it also assists in monitoring progress and identifying typical sequences of behaviour. The very act of recording and objectifying the behaviour, together with the support of a sympathetic and understanding clinician may have a most positive effect.

In much the same way that psychotherapeutic treatments are multiple and highly individual, so too are behavioural methods. These are based on learning theory and include notions of reward and punishment. Unfortunately the oversimplistic application of behavioural approaches has given them a bad name. Behavioural programmes should be individually and creatively developed for each case as a collaborative effort between parent, child and clinician. Certainly drawing up a simple star reward chart is a complex matter and keeping it going is harder still. Common sense is helpful, but not sufficient in itself for dealing with childhood behaviour disorders. The general approach must also be appropriate.

General guidelines for behavioural treatments

- First consider methods of prevention
- Identify probable causes and deal with them as far as possible
- Focus on rewarding appropriate behaviour
- Check that any rewards really are desired
- Avoid punishment – it only works in the short term
- Use restitution – making good whatever has been wrong
- Promote behaviour that is incompatible with the unwanted behaviour
- Encourage training by repetition of the desired behaviour
- Set a good example
- Close supervision is often necessary for the child and the parent
- Keep a sense of humour

Drug treatment

The role of psychopharmacology in the community based treatment of child psychiatric disorders is limited. The use of these drugs should therefore be restricted to those with specialist knowledge who prescribe these drugs in routine clinical practice. There are high risks associated with the use of mind controlling medication in children that relate to the possible long term consequences and to the potential for parents and children to expect drugs to resolve problems while they remain passive and uninvolved.

If treatment fails

If treatment fails to produce the expected result, it should not be immediately discarded as no good. There may be hidden factors that serve to maintain the problem.

Checklist for failed treatment

1 The parents are unco-operative and have not complied with treatment
2 Hidden factors are present that have been missed
   – bullying
   – academic failure
   – parental relationship problem
   – sexual abuse
   – problems with peers
3 The treatment was too brief or too superficial
4 The wrong treatment was used.

Referral to the Child and Adolescent Psychiatry Service

Such is the stigma of psychiatry that the decision to refer a child and family to the Child and Adolescent Psychiatry Service is often delayed until the disorder is so well established that any change will be difficult to achieve. It is therefore better to refer too early than too late. Most child psychiatry services provide assessment, consultation and treatment on a multidisciplinary basis, but there is considerable variation in the level of back up resources in different parts of the country. Child and Adolescent Psychiatry Services are finding new ways of working in the community and in supporting other professionals in their work. Consultation can therefore be requested in the first instance and is always better done before referral of the more complex, multiproblem cases, to ensure that the most efficient and effective approach is taken.

Referrals should be made to a named clinician giving details of the problem, the family background and any other agencies involved. Most important of all is the co-operation of the child and parents and parental motivation to follow things through. These are both greatly influenced by the way the referral is made and the attitude of the referrer. Parental motivation is increased if the referrer appears to value and have confidence in the Child and Adolescent Psychiatry Service.

REFERENCES AND FURTHER READING

Anders T F, Weinstein P 1972 Sleep and its disorders in infants and children: A review. Pediatrics 50: 312–24
Angold A 1988 Review: Childhood depression. British Journal of Psychiatry 152: 601–7
Baker L, Cantwel D P 1987 A prospective psychiatric follow-up of children with speech/language disorders. Journal of the American Academy of Child Adolescent Psychiatry 26: 546–53
Berg I 1985 Management of school refusal. Archives of Disease in Childhood 60: 486–8
Bishop D V M 1987 Causes of specific developmental language disorder. Journal of Child Psychology and Psychiatry 28: 1–8
Bohman M, Sigvardsson S 1979 Long term efects of early institutional care. Journal of Child Psychology and Psychiatry 20: 111–7
Brooksbank D J 1985 Suicide and parasuicide in childhood and early adolescence. British Journal of Psychiatry 146: 459–63
Brunn R D 1984 Gilles de la Tourette's syndrome: an overview of clinical experience. Journal of the American Academy of Child Psychiatry 23: 126–33
Campbell M, Spencer M K 1988 Psychopharmacology in child and adolescent psychiatry: A review of the past five years. Journal of the American Academy of Child Psychiatry 27: 269–79
Cox A 1975 Assessment of parental behaviour. Journal of Child Psychology and Psychiatry 16: 266–70
Clarke R V G 1985 Delinquency, environment and intervention. Journal of Child Psychology and Psychiatry 26: 505–23

Cox et at 1987 The impact of maternal depression in young children. Journal of Child Psychology and Psychiatry 28: 917–28

Duncan M K 1985 Brief psychotherapy with children and their families: The state of the art. Journal of the American Academy of Child Psyciatry 23: 544

Frankel E F 1985 Behavioural treatment approaches to pathological unsocialised physical aggression in young children. Journal of Child Psychology and Psychiatry 26: 525–51

Garralda M E et al 1988 Psychiatric adjustment in children with chronic renal failure. Journal of Child Psychology and Psychiatry 29: 79–90

Gath A 1977 The impact of an abnormal child on the parents. British Journal of Psychiatry 130: 405–10

Golombok S, Spencer A, Rutter M 1983 Children in lesbian and single parent households. Psychosexual and psychiatric appraisal. Journal of Child Psychology and Psychiatry 24: 551–72

Graham P 1985 Psychology and the health of children. Journal of Child Psychology and Psychiatry 26: 333–47

Graham P, Rutter M 1973 Psychiatric disturbance in young adolescents – a follow up study. Proceedings of the Royal Society of Medicine 66: 1226–9

Gratten-Smith P et al 1988 Clinical features of conversion disorder. Archives of Disease in Childhood 63: 408–14

Green R et al 1987 Specific cross-gender behaviour in boyhood and later homosexual orientation. British Journal of Psychiatry 151: 84-8

Herd D 1987 The relevance of attachment theory to child psychiatric practice: an update. Journal of Child Psychology and Psychiatry 28: 25–8

Hetherington E M et al 1985 Long-term effects of divorce and remarriage on the adjustment of children. Journal of the American Academy of Child Psychiatry 24: 518–30

Hoare P 1984 The development of psychiatric disorder among school children with epilepsy. Developmental Medicine and Child Neurology 26: 3–24

Kaszdin A E, Esveldt-Dawson K et al 1987 Problem solving skills training and relationship training in the treatment of anti-social child behaviour. Journal of Consultation and Clinical Psychology 55: 76–85

MacFarlane A C et al 1987 A longitudinal study of the psychological mobidity in children due to a natural disaster. Psychological Medicine 17: 727-38

Macquire J, Richman N 1986 Screening for behavioural problems in nurseries. The reliability and validity of the pre-school behaviour check list. Journal of Child Psychology and Psychiatry 27: 7–32

Marks I 1987 The development of normal fear: A review. Journal of Child Psychology and Psychiatry 28: 667–97

Nicol A R et al 1987 The nature of mother and toddler problems. Journal of Child Psychology and Psychiatry 28: 739–54

Offord D R 1987 Prevention of behavioural and emotional disorders in children. Journal of Child Psychology and Psychiatry 28: 9–19

Patterson G R, Chamberlain T, Reid J P 1982 A comparative evaluation of a parent training programme. Behaviour Therapy 13: 638–54

Pynoos R S et al 1987 Life threat and post traumatic stress in school age children. Archives of General Psychiatry 44: 1057–63

Rapoport J L 1986 Childhood obsessive-compulsion disorder. Journal of Child Psychology and Psychiatry 27: 289–95

Rutter M, Quinton D 1984 Parental psychiatric disorder: effects on children. Psychological Medicine 14: 853–80

Rutter M, Schopler E 1987 Autism and pervasive developmental disorders: Concepts and diagnostic issues. Journal of Autism and Developmental Disorders 17: 159–86

Rutter M et al 1980 School influences on children's behaviour and development (the 1979 Kenneth Blackfan lecture). Pediatrics 65: 208–20

Shafer D 1978 'Soft' neurological signs and later psychiatric disorders in children. Journal of Child Psychology and Psychiatry 19: 63–5

Shafer D et al 1988 Preventing teenage suicide: A critical review. Journal of the American Academy of Child and Adolescent Psychiatry 27: 675–87

Sturge C 1982 Reading retardation and antisocial behaviour. Journal of Clinical Psychology and Psychiatry 23: 21–31

Taitz L S et al 1986 Factors associated with outcome in management of defaecation disorders. Archives of Disease in Childhood 61: 472–7

Thorley G 1986 Hyperkinetic syndrome of childhood: clinical characteristics. British Journal of Psychiatry 144: 16–24

Weissman M M et al 1987 Children of depressed parents: Impaired psychopathology and early onset of major depression. Archives of General Psychiatry 43: 847–53

Werry J 1988 Behaviour therapy with children and adolescents: A 20 year overview. Journal of the American Academy of Child Psychiatry 28: 1–18

Werry J S et al 1987 Attention deficit, conduct, oppositional and anxiety disorders in children. 1. A review of research on differentiating characteristics. 2. Clinical characteristics. Journal of the American Academy of Child and Adolescent Psychiatry 26: 133–43, 144–55

Wolkind S, Renton G 1979 Psychiatric disorder in children in long-term residential care: a follow-up study. British Journal of Psychiatry 135: 129–35

Woolston J L 1983 Eating disorders in infancy and early childhood. Journal of the American Academy of Child and Adolescent Psychiatry 26: 123–6

Yates A 1990 Current perspectives on eating disorders: treatment, outcome and research directions. Journal of the American Academy of Child and Adolescent Psychiatry 29: 129

26 Counselling

This chapter aims to provide some basic and practical advice on how to begin to develop a counselling approach in your work. As such it is primarily aimed at developing a style which will make interviewing and short-term involvement with patients and families more productive and satisfying for all concerned. The counselling approach described is applicable to adults and to adolescents. Work with younger children often needs to proceed at a less verbal level using activities like play and painting and is not covered here.

There are many definitions of counselling but in this context it means talking with people in a way which enables them to express themselves, to help them to understand themselves and their problems better and to develop ways of coping with or ameliorating their difficulties.

Counselling operates on the psychological plane and may at first be thought of as appropriate only for psychological problems, eg anxiety, depression, fears. However it is important to recognise that there is no clear separation between physical and psychological difficulties. A counselling approach to all encounters will enhance the quality and quantity of information you receive and the person is likely to find the encounter to be of positive value to them.

In some cases of physical illness, psychological factors may play a role in their genesis and maintenance. All physical illnesses have a psychological impact and this becomes increasingly important in chronic, incapacitating and life-threatening diseases. People suffering from or caring for those with such diseases often derive considerable benefit from being able to discuss their feelings, fears, practical concerns etc with someone who is knowledgeable in the area. As an example, a counselling-type interview with a parent about a child with diabetes may reveal the difficulties which the special diet creates within the family and explain why relatively poor control is being obtained.

Longer-term counselling

In cases where problems are serious or severe, your role may be to refer on to more specialist services. Such services vary in different parts of the country both in terms of availability and organisation. It would be worth investigating the following services in your locality: clinical psychology (NHS), educational psychology (LEA), psychiatry, social services, self help groups, voluntary agencies.

If you wish to develop your own counselling work, then training in the first place and supervision in the longer term should be considered as essential. Working with people with psychological problems can be both difficult and emotionally draining and access to an experienced supervisor is necessary in your own and your patient's interest.

BASIC REQUIREMENTS FOR EFFECTIVE COUNSELLING

It is a worthwhile exercise to consider what you, yourself, would be looking for if you were seeking counselling and then to contemplate whether you are able to provide that for those you are seeing. It is also a good idea to think about what you would find aversive and make you disinclined to return for a further session.

Physical surroundings. It is usually helpful to be able to see people in an informal room where it is possible to sit in a relaxed way on comfortable chairs. A counsellor sitting behind a desk instantly produces a formal atmosphere which is not conducive to open discussion. A vital ingredient is that the person who is talking should feel that it is private and that they will not be overheard by those in the room next door or in the corridor. Every attempt needs to be made to avoid interruptions during the session and the setting should be relatively quiet and peaceful.

Whilst these seem like relatively simple arrangements they are very difficult to achieve in many community settings where the rooms which are used are often temporarily made available and have been designed for other functions. In many schools, the medical room has been planned for clinical rather than counselling purposes and a sense of privacy may be very hard to achieve. Depending on the physical siting of the room it is often the case that noises in the corridor, phonecalls and conversations next door intrude on the counselling session and if you can hear them, you assume that they can hear you.

Another major physical constraint is the amount of time which you have available to talk to the person. In a busy clinic schedule with patients every five minutes it is not possible to enter into a counselling relationship. A person needs to feel that you do have the time for them and if they are going to talk about matters which have emotional impact they need to be given the time to talk these through. You will not be able to relax and give them this sense of time if you are aware of a lengthening queue developing. Counselling sessions need to be planned accordingly.

Characteristics of the counsellor. Again, it is worth considering what you would be looking for yourself. It is likely that you would want to see someone who you felt was genuinely interested in you and cared about your welfare. You would want to be listened to and understood and to have the sense that what you were saying was accepted, not judged to be good/bad, acceptable/unacceptable, sensible/foolish. You would want to be able to talk at your own pace, to have time to think and not be rushed.

You are likely to be assessing the counsellor and judging their reactions to you. If you felt patronised, interrupted, misunderstood or that the counsellor found you boring or irritating, then you would be unlikely to confide in that counsellor.

Rogers (1961) summarised the basic conditions for effective counselling to take place and described the three essential characteristics in a counsellor as empathy, genuineness and unconditional positive regard.

Three essentials in a counsellor

Empathy. This is the ability to be able to see the world from the other person's perspective, to understand the feelings they have and the meanings they ascribe to their experiences. In order to do this you have to develop an understanding of that person in their context – their life experiences, the nature of their relationships, their belief structures.
Genuineness. This is about being interested and concerned about the other person.
Unconditional positive regard. This is sometimes described in terms of warmth and being non-judgemental, accepting the person as they are and not making value judgements.

Frank (1973) argues that underlying all effective therapeutic relationships there are the following characteristics: warmth, respect, kindness, hope, understanding and the provision of 'explanation'. When people turn to a counsellor in a time of trouble they are usually unhappy and confused. They tend not to understand the nature of their problems and cannot see ways out of it. Within counselling you are working with the person in a *joint* endeavour to try to understand them and their difficulties – 'to provide explanations' and to work out ways forward.

Characteristics of counselling. When people are asked to consider what they might hope to gain if they sought counselling, the initial answers tend to be in terms of problem-solving yet many people have problems for which there is no straightforward solution. An example of this is in bereavement where the counselling is aimed at helping the person through the grieving process towards long-term adjustment to the bereavement.

The supportive element is vital in any counselling relationship and in many cases may be the only thing you have to offer. Being on the person's side, being willing to care, being available for them to share their problems and helping them to find ways to cope are very valuable.

In many cases you may be working towards helping the person to find a way to deal with their difficulties. On occasion this may be purely practical, eg obtaining rehousing, and you are able to use your knowledge and influence to make things happen. In other cases people simply need a piece of factual information to enable them to sort things out for themselves. Even in such cases, your message is more likely to be heard if you have established a relationship in which the person feels valued as an individual by a counsellor who is genuinely interested in them.

THE FIRST SESSION

When you see someone for the first time it is not possible to know whether this will be a one-off occasion or the beginning of a longer relationship. However, there are certain aspects to a first contact which need to be present as they will lay the basis for longer-term work or permit a single session to proceed and be concluded in a satisfying manner. There are three main activities which need to take place.

1. Laying the foundation – introductions, explanation.
2. Beginning the exploration of the problems and their context.
3. Beginning the process of developing a therapeutic relationship

Laying the foundation

It is easy to forget how a person feels when they are coming to see you for the first time to discuss a problem. They are likely to feel anxious and uncertain in what is, for them, an unfamiliar situation. They may not know who they are to see, what will be expected of them, how they will be able to explain their situation. Introducing yourself and explaining how the session will be conducted are useful starting points and every effort should be made to make the situation a comfortable one. You should remember that when people are anxious they are less likely to retain information which is given and failures of communication are a common complaint that people have about their encounters with professionals.

Beginning the exploration of the problems and their context

It is usually helpful to have a flexible structure in which you begin to explore the areas of concern and obtaining a history is a very valuable starting point. The means by which this is done will be covered in more detail later but at this early stage you are trying to develop an understanding of the problems, their history and context. At all stages it is crucial not just to obtain factual information but to explore the person's feelings about events, to understand the meaning that they have for them. It is in this way that you can develop an empathetic relationship and it is at the level of feelings and meanings that counselling should operate. In this process you are not simply recording information but are also looking for clues to help you to develop hypotheses about a person's difficulties. Later you will need to test out your hypotheses.

In any given situation, a person's reaction will be dependent on their past experiences, their present situation and their expectations about the future. Failure to get a job applied for may be a minor setback to someone who has a fairly high level of self-esteem with a history of successful work behind them but may feel like a major disaster to someone with little self-confidence and a history of rejection in social relationships and who expects to fail to achieve what they want in life.

It is therefore very important to get to know about a person's life through taking a history. However, in a first interview only limited information can be obtained and it often takes a considerable length of time before a person can trust you enough to begin to disclose their most sensitive and painful feelings. Thus on a first interview, a person may describe their childhood as wonderful and their family as happy only later beginning to talk about a violent father or a sense of being unloved compared to a sibling.

This first attempt at getting the history should therefore be regarded as a shallow trawl for clues.

Areas which you should aim to cover for an adolescent would be:

School – which ones, experiences at infant, junior, secondary. Favourite and least favourite subjects. Any academic difficulties. Relationships with teachers. Relationships with peer groups. Any social difficulties eg bullying. Plans and expectations for the future. Worries and concerns.
Family – close family, names, ages, occupations, brief descriptions of family members. Who is living at home. In case of separated parents, amounts of contact. Relationships. Extended family, particularly grandparents, including information on those who are deceased.
Background – moves to different houses, schools, changes in family circumstances over time, significant events eg financial problems.
Social relationships – friendships or lack of them. Opposite sex relationships. Nature of any difficulties.
Leisure – what the person is interested in. How they spend their free time.

Developing a therapeutic relationship

Again, the stress is upon feelings and meanings not just upon events. As an example, a child may tell you that he sees his natural father two or three times a year. The immediate response should be to ask how he feels about that – he may wish to see him more/less/not at all. It may or may not be important.

If you refer back to the important characteristics in a counsellor, it is important to establish yourself in that mode from the beginning: as warm, sympathetic and genuine. In doing this, the way in which you listen to the person and respond to them is crucial and listening is an active not a passive process.

Setting the right atmosphere. Within comfortable physical surroundings you should be aiming to make the person aware that you are concerned and interested and have time for them. You should sit in a relaxed way and maintain normal eye contact even if the person does not appear to be looking at you. An atmosphere of relative stillness is helpful and restlessness, doodling etc should be avoided. It is important to allow the person to talk without rushing them or butting in when they may be thinking about what they want to say. Silences are usually helpful – you can use them to give you time to think and decide on your response too.

Taking in what is said. Making sure that you are actually listening rather than thinking about your own concerns, eg what you will say next. It is important to recognise that the ways of talking described here are just as valid in conducting an interview, even one which appears at its outset to be a simple information-gathering session.

Processing the information. In listening to someone's words it is important to be aware of non-verbal communication too and what may not be said. This is part of the looking for clues as you are putting to-gether what is said with other information – non-verbal clues, past statements, putting the current situation into the perspective of the person's past. You should be trying to feel what it would be like to be them and then making hypotheses on the basis of that.

Deciding on your response. You must decide how you are going to respond to what is said. Some ideas are given below on how different types of questions and responses lead to a much fuller understanding.

HOW TO CONDUCT A COUNSELLING SESSION

Open v closed questions

A counselling situation is very different from a conventional medical consultation where the initial concern is to narrow the focus of discussion down to a diagnosis. In counselling it is necessary to open out the discussion, to talk about and explore other areas rather than focus on symptoms. In order to do this it is important to ask more open-ended questions. A simple working definition of a closed question is one that can be answered by Yes or No. An open-ended question requires the person to think and give you their answer in their own terms.

Below are two examples of how a dialogue could progress with two different counsellors. In the first only closed questions are asked whereas the second uses only open-ended questions.

Dialogue using closed questions

Mary	My husband came home drunk again last night and that's why I've got this black eye.
Counsellor	Did you call the police?
Mary	Yes, or at least my neighbour did.
Counsellor	Are they going to prosecute?
Mary	No, I don't want that to happen.
Counsellor	Have you thought any more about going into a refuge?
Mary	Well, I do think about it but I don't think it would really help.

Dialogue using open-ended questions

Mary	My husband came home drunk again last night and that's why I've got a black eye.
Counsellor	How did it happen?
Mary	Well, he came in and started shouting that I hadn't got his supper ready. This woke up our son who came down and told his Dad to shut up and his Dad went for him. I tried to stop him hitting Steven and then he started on me. Steven ran next door and the neighbour called the police.
Counsellor	What happened then?
Mary	When they came he calmed down and said he was sorry and everything and begged me not to let them take him.
Counsellor	How did you feel then?
Mary	Well, I always feel sorry for him when he breaks down like that and I know that it's only the drink which makes him aggressive. I just don't know what to do for the best. I don't think he'd ever really hurt me but I'm worried about the effect on the kids. But I don't think he could manage if I left him.

In the first example, the counsellor is looking towards finding solutions to the woman's problem and so focuses directly on possible ways of dealing with her situation – the police and a women's refuge. In this type of format Mary is constrained in what she talks about by the counsellor's focus on action rather than feelings and has no opportunity to talk about what actually happened to her. The counsellor has gained a small amount of factual information but has no understanding of how the woman feels or what has led her to reject the possibilities of prosecution or a refuge. The counsellor is proceeding towards problem-solving on the basis of his/her own preconceptions of how to deal with a situation rather than trying to develop an understanding of Mary's perspective. Mary is also likely to feel on the defensive following this interchange – with a sense of being pushed, having to account for herself, not being understood.

In the second example, the counsellor uses open-ended questions to explore what happened and how Mary feels about it, allowing her to talk about it in her own way. A considerable increase in the amount of information is noticeable both in terms of the events of the night before and her feelings about it.

The counsellor has begun to understand the conflict of emotions which is preventing Mary from being able to act to change her situation. She is torn between her husband and her child and is also torn in regard to her fear and pity for her husband. This counsellor is able to see why Mary did not prosecute and does not leave the home and has the basis on which to proceed to help Mary with her difficulties.

Mary is likely to feel positive about this counsellor. She has been allowed to express herself without pressure and would not feel judged on what she has done. She would probably feel that the counsellor is interested in her and understands her.

This is not to say that closed questions do not have a place – at times they may be the most efficient way of gaining a particular piece of information. However, in using a closed question the counsellor is doing the work and the person can simply answer Yes or No. An open-ended question means that the person has to think about their feelings or behaviour and put it into words for the counsellor to hear. This should help the counsellor to see the person's perspective whereas closed questions are more likely to come from the counsellor's own perspective.

Reflection

Reflection is a style of talking in counselling which was developed by Rogers in his client-centred therapy. Rogers focuses on the importance of understanding the person from the person's perspective and grasping the meaning for the individual of his experiences – developing an empathetic understanding of that person.

Reflection is a means by which that process can occur. The counsellor needs to listen to what is said, to try to understand what that feels like and then to put a description of that understanding back to the person. Reflection operates at the level of feelings and meanings.

Example

John	Although I go out quite a lot now, to clubs and things, the people I'm with are really my brother's friends. They seem to like me and we have a good time but I just get worried that perhaps they're not really my friends at all. Sometimes I think they just feel sorry for me or have me along as a favour to my brother.
Counsellor	So, even though you are now part of a group, you feel very unsure about whether the others really see you as a friend, as part of the group?
John	Yes – I don't really see why they should want me around unless it was a favour to Michael. He is so confident and cheerful and gets on well with people whereas I'm shy and find it hard to talk.
Counsellor	So you feel that, in comparison to your brother, people would not find it easy to get to know you?
John	It's not really that – it's more that I don't think I'm interesting to people anyway. I can't tell jokes and make people laugh, I can't even think of things to say unless I've had a bit to drink.

In this example, the counsellor is listening to what John has to say, trying to put herself in his place and work out what that place feels like. She then reflects back that feeling – trying to put succinctly the essential aspect which has struck her. This then gives John something to focus his thoughts around – is the counsellor's statement accurate? He then explores the topic further. On the second occasion, the counsellor is somewhat off-beam with the reflection but this serves to get John to analyse and explain what is crucial for him about this uncomfortable situation.

In this way a joint exploration can take place into the underlying causes of John's sense of social unease. Although John knows he is uncomfortable in social situations he does not really understand the reasons for this and the process of counselling is helping to clarify these. He is likely to feel that his counsellor is interested, concerned and understanding following an interchange like this.

Learning to use reflection is often difficult at first as questions tend to leap to mind. It may be helpful to recognise the process by which we arrive at questions. When we listen to someone we are automatically forming an impression of the person and their world. A question will then be based upon that impression which itself remains internal to us. Reflection makes the impression explicit. The counsellor asks him or herself how the person is feeling/thinking/behaving and then puts the answer back to the person in the form of a reflection.

Summarising

In real-life counselling situations, discussions are usually rather more meandering, confused or ill-defined than the examples given so far. It is often helpful for the counsellor to be able to draw the threads of discussions together to refocus attention on aspects which seem particularly relevant. In this way, the person may become aware of contradictions in their statements which have occurred over a session or realise that there are consistencies in their reactions to several seemingly diverse situations which have been discussed over a few sessions.

Making the generalisations specific

People have a tendency to generalise their experiences and to make global statements, eg 'things always go wrong for me' or 'whenever I sit down to a meal with my parents it always ends up in a row'. Such statements are difficult to work from and it is always important to analyse the actual nature of the situations referred to. Taking the example of the rows with the parents, it is useful to ask for a specific example which can be discussed in more detail and then related to other examples.

Example

Paul	Whenever I sit down and have a meal with my parents, it always ends up in a row.
Counsellor	Can you think about the last row like that and describe to me what happened.
Paul	Well, I went to have Sunday lunch and I was determined to avoid the usual topics. It started off OK and we were talking about the holidays. I said that I was going to get a railcard and travel round Europe and that did it. Dad started on his usual thing about how I should get a job for the whole vacation and how was I going to clear the overdraft and on it went.
Counsellor	You seem to be suggesting that the topic of money and your bank balance is something that usually makes your Dad angry.
Paul	Yes – he had to leave school and get a job when he was 16 and he really resents that fact that times have changed and I can do things he never could.
Counsellor	What was your Mum's reaction to this?
Paul	She just got upset and said we were ruining the meal she's spent all morning preparing.
Counsellor	So how did you feel in all this?
Paul	I just can't help answering back when he starts. I can only take so much of it.

The counsellor has now begun the process of helping Paul to analyse the arguments with his parents, to look at what triggers them, how each family member contributes, what feelings are evoked. In the end it would be hoped that this understanding of the pattern would enable Paul to change it.

Advice and strategies for change

Many people will come into a counselling session asking for advice but their response to being given it is often negative. There are obviously times when a straightforward piece of advice, an item of knowledge which the counsellor has access to, is useful but as a general rule it is better for the person to develop their own strategies than to be given them. It is important to discover what types of strategy a person has tried already and what effects they have had. An example – a mother is concerned about the fact that her young son has been taking money from her purse. As part of the history-taking the counsellor will wish to know what her past reactions have been.

Example

Counsellor	What ways have you tried to deal with the stealing so far?
Mum	Well, at first I couldn't be sure it was really happening so I kept a closer check on my money. When I felt sure it was happening, I was so angry that I stopped all his pocket money as a punishment till he'd paid it back. The trouble is that just made him worse and he stole more.
Counsellor	Have you tried anything else?
Mum	I've tried talking to him but he won't tell me why he does it and I just get so angry when all he says is 'don't know'.
Counsellor	What are you doing at present?
Mum	Well I try to keep all my money locked away. He has no pocket money and I don't let him out in case he starts stealing outside.

The counsellor is here gaining a clearer idea of the situation – knowing what has gone before makes it easier to see where to go to next. It is also useful to tap people's own resources and ideas of making changes. As an example, take a boy who keeps arguing with his parents and these arguments just build up often ending in physical violence.

Example

Counsellor	Once you are into an argument, you seem to reach a point where you feel too angry to be in control of yourself. It is important to find a way to stop arguing before you reach that point. Have you any ideas about how you could break the pattern and calm yourself down?
Michael	The only way is to get away and be on my own. I can't get calm when they're still there and on at me.
Counsellor	How do you think you could organise that?
Michael	Well, it would be best if I went up to my room and put some music on.
Counsellor	How do you think your parents would react to that?
Michael	I'm not sure, I think they might agree if we explained it to them.

Moving towards action

In the discussions so far, the emphasis has been upon understanding the predicament of the person being counselled in a joint endeavour to elucidate its meaning. However, insight by itself changes little and change is usually what is being sought. It is important to be aware of how difficult making changes in our lives can be. A person may be in a very unhappy situation but at least it is familiar, making changes means moving out into uncharted territory, taking risks, dealing with the unknown.

Many people who we see have very little room to manoeuvre in their personal circumstances anyway, being limited by poverty, lack of education or lack of resources. The sources of most people's problems are in the world surrounding them, the relationships they have and the past experiences which lead them to construe their world in their own individual way.

People vary in the amount of power that they have to control their world – children and adolescents being among the most powerless. It may be necessary for adults to bring about the necessary changes to enable them to develop. Whilst it may be possible to produce the necessary changes for someone, eg obtaining a day-nursery place for the child of an oppressed single-parent, there are many other social factors which we cannot alter on an individual level. A teenager living in a family in which they are very unhappy but whose treatment does not constitute sufficient grounds to be taken into care may have little prospect of change until they are old enough to leave. If the family are unwilling to become involved in the counselling process then supportive work with the teenager may be the only avenue open.

It is sadly the case that it is not possible to be of help to everyone. You may be aware of how unhappy a person is, but you cannot force them to accept your help. Counselling of this type can only take place when voluntarily entered into.

A positive outcome to counselling would be that a person is able to proceed with their life with a greater understanding of themselves and their world, having been validated in their views through the counselling process. This greater understanding may lead them to direct their energies towards change, solving a problem or accepting and finding ways to live with their situation.

In doing this, the continued understanding, encouragement and support of their counsellor will be a vital ingredient. This may mean that the person becomes dependent on their counsellor during a very vulnerable period. Counsellors may feel rather anxious about such dependence and need to recognise that it is to be expected.

Working towards ending of counselling is a vital part of the process, enabling the person to consolidate what they have learned and gradually grow from dependence to independence. Counselling should therefore be wound down rather than ended abruptly and proceed at a pace which is appropriate for the person concerned, preferably by agreement with them. At the end of this process, it should be the aim of any counsellor that the person ends with a sense of greater self-efficacy, better equipped to deal with the inevitable future difficulties which will come their way.

REFERENCES AND FURTHER READING

Bannister D, Fransella F 1971 Inquiring man. Penguin, Harmondsworth
Bowlby J 1988 A secure base: clinical applications of attachment theory. Tavistock, London
Frank J 1973 Persuasion and healing. The Johns Hopkins University Press, Baltimore
Herbert M 1991 Clinical child psychology. John Wiley, Chichester
McLeod S 1981 The art of starvation. Virago Press, London
Rogers C 1961 On becoming a person. Constable, London
Smail D J 1978 Psychotherapy: a personal approach. Dent, London
Truax C B, Carkhuff R R 1967 Towards effective counselling and psychotherapy: training and practice. Aldine, Chicago

27 Young Adults

Adolescence may be defined as the process or condition of growing up, in the period between childhood and maturity. The age span is variable and not clearly fixed.

The World Health Organization put the ages for adolescence between 11 and 21.

It is a time of becoming independent and establishing a personal identity; a period when many young people question the fundamental values of their parents and other adults, and develop a critical awareness of the world around, and its social injustices. Personality development is associated with changing relationships and feelings towards parents, and hopefully attaining loving, respecting relationships with friends, family members, and sexual partners. It also involves achieving personal control over impulsive behaviour. In order to mask feelings of inadequacy, some young adolescents may be seen to be trying on different roles while struggling with this task of identity. Adopted children may wish to seek out their biological parents.

Cognitive development is characterised by a widening scope of intellectual activity, and a capacity for insight. Disabled and chronically ill children may become increasingly aware of their handicaps, resulting in feelings of aggression, depression or even suicide.

As well as the profound physical and emotional maturational changes, there are the social changes on leaving school – to further education, earning and financial independence, or unemployment. The struggle to become independent is often too threatening to accomplish alone, so adolescents may choose to go through the process in the same way as their peer group with all its pressures. It is a time too of risk taking to imitate adult behaviour and 'test the limits' particularly in relation to smoking, drinking, drugs and sex.

Social status acquisition is also a variable, created by society, which causes further confusion. In this country 16 year olds are allowed to leave school, marry with parental consent, legally have sex, and ride a motor-cycle; but have to wait until 17 to drive a car, and 18 to drive a lorry, vote, and legally buy alcohol.

PUBERTY

Puberty is defined as the stage in life when gonadal maturation occurs. It involves the acquisition of secondary sexual characteristics and an associated growth spurt, and ends with achievement of fertility.

There is a wide variation in the age of onset and duration. The trigger factor which initiates this maturation remains unknown. The hypothalamus is responsible for the synthesis and release of gonado-trophin releasing hormone which in turn stimulates the synthesis and release of follicle stimulating hormone (FSH) and luteinising hormone (LH) from the pituitary. The secreted FSH and LH stimulate the production of gonadal testosterone and oestrogen.

Signs

GIRLS The first signs of puberty in over 85 per cent of white girls are the oestrogenic changes of breast development and in the vagina. Breast budding usually begins around 10.5–11 years and may be initially uni-lateral. Adrenal androgens produce growth of pubic and axillary hair, sweat gland activity and facial acne. Pubic hair development usually occurs about 6 months after the onset of breast development, but may be the first sign in Afro-Caribbean races. Both growth hormone and sex steroids appear to contribute to the growth spurt which occurs early in girls, and is almost complete by the time menstruation begins. From the Tanner series, the mean age of menarche is 13.4 years, the range is 9–16 years. The interval from breast development to menarche is 2.3 years with a range of 0.5–5.75 years. Menarche appears to be associated with a critical body weight. One theory suggests a minimum fatness level of about 17 per cent body weight is necessary for the onset of the menstrual cycle, and a minimum fatness level of about 22 per cent is necessary to maintain regular ovulatory cycles. Gymnasts, ballet dancers and long distance runners with reduced weight often have significant delays in development and menarche, especially if their training began in the pre-pubertal years. Irregular and heavy menses are common in the first year following menarche and require no treatment. Adolescent girls who are not sexually active are less likely to be worried about mildly irregular or late menses. Primary dysmenorrhoea is relatively common and may cause absence from school.

Breast development	
5 stages are described:	Mean age
No development	
Pre-adolescent: Breast and papilla elevated as a small mound; areola diameter increased	11.5 years
Breast and areola enlarged, no contour separation	12.5 years
Areola and papilla form secondary mound	13.5 years
Mature stage: Nipple projects, areola part of general breast contour	

Pubic hair – girls and boys

5 stages are described:	Mean age	
	Boys	*Girls*
No pubic hair		
Sparse growth of slightly pigmented hair along labia or at base of penis	12.5 years	11.5 years
Darker curled hair, increasing in amount	13.5 years	12 years
Coarse, curly hair, small adult configuration	14.5 years	13 years
Adult configuration, complete triangle plus spread to medial surface of thighs		

BOYS The first sign of puberty in boys is testicular enlargement above the pre-pubertal size of 2.0 cm^3. Increasing testosterone secretion produces growth of pubic, axillary and facial hair, enlargement of the penis, deepening of the voice, ability to ejaculate, and acne. The growth spurt is associated with an increase in body size and muscle bulk, and reaches its peak 2 years later in boys than it does in girls. Gynaecomastia occurs in 65 per cent of normal boys. It is usually transient, frequently unilateral, and is thought to be due to increased end-organ sensitivity to normal oestrogen concentrations.

Genitalia – boys

5 stages are described:	Mean age
Pre-pubertal, testes <2 cm^3	
Scrotal enlargement, skin reddens, texture alters, testes >2 cm^3	12 years
Lengthening of penis, further growth of testes and scrotum	13 years
Scrotum enlarges further, and darkens. Penis broadens, glans develops	14 years
Adult male genitalia: testes average 15 cm^3	

Delayed puberty

Delayed puberty is defined as the onset of puberty later than 14 years in a girl, and 14.5 years in a boy. 3 per cent of children have some delay; in 50 per cent of the boys and 15 per cent of the girls it will be constitutional in origin. Of the rest, 30 per cent will have pituitary problems, 10 per cent of boys and 14 per cent of girls will have gonadal failure and in the remaining 10–15 per cent the delay is associated with chronic and severe disease such as cystic fibrosis, coeliac disease or renal failure. Another possible cause is anorexia nervosa.

Precocious puberty

Precocious puberty is defined as the onset of sexual maturation before 9 years in a boy, and 8 years in a girl. It is more common in girls than in boys. In girls, the aetiology is usually idiopathic, whereas in boys it is commonly associated with an intracranial tumour. The precocious development may cause considerable embarrassment to the child and may lead to unrealistic expectations of the child in that emotional and intellectual maturity are not similarly advanced.

Premature thelarche

Premature thelarche or isolated breast development occurs in girls under the age of 3 years. The growth rate is normal. Reassurance only is required.

SEXUAL ASPECTS OF ADOLESCENCE

Surveys among adolescents have shown that there is a trend towards more sexual activity, and from an earlier age, than in the past. Changing attitudes towards premarital sex, changing parental behaviour, increasing divorce, media influence and peer group pressure may all play their part. In the mid 1960s, 2 per cent of girls and 6 per cent of boys reported that they had experienced sexual intercourse before the age of 16; whereas in a recent study the figures had risen to 35 per cent of girls and 46 per cent of boys.

Although 90 per cent of sexually active teenagers appear to have some experience of using contraception, first intercourse and casual relationships are particularly likely to be unprotected. Contraceptives are often not used because sexual intercourse is viewed as an unpremeditated and infrequent act. Alcohol is often an important factor in unplanned teenage pregnancy. Many 14–15 year old adolescents do not seek contraceptive advice until they have been sexually active for six months or more because of the fear of parents finding out and doubts about the confidentiality of any advice they seek.

Associated with sexual activity is the whole range of sexually transmitted diseases, including HIV, and their potential effect on future fertility. The risk of sexual dysfunction in the future is increased if the initial sexual experience is unhappy, for example in cases of sexual abuse.

Teenage pregnancies

In 1985, 56 900 live babies were born in England and Wales to mothers who were under the age of 20. This represented one in 12 births to women of all ages in that year compared with one in 10 in 1970 and one in 15 in 1960. The major change associated with teenage pregnancy since 1975 has been in decision making relating to the outcome of pregnancy. Instead of legitimising the birth by 'shotgun' marriage, teenage mothers are now choosing to co-habit, remain single or terminate their pregnancy. There is also a trend towards joint registration of births.

The 1987 Family Law Reform Act has formally abolished the status of illegitimacy and removed the legal discrimination against children born outside marriage.

The number of teenage pregnancies continues to rise. In 1990 there were over 120 000 such conceptions in England and Wales, approximately 9000 to under 16 year olds. One third of these ended in legal abortion. Termination of pregnancy is likely to have a considerable emotional effect on the pregnant girl, and adverse effects are more likely where the girl has a poor relationship with her parents. Those undergoing termination of pregnancy under the age of 16 years particularly need very careful counselling and support, to help them understand fully the benefits of contraception, as a great many become pregnant again within a year.

There appear to be two distinct groups of pregnant schoolgirls, those who become pregnant inadvertently, and those who become pregnant deliberately, and who want to continue their pregnancies and to keep their babies. Teenage mothers are more likely to come from large families (more than 4 children), broken homes and be low achievers educationally. Siblings of teenage mothers are also affected; loss of bedroom, noise, added family financial strains and emotional upheavals, and the time devoted to sharing baby care, all impinge on their study time, with lowering of achievements and expectations.

Young people most at risk from pregnancy

1   Those who have started to be sexually active in their early teens. They may not have developed the skills to talk about sex with a partner, negotiate a contraceptive method, and use it effectively.
2   Those with lack of self-esteem and poor self-image. They may seek to become pregnant as a reassurance of their femininity and fertility.
3   Those from unhappy or unstable backgrounds. A baby is seen as someone who will give the love denied them by others and the pregnancy may be a means of establishing independence and gaining state benefits and housing.
4   Those in care; the complexity of their problems making them a particularly vulnerable group.

Consequences of teenage pregnancy. In 1985 the perinatal mortality rate in England and Wales for babies born to teenage mothers was 12.1 per 1000 compared with 9.8 per 1000 for mothers of all ages. The infant mortality rate for the same year was 14.1 per 1000 for babies of teenage mothers compared with 9.2 per 1000 for mothers of all ages. The highest perinatal mortality rates were found among infants of mothers under 16 years of age.

Teenage maternal morbidity. In early teenage pregnancies some investigators have reported an increased risk of obstetric complications such as pre-eclampsia, prematurity, pelvic insufficiency and prolonged labour. Contributing factors are late booking for antenatal care, poor nutrition and poor attendance at antenatal clinic and mothercraft classes. There appears to be an increased risk of post-natal depression, and even suicide, in this group, particularly in those who have little support from family and friends.

Impact on children of teenage mothers, more at risk of:

• Sudden infant death syndrome
• Low birth weight both pre- and post-term
• Hospital admissions for gastrointestinal problems
• Hospital admissions for accidental and non-accidental injury
• Behaviour problems and poorer verbal, intellectual and motor performance

HEALTH PROBLEMS OF ADOLESCENTS

The incidence of illness in this age group is lower than that at any other time in life. There is evidence from life style surveys that teenagers are at risk from harmful behaviours such as smoking, alcohol consumption, drug abuse and unsafe sex, even though most feel responsible for their own health and agree that good health is mainly due to sensible living. There appears little interest in discussing these topics with health professionals, and a failure somehow in this age-group to be convinced of the link between smoking and carcinoma.

Little information is available about the general health concerns of adolescents themselves, but from questionnaire surveys they do seem to have many worries regarding weight, acne, nutrition and exercise, as well as unmet needs to discuss sexual development, sexually transmitted diseases and contraception. The extent of these worries may be greatly underestimated by school teachers, school nurses and doctors.

Although concerns about unemployment and nuclear war predominate throughout adolescence, the prospects of marriage and motherhood may cause concern in many girls.

> **The major causes of death in the 15–19 year age group are:**
>
> - Accidents, poisoning and violence
> - Neoplasm
> - Suicides and self-inflicted injuries

Many of the accidents are the result of some risk-taking behaviour, for example excess alcohol consumption and driving, dangerous sports, or not wearing protective clothing.

Alcohol

Under-age drinking is on the increase. Surveys show that children are becoming familiar with alcohol at an early age, and by their teens, drinking is a regular part of their lives. 90 per cent of girls and 95 per cent of boys of 13 years have tried alcohol. By the age of 15 years, 77 per cent of boys drink up to 10 units a week, and 66 per cent of girls drink up to 6 units a week. Home is the major source of the alcohol. The way alcohol is used at home influences the development of their drinking behaviour as young people mature. Young inexperienced drinkers have a lower tolerance to alcohol and even small amounts of alcohol significantly lower their judgement and control.

Smoking

Smoking is a well recognised health hazard. The earlier a person begins to smoke, the greater the risk of chronic bronchitis, emphysema, cardiovascular disease and lung cancer. Prevalence is decreasing in all age groups except the young. 10 per cent of 11–15 year olds smoke regularly. Although girls are more likely to be smokers than are boys, they smoke fewer cigarettes. Girls' smoking habits are closely related to those of their mother and are strongly influenced by the attitudes of older siblings, 'best' friend and boy friend. Peer influence is a stronger influence among boys. Girls who smoke are more likely to try other drugs, sniff solvents, drink alcohol and go to discos. They are often under-achievers and truants.

Drug and solvent abuse

Studies of drug and solvent misuse amongst secondary school children suggest misuse levels of about 16 per cent, of which 5 per cent represent 'hard' drugs (hallucinogens).

Misusers are not confined to any particular group, but are more likely to come from single parent families, have unemployed fathers, or have parents who smoke (especially mothers). They are also more likely to be involved in truancy, fighting, vandalism, smoking and drinking. Peer group influence is important in experimentation, and youth club membership often provides the means of distribution. Most involvement is temporary, but a minority progress to multiple drug use, chronic use and addiction. Chronic drug users are more likely to come from families where adults are dependant on drugs such as alcohol or tranquillisers. The general effects of substance abuse are alteration of mood, perception (visual and auditory) and lessening of personal and social inhibitions.

Illegal drugs may be unpredictable in strength and quality, with a variable individual response to them. Doctors are required to notify the Home Office of any opiate or cocaine addicts they treat for addiction.

Signs of drug taking

- Sudden changes of mood, unexpected irritability or aggression
- Loss of appetite
- Loss of interest in appearance, school work and hobbies or sport
- Bouts of sleeplessness and drowsiness
- Furtive behaviour, often associated with disappearance of money and belongings
- Unusual stains or smells on body and clothing

Solvent abuse

Solvent abuse is the deliberate inhalation of a volatile compound to achieve a change in mental state – intoxication. The four groups of products which are commonly abused are toluene based adhesives, aerosols, fuel gases and solvents. Solvent abusers are mainly boys between the ages of 11 and 17. About one in ten secondary school children try sniffing. Most will only experiment a few times, but others may go on sniffing regularly for some time, usually with friends. A few may become dependent and sniff heavily for several years.

Signs and symptoms are those of intoxication. These may include excitement and euphoria, hallucination, disorientation, slurred speech and blurred vision. There is a rapid onset, and recovery, with little hangover. There may be evidence of skin irritation or low grade infection around the mouth and nose, and solvent-smells on breath or clothing.

In 1983, 134 people died as a result of sniffing; more young people now die from solvent abuse than from 'hard' drugs. 74 per cent of deaths are associated with fuel gas or aerosol abuse. Over 75 per cent of the deaths are sudden with 53 per cent caused by heart failure (direct toxic effect on the heart due to increased sensitivity to adrenaline). Of the rest, 10 per cent are caused by suffocation in plastic bags, 14 per cent by choking from vomit or acute laryngo-spasm, and 12 per cent through injury or accident while intoxicated. More than half the deaths occur at home or in the house of a friend.

It is not illegal to possess or to sniff substances, but it is an offence for retailers to supply such products knowingly to a person under the age of 18 (1989 Intoxicating Substances Supply Act).

Drug abuse

Cannabis is the most widely used of the drugs controlled under the 1971 Misuse of Drugs Act. It usually precedes the use of other illegal drugs, but has not been proven to lead to their use. 13–28 per cent of 15 year olds have tried it. Generally smoked as a hand-rolled cigarette, it causes pleasurable feelings of relaxation. Larger doses may cause altered sensory perception, red eyes and tachycardia. There is no conclusive evidence of long term dependence or damage from its usage.

Cocaine is usually sniffed through a tube, but can be injected. It is a powerful stimulant causing exhilaration, and indifference to pain and hunger. The peak effect, after 15–30 minutes, is of short duration leaving residual depression and fatigue.

Opiates may be self-administered by swallowing, dissolving in water and injecting, sniffing, or smoking. In moderate dosage they cause euphoria and contentment, but in higher dosage produce sedation and depression of the respiratory centre, cough reflex, heart rate and bowel activity. Tolerance and dependence quickly develop. The serious consequences of injecting opiates, and the associated life-style, are the risks of Hepatitis B, AIDS, thrombophlebitis, heart disease and lung disorders.

LSD is taken orally. The effects are unpredictable, ranging from ecstacy to disorientation and panic, commencing after about 30 minutes with a late peak around 6 hours.

Other drugs. Misuse of prescribed drugs, particularly benzodiazepines, is common.

Drug education. In 1989 the Department of Education supported local initiatives to develop Drugs education and appoint Drug education co-ordinators. In April 1990 the scheme expanded so that Local Education Authorities could appoint health co-ordinators to provide health education and in-service training on the misuse of drugs, tobacco, solvents and the transmission of HIV. Peer group education initiatives are also being developed. As well as providing information, education should aim to promote a climate of respect and understanding, the development of self esteem, decision-making skills and the ability to cope with adverse situations when they arise.

TRUANCY AND DELINQUENCY

Truancy and delinquency are expressions of antisocial behaviour which extend outside school and where police and legal authorities may become involved. It is found more commonly in boys than girls, in those from large families and from those in social classes IV and V. There is frequently a family history of truancy and a negative attitude of the family towards education. Families may have a history of criminality and maternal depression. The families themselves may often be single parent families, or families in which there is considerable discord. There is a noticeable lack of communal family leisure activities. In areas with a high adult crime rate, it has been suggested that the low level of social disapproval attached to delinquency is a direct factor in its causation.

Delinquency has been divided into the solitary delinquent where psychiatric factors are more likely to be present, and group delinquent behaviour. As well as stealing and aggressive activities, other problems such as glue sniffing or more serious drug abuse may be found.

Factors associated with delinquency

- Unhappy homes
- Single parent families
- Parental criminal records
- Low intelligence
- Poor self-image
- Aggression

HOMELESSNESS

The Department of the Environment defines homelessness as 'a person is homeless if they are without adequate shelter now, or if they are to be so within the next month, for example people staying in reception centres, squats, hostels, lodgings and other people's homes.'

Adolescent homelessness is a fast growing problem. Recent estimates by 'Shelter' suggest that there are 150 000 homeless young people in Britain. Children leaving local authority care are all provided with accommodation but many lose that accommodation within a short period of time – they then often turn to hostels or bed and breakfast accommodation. For adolescents leaving family houses the situation is similar; they stay with friends or relatives for a time until they are finally turned out and then turn to hostels or bed and breakfast accommodation.

From September 1988 entitlement to Income Support was abolished for most 16 and 17 year olds, who were instead expected to remain in full-time education, find a job or go onto a training scheme. The withdrawal of social security was supposed to be compensated for by the government's guarantee of a Youth Training place.

Child Benefit was extended for a limited transitional period after school leaving to allow time to find a Youth Training place. Some unemployed 16 and 17 year olds having to live independently retained entitlement to Income Support during this period; others not required to work or train (eg single parents, carers, people with disabilities) were able to claim benefit indefinitely. Discretionary payments were to be provided in case of severe hardship.

These restrictions in benefit have been identified as the major factor contributing to the steady rise in homelessness and destitution amongst young people.

The benefit changes have also decreased the amount of bed and breakfast accommodation available – it is no longer a good financial proposition for landlords. Hostels have also suffered a large loss of income resulting in less places being available.

SERVICES FOR ADOLESCENTS

In 1976 the Court Report stated 'adolescents have needs and problems sufficiently distinguishable, from those on the one hand of children, and on the other of adults, to warrant consideration as a distinct group for health care provision.'

In 1985 the British Paediatric Association's Working Party on the needs of adolescents said 'physical illness was not the predominant problem, but there was a need for self-referral clinics to provide advice on: a) growth and development, b) sexual problems, c) emotional difficulties including drug abuse.'

Services for adolescents need to be relevant and specific to their particular needs, be they physical, mental or emotional. The aim is to promote happy, healthy adolescents who can benefit from the education offered and develop into well-adjusted adults. Services need to be multidisciplinary, friendly, discrete, attractive and easily accessible to them. All adolescents should be catered for, but in particular those whose life experiences are adversely affecting their development.

Vulnerable adolescent groups

- Those with chronic illness
- Those with a physical handicap
- Those with a mental handicap
- Those with visual or hearing impairment
- Those with language development problems
- Those whose parents suffer chronic physical or mental illness
- Victims of physical, emotional or sexual abuse
- Those who are sexually exploited
- Those who are homeless, unemployed or experiencing poverty
- Pregnant adolescents, and young teenage parents
- Those who are bereaved, from disrupted homes or who are unwanted
- Minority groups

School Health Service for adolescents. The foundations for involving children in their own health are laid down during health appraisal at primary school. This continues during the adolescent years, the emphasis being on explanation of health indices, self-awareness and accepting responsibility for one's own health. Secondary school children should be able to self-refer to the school nurse or doctor to discuss any health, personal or social problems which may be worrying them.

Sex education. Certain aspects of sex education are a statutory part of the national school science curriculum. Under the 1986 Education Act the governing bodies of schools are responsible for determining what other, if any, sex education should be provided. Parents have no legal rights to withdraw their children from sex education classes.

The importance of sex education has been increasingly recognised. As well as providing biological information, it should promote sexual health covering personal relationships, values and attitudes. A flexible curriculum is necessary, and should be an ongoing part of the general subject of Health Education, and not dealt with as a separate subject on one occasion. Teachers need appropriate training and advice.

Adolescents need to be provided with adequate information and easy access to confidential services to promote a responsible approach to sexual relationships and contraception. Information needs to be directed at both boys and girls, and to be easily understood by youngsters of all abilities. Young people should be helped to understand the implications of sexual activity without moralising or censuring, but with obvious concern for their future happiness. Although behaviour is much more strongly influenced by family attitudes and experience than by formal teaching, a great many parents prefer someone else to teach their children about sex. Most young people learn from their friends or books.

Teenage Health Clinics

These need to be able to provide:
- Immediate help and advice on all health matters
- Counselling for emotional and personal problems
- Contraceptive advice and supplies
- Emergency contraception
- Pregnancy testing and pregnancy counselling.
- Advice about sexually transmitted diseases, and safer sex

Ideally the clinics should be open two to three times a week at times when young people can call in on their way home from school, college or work. They need to be held in discrete, central, easy to find premises, providing anonymity. 'Drop-in' facilities should be available, as well as an appointment system – making an appointment can often be a deterrent to seeking help.

The atmosphere of the clinic must be welcoming and informal, with a sympathetic, non-judgemental approach by staff. The surroundings should be relaxing and non-clinical, with background pop-music and refreshments available. The staffing levels should be adequate to keep waiting times to a minimum, and allow sufficient consultation time. The staff should consist of nurses, doctors, counsellors, plus clerical support.

Publicity of the service should be aimed at both young people and professionals; for example posters and leaflets in schools and leisure centres, and local media coverage. Within the legal guidelines of prescribing contraception to those under 16 years, confidentiality should be assured to those attending.

REFERENCES AND FURTHER READING

Abortion review, no. 38, 1990 Birth Control Trust
Balding J 1987 Alcohol consumption and alcohol related behaviour in young children. University of Exeter
Bancroft J, Reinisch J 1990 Adolescene in puberty. Oxford University Press, New York
Belfield T, Guillebaud J 1990 Contraception and sexuality in health and disease. McGraw Hill, London
Benefit rights for 16 and 17 year olds, no. 80 1991. Childright
Birch D 1991 Journal of Adolescent Health and Welfare 4 (2)
Bury J K 1984 Teenage pregnancies in Britain. Birth Control Trust
Charlton A 1986 Why do girls smoke? Department of Epidemiology and Social Oncology, Manchester
Christopher E 1980 Sexuality and birth control in social and community work. Maurice Temple Smith, London, pp. 196–202
Court D 1976 Fit for the future. Report of the Committee on Child Health Services, London
Drug notes 1989 1, 2, 3, 5, 6. Institute for the Study of Drug Dependence, London
Emans S, Goldstein D 1990 Paediatric and adolescent gynaecology, 3rd edn. Little, Brown, Boston, pp. 95–114
Epstein R, Rice P, Wallace P 1989 Teenage health concerns. Implications for primary health care professionally. Journal of the Royal College of Practitioners 39: 247–9
Family Planning Information Service 1989 Pregnancies in Britain, Fact Sheet H3
Goddard E 1989 Smoking among secondary school children in 1988. OPCS, London
Harvey D, Kovar I 1991 Child health. A textbook for the DCH, 2nd edn. Churchill Livingstone, Edinburgh
Ives R 1990 Working with solvent sniffers. Institute for the Study of Drug Dependence, London
Lewis M, Volkman F 1990 Clinical aspects of child and adolescent development, 3rd edn. Lea and Febiger, Philadelphia, pp. 211–47
MacFarlane A et al 1987 Teenagers and their health. Archives of Disease in Childhood 62: 1125–9
Modell M, Boyd R 1988 Paediatric problems in general practice, 2nd edn. Oxford Medical Publications, Oxford
Polnay L 1988 Manual of community paediatrics. Churchill Livingstone, Edinburgh
Pritchard C, Cox M 1990 Drug and solvent misuse and knowledge of HIV infections in 14–16 year old comprehensive school students. Public Health 104: 425–35
Report of the British Paediatric Association Working Party 1985 The needs and care of adolescents. BPA, London
Report of the RCOG Working Party on Unplanned Pregnancy 1991. RCOG, London
Report of the Working Party of Community Unit Services for Adolescents in Nottingham 1990
Stanhope R, Brook C 1990 Disorders of puberty. Update April
Steinberg D 1987 Basic adolescent psychiatry. Blackwell Scientific, Oxford
TACADE 1991 Solvents facts leaflets

28 Genetic Counselling

Genetic contributions to handicap (%)	
Mental handicap	35%
Physical handicap	25%
Young chronic sick	30%
Visual handicap	40%
Childhood deafness	50%

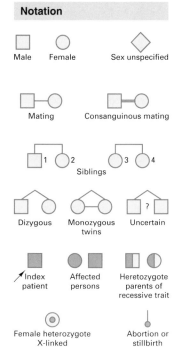

Clinical genetics has developed rapidly in the past two decades, particularly so in the last few years. The gene causing Duchenne muscular dystrophy was characterised in 1987 and its protein product, dystrophin, identified (Koenig et al 1987). In 1989 the cystic fibrosis gene was identified and its major mutations revealed (Kerem et al 1989). Recently the FMR1 gene was cloned (Oberle et al 1991). This X-linked gene is the cause of the fragile X syndrome (FRAX A). The molecular studies which led to this cloning showed that FRAX A was associated with excessive repetition of a triplet of bases (cytosine, guanine, guanine, or CGG) in affected people. Still more recently the gene for myotonic dystrophy has been identified (Brook et al 1992); it also has triplet repeats but with different bases being involved (cytosine, thymine, guanine or CTG).

The aim of this chapter is to set out the developments in modern genetics in the context of community paediatrics. One consequence of rapid genetic progress has been that clinicians feel intimidated by the subject. They may be tempted to avoid considering the new concepts, and the jargon of molecular genetics. However, with the increased experience and knowledge of genetic counselling techniques (as much changed as is our knowledge of genes!), molecular genetic, clinical genetic and cytogenetic techniques have vast potential, especially within the community. The powerful tools available can now facilitate diagnosis, screening for carriers, presymptomatic detection of abnormal genes and prenatal diagnosis. Examples have been chosen to illustrate the genetic approach to each different mode of inheritance.

With the decrease in infectious diseases, genetic disorders have assumed increasing importance over the years and now make a major contribution to the total burden of community disease (World Health Organization 1972, Modell et al 1991). Congenital malformations, including those due to genetic factors, occur in 4–5 per cent of all live births, are responsible for 30 per cent of the admissions to paediatric hospitals and are the primary cause of 50 per cent of all deaths under the age of 15. Congenital abnormalities account for about 25 per cent of the total stillbirths, 20 per cent of deaths in the first week of life, and 1 in 4 deaths in the first year of life. More than one in 5 of the total population will suffer from genetic disease at some time in their lives (Alberman 1982, Royal College of Physicians 1989).

Incidence of genetic diseases	
	Number/ 10 000 at birth
Cystic fibrosis	4.2
Huntington's disease	5.0
Duchenne muscular dystrophy	2.0
Serious congenital malformation	30.0
Ischaemic heart disease	20.0
Serious mental handicap	25.0

The tables give an estimate of the proportion of certain types of disability due to genetic factors and lists 3 examples of single gene disorders and three groups of disorders which are multifactorial (congenital malformations, ischaemic heart disease and mental handicap). The birth incidence estimates shown indicate the much larger problem in our community of multifactorial disorders. However in a family in which single gene disorders occur the recurrence risk, and the number of family members affected will usually be much greater. It is obvious that the rarity of a disease will not be of comfort to the affected family, who will consider not the population frequency, but the 100 per cent involvement of some of their closest relatives.

PATTERNS OF INHERITANCE

The genetic contribution to a condition can be grouped into 3 main categories, single gene, chromosomal and multifactorial disorders. In addition there is a fourth group, in which somatic mutations must occur in addition to the genetic predisposition for the disease to be expressed. Certain cancers are due to somatic cell mutations but this group will not be discussed.

Single gene

Autosomal dominant (AD) disorders. A large number of conditions are transmitted in this way (see Emery & Rimoin 1990). Individually rare, most having a frequency of less than 1 in 5000, they are important because several generations of a family may be affected. In approximately 1 in 1000 births there is a dominant gene present which could cause handicap in childhood (Royal College of Physicians 1989). In dominant inheritance both males and females are affected. Each offspring of an affected parent has a 50 per cent (or 1 in 2) chance of inheriting the abnormal gene and of thus manifesting the disease. This chance is the same for each pregnancy, irrespective of the outcome of the preceding one. This feature must be clearly explained to couples who might otherwise consider that having had one affected child the next would always be unaffected.

The severity, or expressivity, of an autosomal dominant condition may vary to a great extent. This fact emphasises the importance, in a family known to have an AD disorder, of a careful examination of each individual in order to exclude minor features of the affected phenotype. For example in Marfan syndrome, a teenage child might have clear diagnostic signs whilst both parents are reported as normal. Investigation of the wider family could show that a grandparent of the affected child died in early adult life due to 'a heart attack'. Examination of the intervening parent might then identify minor features of Marfan's syndrome, possibly asymptomatic, but significant, aortic valve pathology requiring treatment (Pyeritz 1991). In other situations the gene may be present in an individual without any phenotypic manifestation. Such genes are referred to as non-penetrant; the phenomenon of variable (or non) penetrance can greatly complicate genetic counselling.

An example of an AD pedigree illustrating a family with Waardenberg's syndrome, a condition in which the gene location, and the probable candidate gene, has recently been identified on the long arm of chromosome 2

Note:
- Each child, either sex, born to I1 has 50/50 or ½ risk of inheriting the gene
- Variation in clinical severity of affected offspring II1, II2, II3, II6
- Individuals II1, II2, II3, II6 have 50/50 risk of affected offspring
- II4 and II5 have no evidence of disease and cannot pass the abnormal gene to offspring
- Deafness occurs in 1:6 (approx.) of those who inherit the gene

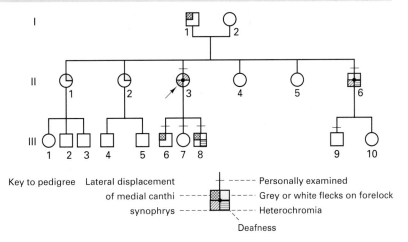

In other families there may be only a single affected member with the AD disorder. In such families the likely cause is that a new mutation has caused the dominant abnormality, which has arisen 'de novo' in the sperm or egg of the affected individual. Although siblings and others in the family then have a low risk of involvement, the offspring of such an individual have a 50 per cent chance of inheriting the condition. Distinction between a new mutation and a gene which is incompletely expressed in a parent or is non-penetrant, is an important aspect of genetic counselling which determines whether investigation and counselling in the wider family is necessary.

Summary of characteristics of autosomal dominant inheritance

1. Normally an affected individual has an affected parent (the exception being a new mutation).
2. Affected persons have, on average, affected and normal offspring in equal proportion.
3. Both sexes are affected.
4. There may be considerable variation in the severity of the disease.
5. Affected males can transmit the disorder to their sons.

Autosomal recessive inheritance. More than 500 autosomal recessive disorders are recognised and overall they occur in 2.5 per 1000 live births (McKusick 1990). In many there is a biochemical abnormality, due to a gene defect of a specific enzyme system or metabolic pathway, eg. phenylketonuria where a defect of phenylalanine hydroxylase in hepatocytes, leads to a build-up of toxic levels of that amino acid in the plasma. The principle of autosomal recessiveness is that the affected individual has inherited an abnormal recessive gene from each parent, thus having a double dose and being an abnormal homozygote. The parents each have the gene in a single dose and are therefore carriers (heterozygotes). The pedigree pattern of autosomal recessives will usually show several affected individuals in one sibship without there being affected people in the wider family. Also, since it is more likely that the offspring of a consanguineous relationship receive an identical recessive gene from each parent leading to homozygosity, autosomal recessive disorders occur more frequently in cousins and other consanguineous marriages.

The carrier rate for autosomal recessive conditions is far higher than the prevalence of the disease itself. For example, in the case of cystic fibrosis (CF), with a birth incidence of 4.2 per 10 000, the carrier frequency is about 1 in 24. For an autosomal recessive condition with a birth incidence of 1 in 10 000, the carrier (heterozygote) frequency will be 1 in 50, high enough for population screening for carriers to be considered. It has been calculated that on average everyone carries up to 4 to 6 recessive genes that, in a homozygous situation, would have been lethal.

Summary of characteristics of autosomal recessive inheritance

1. The disease tends to appear only in siblings; parents and most other relatives are phenotypically normal.
2. The risk of an affected child if both parents are carriers is 1 in 4 (25 per cent).
3. If there is consanguinity there is a greater chance of an individual being homozygous for an autosomal recessive gene, because the parents, being related, are more likely to be heterozygotes for the same recessive.
4. If the gene is common the condition can occur in the absence of consanguinity.
5. Both sexes are affected.

Sex-linked disorders. The principle of this type of inheritance is that the abnormal gene is located on the X chromosome. If, as is usual, the gene is recessive (ie. it is not expressed if present in a female in a single dose) then females are completely healthy despite carrying the gene. However their sons have a 50 per cent chance of in heriting the X chromosome which includes the abnormal gene. They will be hemizygous. The Y chromosome does not have genes which are homologous to the X chromosome. Thus males inheriting an X-linked recessive gene from their mother will manifest the disorder which can be extremely serious, eg Duchenne muscular dystrophy, retinitis pigmentosa, the Lesch-Nyhan syndrome or Hunter's syndrome, an X-linked form of mucopolysaccharidosis.

If a male with an X-linked disorder is diagnosed for the first time in a family then there are different possibilities. He may represent a new mutation on the X chromosome, not present in the mother or anyone else in the family. Or the mother may carry the condition, either herself being the person with a new mutation or having inherited it from one of her parents, usually the mother. Another possibility is that the mother may have gonadal mosaicism, with some oogonia carrying the mutation and others not. This is a problem for genetic counselling as it can be extremely difficult to identify or exclude. However new molecular techniques can sometimes clarify the situation.

An exception to the rule that female carriers do not show features of the disease occurs sometimes in X-linked recessive disorders (including

Duchenne muscular dystrophy, DMD) where females may be seen with mild symptoms. The explanation is that in each female cell one of the X chromosomes is inactivated, therefore the woman will show characteristics of only the active X. If the active X happens to be the one with the Duchenne deletion then that cell will show the abnormalities associated with DMD. Such 'manifesting carriers' are a problem in several X-linked conditions; in the case of DMD the manifesting carrier may be mistakenly diagnosed as having an autosomal recessive form of muscular dystrophy.

Summary of the characteristics of X-linked recessive inheritance

1. Sons of a carrier female have a 50 per cent chance of inheriting the abnormal gene and being affected.
2. Daughters of a carrier female have a 50 per cent chance of inheriting the gene in which case they too will be carriers.
3. All the daughters of an affected male will be carriers.
4. None of the sons of an affected male will inherit the gene.

X-linked dominant disorders. Rarely an X-linked condition can be expressed to the same extent in the heterozygous female as in the hemizygous male, indicating dominant inheritance. These conditions are uncommon but X-linked dominant inheritance may be suggested when a condition is only present in females. In such circumstances it is thought that males hemizygous for the X-linked gene cannot survive beyond the early stages of pregnancy. Examples are Rett's syndrome and incontinentia pigmentiae.

CHROMOSOME ABNORMALITIES

Around 0.5 per cent of all liveborn babies have a chromosome abnormality. At older maternal ages this proportion is increased. If a woman of 45 years conceives, the risk of any type of chromosome anomaly is almost 5 per cent. Unlike single gene disorders in which only one genetic locus is involved, a chromosome abnormality involves either excess or absence of a whole chromosome (numerical abnormalities) or of missing or duplicated chromosomal parts (structural chromosome anomalies). In both situations many genes are unbalanced as a result. Thus chromosome disorders are usually more severe and almost always cause mental handicap as well as many physical abnormalities. For many chromosome anomalies life beyond the first few weeks of fetal life is impossible and they lead to early spontaneous abortion. An excellent brief account of the genetic counselling aspects of chromosome anomalies is given in Harper (1988).

Alterations of chromosome number (aneuploidy). Down's syndrome is the most important and commonest numerical chromosome abnormality and the most likely to be compatible with independent life. Nevertheless the majority of Down's syndrome conceptions miscarry and do not survive to term. Aneuploidy is due to nondisjunction, ie the homologous pairs of chromosomes do not separate (disjoin) after alignment during meiosis; thus both of a pair pass to the one gamete, leading to a gamete which has an extra chromosome and one with a chromosome missing. There are specific features in many chromosome abnormalities, an indication perhaps of the major genes located on the chromosome which is involved. However, most autosomal aneuploidies are incompatible with extra-uterine life.

Sex chromosome abnormalities may be compatible with survival to term – the main ones being Klinefelter's (47,XXY) and Turner's (45, X) syndromes. In the case of Turner's syndrome there is a very high fetal mortality; 40 per cent of spontaneous abortuses have been shown to have this chromosome pattern.

Structural chromosome abnormalities. If a portion of a chromosome is deleted then the imbalance produced leads to a variety of abnormal features. As with aneuploidies the features depend on the genes involved in the abnormal chromosome. In terms of size, the changes in structural abnormalities are much smaller than whole chromosome anomalies and may be less disabling and are more likely to be compatible with independent life. However the great majority of chromosome abnormalities cause mental handicap along with a variety of serious physical abnormalities such as congenital heart disease, renal anomalies or skeletal defects. Small deletions of the terminal part of the short arm of chromosome 4 appear to be especially likely to be viable but with major handicaps.

Portions of two different chromosomes may interchange so that a fragment of one is attached to the main part of another and vice versa. Such translocations can occur without any abnormality if there is no net chromosome gain or loss. However the offspring of such a person with a balanced translocation may be unbalanced in that there is excess of one and partial loss of the other chromosome involved. When a balanced chromosome translocation is present it may be difficult to estimate the risk of unbalanced offspring occurring and being viable. Several different methods are now available to tackle this problem but specialist referral for this type of genetic counselling is recommended (Gardner & Sutherland 1989, Young 1991). A careful family history is most important because a mathematical calculation based on the number of spontaneous abortions of conceptions involving carriers and the number of liveborn abnormal offspring can be a guide to the future likelihood of such events.

Sub-microscopic chromosome disorders/contiguous gene syndromes. Until recently chromosome anomalies were only detectable if there were clear numerical or structural changes at the microscopic level. The combination of molecular and cytogenetic methods has now made it possible to identify much smaller lesions than can be seen with high power microscopy. Thus most individuals who had the rare combination of thalassaemia and mental handicap were shown to have a sub-microscopic lesion of chromosome 16 which included the alphaglobin locus (Wilkie et al 1990 a, b) whilst others have an X-linked disorder (Anon 1991). An example involving another chromosomal site is the dysmorphic, delayed development syndrome first described by Smith and Magennis in 1982 and showing deletion of the proximal short arm of chromosome 17. Molecular and cytogenetic analyses combined have shown, in at least 35 cases, that a contiguous segment of chromosome 17 is deleted in all patients with this particular phenotype (Magenis et al 1986, Smith et al 1986, Greenberg et al 1991, Moncla et al 1991). Although these conditions are rare, the mechanism is of great importance. In the next few years there will be many other sub-microscopic deletions identified using the combination of molecular and cytogenetic techniques.

MULTIFACTORIAL DISORDERS

The single gene and chromosomal disorders are recognised either by the characteristic family tree pattern, which suggests a Mendelian mode of inheritance, or by microscopic or molecular evidence of chromosome imbalance. There remain many other common disorders in which the inheritance is not simple and yet family members are affected more often than could occur by chance. Mathematical techniques may show that a high proportion of these conditions are caused by genetic factors, albeit in a complex way.

The likely explanation for multifactorial disorders is that one or more genes interact with environmental influences to produce the phenotype. Thus neural tube defects have a genetic basis such that a couple who have had one affected child or fetus are at increased risk (1 in 20) of having further affected offspring. The genes responsible have not yet been identified but a large multicentre study has shown that a further factor in the aetiology is a relative deficiency of folate in the diet. Replacement with folic acid supplementation, preconceptually and in early pregnancy, reduces the recurrence risk to around 1 in 100 (MRC Working Party 1991), a finding which confirms earlier work referred to in the previous edition (Smithells et al 1983). Neural tube defects in this respect illustrate the importance of identifying conditions which are multifactorial. Once identified, and if the environmental trigger can also be shown, then a very direct approach to prevention is possible.

A considerable proportion of congenital malformations are caused by multifactorial inheritance or perhaps by the combined action of many genes (ie polygenic disorders). Within the past 5 years, genes which affect development have been identified in animals which show a great deal of homology in man. It is confidently expected that this new area of developmental genetics will help our understanding of many multifactorial disorders.

ILLUSTRATIONS

Genetic syndromes causing mental handicap

Syndrome	Mode of inheritance
Congenital myotonic dystrophy	AD
Hunter	XR
Lesch-Nyhan	XR
Menke's	XR
Microcephaly	Usually AR
Tuberous sclerosis	AD
Seckel's	AR

* For a fuller classification, refer to Harper 1988 or Emery & Rimoin 1990

Genetics of mental handicap. When there is a mentally handicapped child in the family and the parents have fully appreciated the significance of this disorder, they may often worry about the genetic basis and the recurrence risk even though they do not request genetic counselling. If the cause of the handicap is environmental then not only should it be fully explained but also the lack of a genetic basis and low recurrence risk must be emphasised. To elucidate the genetic basis of mental handicap may necessitate the identification of specific syndromes, some of which are listed in the table. A careful preparation of the family tree often with examination of the parents and other individuals in the family (Raeburn 1984) is also important. Even if it is impossible to achieve a specific diagnosis, some estimate of the recurrence risk can be based on empirical data (Bundey et al 1989).

Visual disorder. A large proportion (40 per cent) of childhood visual disorders have a genetic basis. Ophthalmological genetics is however a most complex specialty; there is a strong case for specialised centres to be set up supra-regionally to provide both treatment and genetic information.

Some single gene eye disorders

Condition	Mode of inheritance	Incidence
Aniridia	AD or chromosomal	1/80 000
Cataracts	Different causes	1/250
Colobomata	Usually AD	1/40 000
Leber's optic atrophy	Mitochondrial	1/50 000
Retinoblastoma	AD	1/20 000

Deafness. When a young child has severe deafness, there is a high risk that there is a genetic basis. The approach here is to identify all other clinical features present, besides deafness, which might lead to the diagnosis of a specific syndrome (eg Waardenberg syndrome or Usher syndrome, a condition which combines both sensorineural deafness and retinitis pigmentosa). If there are no features which distinguish a specific single gene disorder (with a probable high recurrence risk), then the empirical risks shown can be used to indicate to the parents the likelihood of recurrence in the family.

Recurrence risks in undiagnosed childhood deafness (based on Harper 1988)

Family history of deafness	Recurrence risk
Parents normal, 1 child affected	1 in 6
Consanguineous parents, 1 child affected	1 in 4
1 parent and 1 child affected	1 in 2
Parents normal, 1 child affected and 2 children normal	1 in 10
1 parent affected	1 in 20

Duchenne muscular dystrophy. This is a severe X-linked recessive disorder which affects 1 in 3000 males. Symptoms are not usually evident until aged 2 or 3 but over the subsequent few years there is progressive muscle weakness such that the affected boy needs to use a wheelchair some time between the age of 10 and 14 years. Death almost always occurs before the age of 25. After the initial provisional localisation of the relevant gene to the short arm of the X chromosome in the early 1980s, the methods of reverse genetics were used to locate the gene very precisely. Subsequently the gene was cloned and sequenced (Koenig et al 1987, 1989). With the knowledge of the gene sequence it was possible to identify the exons which were deleted in particular patients. It was then possible to screen pregnancies of known carriers for the type of deletions known to occur in the index patient. In some circumstances this has made carrier detection possible.

Another development from the knowledge of the Duchenne gene sequence was that a prediction could be made about its protein product. Subsequently that protein was identified and named 'dystrophin'. This protein is missing in Duchenne muscular dystrophy or altered in Becker muscular dystrophy and plays a very major role in muscle function. Using measurements of dystrophin levels or by identifying the exons deleted in specific patients it is possible now to provide prognostic information in individual patients (Bulman et al 1991).

Fragile X syndrome. The discovery of the FMR1 gene in 1991 revolutionised the genetic approach to this condition. Fragile X is the most common inherited cause of mental handicap and second in frequency only to Down's syndrome as a cause of individual retardation. Until the molecular basis was identified, methods for carrier detection or to make the initial diagnosis in the family were based on careful cytogenetic studies using special media to culture cells. The molecular basis was identified as a result of systematic investigations which, having shown the location of the fragile X gene approximately, with a combination of cytogenetic and molecular methods, made it possible to note the base sequences closer to and within the gene. The finding that abnormal people who had the condition showed an abnormal smear led to an understanding of the repeated sequence (CGG) which has already been mentioned (Oberle et al 1991). Normal people have up to 50 CGG repeats, carriers have up to 100 and affected persons, with mental handicap, have over 200. The important consequence of the gene discovery, and of the applications explored in the past year, is that individual members of families in which the condition occurs can now receive much more accurate indications of their carrier status. Also, provided some ethical and practical questions can be answered, there may be a possibility of carrier screening for fragile X in the general population.

Cystic fibrosis. The autosomal recessive basis of cystic fibrosis has already been mentioned; the condition is one of the most frequent causes of chronic ill health and mortality in child and adult life. In the UK there around 6500 people who suffer from CF. This figure is dwarfed though by the number, approximately 2.2 million, who are heterozygotes for one of the CF gene mutations. This number is based on the estimated carrier frequency which would lead to the known birth incidence of 1 in 2500 live births.

The identification of the CF gene in 1989 was accompanied by strong evidence which showed that the most frequent CF mutation (known as the delta F 508 mutation) accounted for about 75 per cent of CF chromosomes in the UK population (ie about 56.25 per cent of CF people have both CF chromosomes with delta F 508). The possibility that there may be only a small number of different CF gene mutations to account for all the individuals with CF has since been disproved. There are at least 150 different mutations known which together with those yet to be identified, will collectively account for the remaining 25 per cent of CF chromosomes.

The fact that 75 per cent are due to delta F 508 does however give rise to the possibility of performing carrier screening for cystic fibrosis in the general population. Research into this aspect is under way but the community paediatrician should be aware of the practical and ethical issues which must be resolved.

At what age is screening advisable? To do so in childhood would remove some of a child's autonomy. If screening is not performed before a pregnancy then high risk couples identified when the mother is at, say, 12 weeks gestation do not have a choice between all the options. The Nottingham approach has been to offer carrier screening to first degree relatives of a person with CF by means of publicity through the specialised clinics as well as in the Cystic Fibrosis Trust's literature. We believe that a good time to make an offer of testing is in the later years at secondary school and are investigating the pros and cons of such a policy. The individual must be able to reach an informed decision about such testing, without any coercion from professional groups.

GENETIC COUNSELLING

It is often forgotten that genetic counselling techniques have evolved just as rapidly as have molecular genetic investigations! The early approaches of emphasising a specific risk have now been augmented by a good knowledge of the impact of genetic findings within a family and the various factors that influence an individual's or a couple's decisions about genetic tests (Kessler 1979, Raeburn 1984). Whilst genetic counselling is always hoped to be non-directive, there are situations in which the counsellor is unwittingly influencing the consultand; these are now much better understood.

In Nottingham, the genetic counselling provision has evolved to a team effort in which genetic nurse specialists make initial contact within the family home and acquire important pedigree and psychosocial/family information prior to attendance at the clinic. Subsequently, it is much easier to carry out genetic counselling and the necessary family investigations using this background knowledge. The sequence of this genetic counselling strategy is shown in the table; preliminary evaluations have shown that this system is appreciated by the consultands who come for counselling. In the future it is likely that the family doctor will play a greater part in genetic counselling and even in the supervision of certain forms of genetic screening (Harris et al 1992).

The Nottingham approach to genetic counselling

Stages of the process:

1. Home visit by a genetic nurse specialist for pedigree, psychosocial assessment and prioritisation (within 4 weeks of referral).
2. Genetic clinic appointment (clinical geneticist plus the genetic nurse specialist who knows family). Genetic assessment and investigations, diagnosis, initial counselling.
3. Further appointment or letter for disclosure and discussion of results. Preparation of a list of options).
4. Follow-up of at risk relatives.
5. Review of specific families (1, 2, 5 years later) as relevant.
   (Counselling of new family members who wish this).
   (Letters to referring doctors and family doctors after stages 2, 3, 4 and 5).

Calculation of genetic risks The main requirement for the calculation of a genetic recurrence risk is an accurate family tree and information about the mode of inheritance of the disorder. Thereafter the probability of an individual being affected can be calculated using the genetic risks (or prior probabilities) coupled with the results of specific measurements or pedigree data (known as the posterior probabilities). The technique is based on a method suggested by the Reverend Bayes 200 years ago which combines the prior and posterior probabilities mathematically (Bayes 1763).

The example shown below indicates the use of the method in estimating the residual risk of being a cystic fibrosis carrier if one is a healthy person, negative for the common CF mutations and unrelated to anyone with CF (Young 1991).

Bayes' approach to estimating risk, example cystic fibrosis

		Carrier	Non carrier	Carrier risk
Problem	A Caucasian person who has no family history of CF wishes to know their carrier status (eg because their partner is a known carrier).			
Background data	Empirical chance of being a carrier is approx. 1 in 25. Percentage of carriers who are identified by tests for common mutations = 80%.			
Prior probability		0.04	0.96	1 in 25
Conditional probability (of being found to be mutation negative if a carrier or if not a carrier)		0.2	1.0	—
Combined probability		0.008	0.96	$\dfrac{0.008}{0.96} = 1$ in 121

ORGANISATION OF CLINICAL GENETIC SERVICES

Not every Regional Health Authority has provided resources for a Regional Genetic Service, but already there is a very considerable genetic network throughout the UK. Because each Regional Genetic Service has knowledge of how best to contact individual families in their own community and, through the Clinical Genetic network, the opportunity to identify distant family members, arranging their cooperation for family-wide investigations, eg DNA sampling, can be much simpler. We should never forget that members of the wider family who are asked to provide a blood sample, or information about a genetic disease, will themselves have counselling needs; time must be allowed not just for collecting DNA etc but to identify their questions and ensure that these are adequately answered.

Genetic registers

Many Regional Genetic Services coordinate the genetic follow-up of families with single gene disorders by means of a computerised genetic register. Such registers are of special value for AD disorders which have onset later in childhood or in adult life or for conditions in which inheritance is X-linked recessive. In both situations the possibility of genetic testing either for carriers or for those who wish testing presymptomatically needs to be delayed until the individual can decide for themselves. Registers can alert the genetic team to individuals in affected families who are reaching adult life and the reproductive age groups. Genetic registers have been invaluable tools for the genetic management of particular diseases and families and in the recording of epidemiology of genetic diseases in the community. The many practical, genetic, ethical and theoretical issues are discussed in a recent review (Newbury-Ecob & Raeburn 1993).

ETHICAL ISSUES

Since genetic investigations often provide information about the risk of a child or adult suffering from a life-long illness, it is obvious that the attitude to affected patients and families is extremely important. The value judgement of the professional, eg about the significance of mental handicap or of a physical handicap, must not be made to influence families where different judgements are made. Clearly if a genetic disorder can be detected prenatally, and there is the possibility that a termination of pregnancy would be considered, the choice about such action must remain with the individual couple. Unless they receive clear, accurate, up-to-date information, that choice will not be based on the most reliable facts. Nevertheless, it is important for a couple to realise that their feelings should be taken into account as well as the facts.

In any situation where ethical issues arise, it is very important to allow time for an individual's or couple's decision to be made. For that reason, screening in pregnancy and subsequent urgent counselling may not be the best model for management of certain genetic disorders. Informed choice, with options being offered at appropriate stages for each person, must be the mainstay of an ethical approach to medical genetic knowledge (see RCP report 1991 – ethical issues in clinical genetics).

GENETIC SCREENING IN THE COMMUNITY

The most exciting developments in medical genetics of the past five years have widespread implications in the community. The development of these services has been discussed by an important report of the Royal College of Physicians (1989). For example, it is now possible, and economically feasible, to screen in the population for the carrier state of the main mutation of cystic fibrosis. In theory therefore, a proportion of couples who are both carriers of that condition, could be identified prior to any pregnancy so that their options can be considered. This mode of screening arose because of the identification of the cystic fibrosis gene as detailed above. In many other single gene conditions, screening for the carrier state and then specific mutation screening is possible or is likely to be possible soon.

Other screening techniques have been developed empirically. Of these the most important development was the recognition that pregnancies with a much higher risk of the baby having Down's syndrome, frequently had low levels of maternal serum alphafetoprotein. In due course, this was linked with abnormalities of human chorionic gonadotrophin. Together with age, this provides a triple screening technique which can identify up to 65 per cent of at risk pregnancies (Cuckle & Wald 1990). After screening, amniocentesis can be offered to identify whether or not the higher risk is associated with an affected baby.

One of the challenges of the new genetic screening techniques is to ensure that the wider community are aware of the possibilities and that screening is not carried out as a secret medical procedure only discussed by those who have been screened and found to have abnormalities. The development of genetics in the community requires widespread community education. Doctors have been slow to take advantage of the many disorder-orientated self-help groups in which there are many individuals who will happily give talks, produce literature for lay people and provide other helpful advice on the development of community genetics. Surprisingly, it is the community education element which has often been missing in some of the early screening programmes. If screening services were to be offered using the model of the business community, the consumers in the community would be first to know of innovations, not the last.

REFERENCES AND FURTHER READING

Alberman E 1982 The epidemiology of congenital defects: a pragmatic approach. In: Paediatric research: a genetic approach. Spastics International Medical Publications

Anon 1991 More bad luck for the X chromosome: alphathalassaemia/mental retardation. Leading article. Lancet 338: 1562–3

Anon 1992 Screening for cystic fibrosis. Leading article. Lancet 340: 209–10

Bayes T 1763 An essay towards solving a problem on the doctrine of chance. Philosophy Transactions 53: 376

Brook J D, McCurrach M E, Harley H G et al 1992 Molecular basis of myotonic dystrophy: Expansion of a trinucleotide (CTG). Repeat at the 3' end of a transcript encoding a protein kinase family member. Cell 68: 799

Bulman D E, Murphy E G, Zubrzycka-Gaarn E E et al 1991 Differentiation of Duchenne and Becker muscular dystrophy phenotypes with amino- amd carboxy-terminal antisera specific for dystrophin. American Journal of Human Genetics 48: 295–304

Bundey S, Thake A, Todd J 1989 The recurrence risks for mild idiopathic mental retardation. Journal of Medical Genetics 26: 260–6

Cuckle H S, Wald N J 1990 Screening for Down's syndrome. In: Lilford R J (ed) Prenatal diagnosis and prognosis. Butterworths, London, pp. 67–92

Dolk H, Bertrand F, Lechat M F et al 1992 Chorionic villus sampling and limb abnormalities. Lancet 339: 876-7

Emery A E H, Rimoin D L (eds) 1990 Principles and practice of Medical Genetics, 2nd edn. Churchill Livingstone, Edinburgh

Firth H V, Boyd P A, Chamberlain P et al 1991 Limb abnormalities and chorion villus sampling. Lancet 338: 51

Gardner R J M, Sutherland G R 1989 Chromosome abnormalities and genetic counselling. Oxford University Press, Oxford

Greenberg F, Guzzetta V, Montes de Oca-Luna R et al 1991 Molecular analysis of the Smith-Magennis Syndrome: A possible contiguous-gene syndrome associated with del (17) (p11.2). American Journal of Human Genetics 49: 1207-18

Harper P S 1988 Practical genetic counselling. Wright, London, pp. 49–62

Harris H J, Scotcher D, Craufurd D, Wallace A, Harris R 1992 Cystic fibrosis in carrier screening at first diagnosis of pregnancy in general practice. Lancet 339: 1539

Holtzmann N A 1989 Proceed with caution: Predicting genetic risks in the recombinant DNA era. Johns Hopkins University Press, Baltimore

Kerem B-S, Rommens J M, Buchanan J A et al 1989 Identification of the cystic fibrosis gene: genetic analysis. Science 245: 1073–80

Kessler S (ed) 1979 Genetic counselling: psychological dimensions. Academic Press, New York

Koenig M, Beggs A H, Moyer M et al 1989 The molecular basis for Duchenne versus Becker muscular dystrophy: correlation of severity with type of deletion. American Journal of Human Genetics 45: 498–506

Koenig M, Hoffman E P, Bertekson C J et al 1987 Complete cloning of the Duchenne muscular dystrophy (DMD) cDNA and preliminary genomic organisation of the DMD gene in normal and affected individuals. Cell 50: 509–17

Magenis R E, Brown M G, Allen L et al 1986 De novo partial duplication of 17p: clinical report. American Journal of Medical Genetics 24: 415–20

McKusick V A 1990 Mendelian inheritance in man, 9th edn. The Johns Hopkins University Press, Baltimore

Modell B, Kuliev A M, Wagner M 1991 Community genetics services in Europe. WHO Regional Publications, European Series, no. 38

Moncla A, Livet M O, Auger A et al 1991 Smith-Magennis syndrome: a new contiguous gene syndrome. Report of 3 cases. Journal of Medical Genetics 28: 627–32

MRC Vitamin Study Research Group 1991 Prevention of neural tube defects: Results of the Medical Research Council Vitamin Study. Lancet 338: 131–7

MRC Working Party 1991 Medical Research Council European Trial of chorion villus sampling. Lancet 337: 1492–9

Newbury-Ecob R, Raeburn J A 1993 Genetics in the family and the community. The use of registers and screening. In: Young I D (ed) Genetics in paediatrics. Balliere, London

Oberle I, Rousseau F, Heitz D et al 1991 Instability of a 550 base pair DNA segment and abnormal methylation in fragile X syndrome. Science 252: 1097–102

Pyeritz R E 1991 Marfan syndrome. In: Emery A E H, Rimoin D L, Dofaer J A (eds) Principles and practice of medical genetics, 2nd edn. Churchill Livingstone, Edinburgh, pp. 1047–63

Raeburn J A 1984 Mental handicap. In: Emery A E H, Pullen I M (eds) Psychological aspects of genetic counselling. Academic Press, London, pp. 95–105

Royal College of Physicians 1989 Prenatal diagnosis and genetic screening. Community and service implications, report. RCP, London

Royal College of Physicians 1991 Ethical issues in clinical genetics. A report of the Working Group of The Royal College of Physicians' Committee on Ethical Issues in Medicine and Clinical Genetics. RCP, London

Smithells R W, Nevin N C, Sellar M J et al 1983 Further experience of vitamin supplementation for prevention of neural tube defect recurrences. Lancet ii: 1027–31

Smith A C M, McGavran L, Robinson J et al 1986 Interstitial deletion of (17) (p11.2p11.2) in 9 patients. American Journal of Medical Genetics 24: 393-414

Weatherall D J 1991 The new genetics and clinical practice, 3rd edn. Oxford University Press, Oxford

Wilkie A O M, Buckle V J, Harris P C et al 1990a Clinical features and molecular analysis of the alpha thalassaemia/mental retardation syndromes. I Cases due to deletions involving chromosome band 16p13.3. American Journal of Human Genetics 46: 1112–6

Wilkie A O M, Zeitlin H C, Lindenbaum R H et al 1990b Clinical features and molecular analysis of the alpha thalassaemia/mental retardation syndromes. II Cases without detectable abnormality of the alpha globin complex. American Journal of Human Genetics 46: 1127–40

World Health Organization 1972 Genetic disorders: prevention, treatment and rehabilitation. Technical Report Series, no. 49. WHO, Geneva

Young I D 1991 Introduction to risk calculation in genetic counselling. Oxford University Press, Oxford

GLOSSARY

Aneuploidy: when the chromosome number is not an exact multiple of the haploid number.

Autosomal: relating to the chromosomes, numbers 1 to 22, which are not sex chromosomes.

Base: short for the nitrogenous bases in nucleic acids (A=adenine; C=cytosine; G=guanine; T= thymine; U=uracil)

Candidate gene: a gene whose location and function suggest that the gene may be abnormal in a specific disease.

Cloning: identification of a gene sequence so that it can be replicated using recombinant DNA techniques.

Congenital: any defect present at birth.

DNA polymorphisms: the variations which occur in the DNA extremely frequently along the length of each chromosome. They are useful in localising the position of disease genes.

Dominant: a gene which is expressed when present in a single dose, being dominant to the homologous gene at the same locus on the partner chromosome.

Empirical: the observed facts frequently expressed in numbers (eg it has been shown empirically that the recurrence risk of a neural tube defect for a couple who have had one affected pregnancy is about 1 in 20).

Exon: the part of a gene which is active (ie it remains after splicing of DNA fragments to be transcribed into the RNA).

Expressivity: the degree to which a specific gene is manifest in an individual. When this varies it makes it difficult to ascertain if an individual is likely to transmit a condition.

Gametes: eggs or sperm.

Genotype: the genetic constitution of an individual.

Haploid: the normal chromosome number in the eggs or sperm.

Hemizygous: the genes present in only one dose, usually referring to the genes on the X chromosome in the male.

Heterozygote: an individual with different genes on a locus at a specific site of a given pair of chromosomes.

Homologous: identical or matched.

Homozygote: an individual with identical genes at a specific locus on a given pair of chromosomes.

Locus: the precise gene location on the chromosome.

Mendelian: the type of inheritance described by Gregor Mendel, ie single gene inheritance.

Multifactorial: the type of inheritance in which genetic factors (several genes) combine with environmental factors to give the observed disease.

Mosaicism: when an individual has cells from more than one genotype.

Mutation: alteration in genetic material which can occur either spontaneously or in response to environmental agents.

Non-penetrant: a gene which in a particular person is not expressed, despite being proven to be present.

Penetrance: the degree to which a particular genotype is expressed.

Phenotype: the observed features in an individual.

Posterior probability: the likelihood of an event happening based on specific conditions (eg the results of laboratory tests).

Prior probability: the likelihood of an event happening (eg of inheriting an abnormal gene), expressed mathematically.

Probe: a labelled DNA or RNA fragment which is used to identify sequences complementary to it.

Recessive: a gene which is not expressed in a single dose; to be affected an individual must have two copies of the gene, one from each parent.

Somatic: all body cells except those of the gonads, which produce gametes.

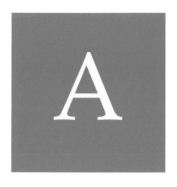

Common Problems

In this appendix aspects of a number of common clinical problems are discussed from the viewpoint of community paediatrics, particularly information related to educational, social or emotional implications. Details of therapy are not included here and the reader should refer to other publications such as Hospital Paediatrics (Milner & Hull) or Manual of Community Paediatrics (Polnay).

ASTHMA AT SCHOOL

Asthma is the most common longterm medical problem in the school age child, with 1 in 10 to 1 in 20 children being affected. It is a common cause of loss of schooling, but rarely now would lead to a need for special education, because of advances in therapy. In spite of greater awareness, many children with asthma go unrecognised and hence do not receive appropriate treatment. Children who cough at night, cough or wheeeze in the cold or who cough or wheeze with PE at school are highly likely to have asthma.

Education of teachers about asthma is as important as education of parents and children. Every year at least one child in school dies because they have not been able to use their inhaler before activities such as cross country running. The other side of the coin is excellent attendence and an Olympic Gold. Children at school should be able to keep their inhalers on them and learn to take responsibility for their use. School non-attendance for asthma may be due to poor control; it may also be due to parental worry, emotional or behavioural problems. Careful assessment is needed and liaison with the GP, school nurse, teacher and education welfare officer.

The school leaver with mild or well controlled asthma has very little problem with choice of career. However, for some children, occupations where there is exposure to dust and cold, would not be suitable.

COT DEATH

Every year there are 1200–1400 cot deaths in England. The risk of cot death is decreased by babies sleeping supine and this advice should be given to all parents. When they are old enough to roll over for themselves, then it is safe for them to choose their own sleep position. Other important avoidable factors in cot death are exposure to smoke from cigarettes, cigars or pipes and overheating. Common problems are for extra layers of clothing or blankets to be put on babies who are unwell and pyrexial. 65°F is the recommended temperature for a baby's bedroom.

Where a cot death has occurred, it is important to exclude non-accidental injury by careful clinical examination. A paediatric pathologist's report is valuable in excluding other medical causes.

Parents should be given the opportunity to see and hold their baby. Medical staff have to offer this as often parents will not ask. Parents must be warned that all sudden deaths are reported to the police and the coroner and that these are legally required arrangements. Both parents should be seen to explain the cause of death and to provide counselling and support. Siblings may also need help. It is important to inform the family doctor and health visitor as soon as possible. A second appointment to see the parents should be made when the results of the post mortem examination are available. Parents should be given the address of the local support group and the Foundation for the Study of Infant Deaths. Counselling and support in subsequent pregnancies will be needed.

CYSTIC FIBROSIS

Most children will attend ordinary school and take part in a full educational programme. They should not be restricted from taking part in sport and school social activities. Teachers will need to know about the illness, medication, diet and need for physiotherapy. A flexible approach to physiotherapy at school should be adopted depending upon who is available and who is willing, eg parent, teacher, classroom assistant, school nurse. A private space also needs to be negotiated for this. Support and communication with all those involved, parents, teachers, the primary health care team and the cystic fibrosis clinic are essential in order to cope with the ups and downs of the condition. Deterioration may lead to the need for part-time schooling or home tuition, but with modern treatment this is now needed much less often. Deterioration or the death of the child must be coped with not only by the family but also by school friends and teachers.

DIABETES MELLITUS

The keys to success in management are a team approach, patient education and support. For the child at school this means a child and teachers who are informed and who share common knowledge, and flexibility and understanding built into the school day in terms of meals and exercise.

In some adolescents diabetes provides a formidable weapon with which to attack parents and sometimes the school. Fear and lack of confidence is far less likely to occur if teachers are well informed. The diabetic liaison health visitor may be invaluable in this respect. For a few children residential schooling is necessary, though this option is taken increasingly rarely.

ECZEMA

Eczema can cause distress because of the symptoms that it causes or because of the physical appearance of the child and the reaction from others at school. It may be worse at times of stress such as examinations. 80% of infants with eczema will be fine by the age of 10 years. However, an uncanny proportion of the remainder seem to want to go into unsuitable jobs such as hairdressing and motor mechanics.

EPILEPSY

Epilepsy is not one condition, but a very broad range of conditions which vary in severity and in their implications for learning and employment. Teachers are now better informed, but often still lack confidence in managing the child at school. The diagnostic label is often loosely applied without convincing clinical evidence. For others a whole series of inappropriate restrictions remain in force years after the last convulsion in a child who is also off all medication.

Overall, one third of the children will require special education because of mental handicap: this is where the epilepsy is part of a wider neurological problem. One third may have more specific learning difficulties in reading or arithmetic. Children with reading difficulties may show earlier delay in language development and foci in the dominant hemisphere for language. Others may fail to reach their potential because of low expectations from teachers. Poorly controlled petit mal will lead to 'gaps' in lessons and explanations, leading to poor achievement especially if the attacks go unrecognised. Boredom in the classroom will increase the likelihood of fits occuring. Medication can also produce side effects of poor concentration and drowsiness in the classroom. The educational problems can be complex and must be assessed jointly by teacher, doctor and educational psychologists.

Behaviour problems can be a result of neurological impairment or as a consequence of not keeping up with the attainments of their peer group. They may also arise because of undue anxiety from parents. Some children may be aggressive, impulsive and over-active; others may be apathetic, quiet, withdrawn and lacking in confidence.

Many children with epilepsy have none of these difficulties, have no behaviour problems and excellent educational attainments.

The school health team needs to provide information and support for teachers, particularly on the correct first aid procedure if the child should have a fit in school. There may be concerns about the risks associated with physical education, science and technology. It is not useful to place uniform restrictions on all children with epilepsy. Each child must be considered separately and in general children should take part in all activities in the curriculum. Decisions rest upon the degree of control, the pattern of fits, (for example only at night), and the warning that the child gets. Swimming with proper supervision, (which is what should be provided for all children), is safe. Cycling in the road is generally not recommended. Restrictions and fears can impede the normal development of confidence and independence. After discussion with parents, it might be preferable to take a small risk than deny the child opportunities for participation and development. The employment situation is complex and expert advice should be obtained. Some occupations are excluded by statute and, for example, a single febrile convulsion as an infant will prevent that person holding a public service vehicle licence.

HAEMOGLOBINOPATHIES

Many Districts now provide a screening and counselling service for heamoglobinopathies. Very successful programmes for prevention have been reported for thalassaemia through a combination of health education, screening and genetic counselling. The community paediatrician should always be alert to this need. Nearly all children with haemoglobinopathies will attend ordinary school. Teachers need support and information for example on crises in children with sickle cell anaemia. The child's treatment programme, for example transfusions in thalassaemia, should be organised to cause the minimal disruption to his education.

HAEMOPHILIA

This affects 1:30000 boys. Most will now attend ordinary school. Any restrictions on physical activity should be decided on an individual basis between parents, the school, the haematologist and the school doctor. Teachers should be made aware of what to do if there is external bleeding or more commonly, if there is a haemarthrosis. Many schools will be anxious (but will not say so), as to whether the child is HIV positive. The school will need information, reassurance and support. Regular dental care and prophylactic fluoride are important.

HAYFEVER

Hayfever is not regarded by many as a handicapping condition, yet symptoms are usually worst at examination times and can impair performance. It is important to start treatment ahead of the onset of high pollen counts and emphasise the importance of compliance. There is no place for using older antihistamines which produce drowsiness.

HEART PROBLEMS

Innocent heart murmurs are common and are heard in over 50% of children. The community paediatrician must be skilled in distinguishing the innocent from the pathological or else run the risk of blocking the cardiac clinic with referrals! In one series a systolic murmur was heard in 90% of children with only 0.3% being clinically significant. Most of the 'significant' murmurs represent minor problems, such as a small VSD or ASD which are functionally insignificant and should have no effect upon the child's activities. Often the stethoscope causes more anxiety and finds few important problems. The children with significant heart problems will have symptoms such as shortness of breath and poor growth. Children with innocent murmurs are asymptomatic, the peripheral pulses are normal and not delayed, the heart sounds are normal, the murmur is only systolic and does not radiate into the neck, and varies in intensity with posture and respiration. The chest X-ray and ECG are normal. With advances in cardiac surgery, more and more children are benefitting from total corrections of their defects. It is important not to label these children as impaired just because they have a large thoracic scar.

LEUKAEMIA AND OTHER ONCOLOGICAL CONDITIONS

Their treatment is provided by the Oncology Clinic, however loss of schooling is very important. This is often far greater than can be accounted for by treatment. Reintegration to school after a period of intensive treatment can be difficult. The community paediatrician and oncology team should work closely together.

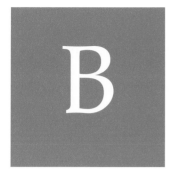

Support Organisations

Aid for Children with Tracheostomies Station House, Station Road, Market Bosworth, Nuneaton, Warwickshire CV13 OPE. 0455 290718

Arthrogryposis Group 1 The Oaks, Common Mead Lane, Gillingham, Dorset SP8 4SW. 0747 822655

Association for All Speech Impaired Children 347 Central Markets, Smithfield, London EC1A 9NH. 071 236 3632

Association for Children with Hand or Arm Deficiency 13 Park Terrace, Crimchard, Chard, Somerset TA20 1LA. 0460 61578

Association for Glycogen Storage Disease (UK) 9 Lindop Road, Hale, Altrincham, Cheshire WA15 9DZ. 061 980 7303

Association for Spina Bifida and Hydrocephalus (ASBAH) 42 Park Road, Peterborough, Cambs PE1 2UQ. 0733 555988

Barnardo's Tanners Lane, Barkingside, Ilford, Essex IG6 1QG. 081 550 8822

British Agencies for Adoption & Fostering 11 Southwark St, London SE1 1RQ. 071 407 8800

British Diabetic Association 10 Queen Anne Street, London NW1 4LB. 071 580 1155

British Dyslexia Association 98 London Road, Reading, Berkshire RG1 5AU. 0734 668271/2

British Epilepsy Association, Anstey House, 40 Hanover Square, Leeds LS3 1BE. 0532 439393

Brittle Bone Society Unit 4, Block 20, Carlunie Road, Dundee DD2 3QT. 0382 817771

Child Health Prevention Trust (CAPT) 28 Portland Place, London WIN 4DG

Child Poverty Action Group 4th Floor, 1-5 Bath Street, London EC1V 9PY. 071 253 3406

Coeliac Society of the United Kingdom PO BOX 220, High Wycombe, Bucks HP11 2HY. 0494 437278

Contact a Family 16 Strutton Ground, London SWIP 2HP

Cornelia de Lange (or Amsterdam Dwarf Syndrome) Self Help Group 46 Victoria Street, Staple Hill, Bristol. 0272 573046

Crohn's in Childhood Research Association Parkgate House, 356 West Barnes Lane, Motspur Park, Surrey KT3 6NB. 081 949 6209

Cystic Fibrosis Research Trust Alexandra House, 5 Blyth Road, Bromley, Kent BR1 3RS. 081 464 7211

Cystic Hygroma and Haemangloma Support Group Villa Fontaine, Church Road Worth, Crawley, West Sussex RH10 4RS. 0293 885901

The Disability Alliance ERA Universal House 88-94 Wentworth Street, London E1 7SA 071 247 8776

Down's Syndrome Association 12-13 Clapham Common Southside, London SW4 7AA. 071 720 0008

Dystrophic Epidermolysis Bullosa Research Association 1 Kings Road, Crowthorne, Berks RG11 7BG. 0344 771961

EPOCH (End Physical Punishment of Children) 77 Holloway Road, London N7 8JZ

Family Fund PO Box 50, York Y01 2ZX. 0904 621115

Foundation for the Study of Infant Deaths (Cot Death Research and Support) 15 Belgrave Square, London SW1X 8PS. 071 235 0965/1721

Friedreich's Ataxia Group Copse Edge Thursley Road, Elstead, Godalming, Surrey GU8 6DJ. 0252 702864

Haemophilia Society 123 Westminster Bridge Road, London SE1 7HY. 071 928 2020

Hyperactive Children's Support Group 71 Whyke Lane Chichester, West Sussex PO19 2LD. 0903 725182

Leukaemia Care Society PO Box 82, Exeter, Devon EX2 5DP. 0392 218514

Leukaemia Research Fund 43 Great Ormond Street, London WC1N 3JJ. 071 405 0101

Lifeline – Family help for abuse within the home PO Box 251, Marlborough, Wilts SN8 1EA. 0793 731286

LINK, the British Neurofibromatosis Patients Association Office BO3, Surrey House, 34 Eden Street, Kingston KT1 1ER

Muscular Dystrophy Group of Great Britain and Northern Ireland Nattrass House, 35 Macauley Road, London SW4 0QP. 071 720 8055

Myotonic Dystrophy Support Group 175 Carlton Hill, Carlton, Nottingham. 0602 870080

National AIDS Trust 14th Floor, Euston Tower, 286 Euston Road, London NW1 3DN. 071 388 1188

National Association of Citizen's Advice Bureaux 115/123 Pentonville Road, London N1 9LZ. 071 833 2181

National Asthma Campaign 300 Upper Street, London N1 2XX. 071 226 2260

National Autistic Society 276 Willesden Lane, London NW2 5RB. 081 451 1114

National Council for One Parent Families 255 Kentish Road, London NW5 2LX. 071 267 1361

National Deaf Children's Society 45 Hereford Road, London W2 5AH. 071 229 9272

National Eczema Society Tavistock House East, Tavistock Square, London WC1H 9SR 071 388 4097

National Federation of the Blind in the Kingdom Unity House, Smyth Street, Westgate, Wakefield, W Yorks WF1 1ER. 0924 291313

National Foster Care Association Francis St, London SWIP IDE

National Gypsy Council (Romany Kris) Greengate Street Oldham, Greater Manchester. 061 665 1924

Network for the Handicapped: law and advice centre for the handicapped and their families 16 Princeton Street, London WC1R 4BB. 071 831 8031

Neuroblastoma Society Woodlands, Ordsall Park Road, Retford, Notts DN22 7PJ. 0777 709238

Organic Acidemia Association UK 5 Saxon Road , Ashford, Middlesex TW15 1QL. 0784 245989

Perthes Association 49 Great Stone Road, Northfield, Birmingham B31 2LR. 021 4774415

Prader Willi Syndrome Association (UK) 30 Follett Drive, Abbots Langley, Herts ED5 OLP. 0923 674543

Research Trust for Metabolic Diseases in Children 53 Beam Street, Nantwich, Cheshire CW5 5NF. 0270 629782/0270 626834

Royal National Institute for the Blind 224 Great Portland Street, London W1N 6AA. 071 388 1266

Royal Society for Mentally Handicapped Children and Adults (MENCAP) MENCAP National Centre, 123 Golden Lane, London EC1Y ORT. 071 253 9433

Royal Society for the Prevention of Accidents (ROSPA) Privy Common House, The Queensway, Birmingham BE4 6BJ

Scoliosis Assocation UK 380-384 Harrow Road, London W9 2UH. 071 289 5652

Share a Care 8 Cornmarket, Faringdon, Oxon

Sickle Cell Society Green Lodge, Barretts Green Road, London NW10 7AP. 081 961 8346, 081 961 7795, 081 961 4006

Society for Mucopolysaccaride Diseases 30 Westwood Drive, Little Chalfont, Bucks. 02404 2789

Sotos Group for Families affected by Sotos Syndrome Kilndown House, Kilndown, Cranbrook, Kent TN17 2SG. 0892 890397

Spastics Society 12 Park Cresent, London WIN 4EQ. 071 636 5020

Tourette Syndrome (UK) Association 169 Wickham Street, Welling, Kent DA16 3BS. 081 855 7478

Tuberous Sclerosis Association of Great Britain Little Barnsley Farm, Catshill, Bromsgrove, Worcs B61 ONQ. 0527 71898

United Kingdom Rett Syndrome Association Freepost, Orpington, Kent BR5 1SZ. 0689 74817

United Kingdom Thalassemia Society 107 Nightingale Lane, London N8 7QY. 081 348 0437

Williams Syndrome/Infantile Hypercalcaemia(WS/IHC) Parents Association Mulberry Cottage, 37 Mulberry Green, Old Harlow, Essex. 0279 27214

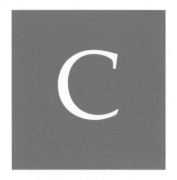

C   Sources of Information

This list of centrally available statistics on child health is taken from *Population Trends* 1990.

Indicators	Description of data available	Publication	First available	Frequency
Stillbirths	Numbers and rates by sex, month of occurence, cause, place of confinement, gestation, birthweight, area	DH3, Mortality – perinatal and infant DH6, Mortality – childhood		Annual
Early neonatal deaths	Numbers by sex, cause, month of occurrence, area			
Perinatal deaths	Rates by sex, cause, month of occurrence and area			
All infant deaths	Numbers and rates by sex, age-group, cause, month of occurrence and area			
Stillbirths Perinatal deaths Neonatal deaths Post neonatal deaths All infant deaths Live births	Linking of information from birth and death registration allows a wide range of tabulations by age of mother, parity, legitimacy, social class, country of birth of mother, month of birth, and birthweight	DH3, Mortality – perinatal and infant	1975	Annual
Trends in infant mortality	Deaths, numbers and rates, from selected causes in infants under one year are given for each of the previous ten years	DH3, Mortality – perinatal and infant		Annual
Birthweight	Since 1975 birthweight provided by health authorities has been added to birth registrations. This process has been virtually complete since 1983. Mortality of infants of different birthweights can be monitored as described above. In addition the birthweight of all live births can be tabulated by social class, age of mother, parity, and country of birth	DH3, Mortality – perinatal and infant	1975	Annual
Low birth weight babies	Number, number of deaths by time of death	DH Summary (Form LHS27/1)	1953	Annual to 1987
Childhood deaths at ages: 1, 2, 3, 4, 5–9, 10–14 and all ages under 15	Numbers of deaths by sex for each cause	DH3, Mortality – perinatal and infant		Annual

Childhood deaths at ages: under 1, 1–4, 5–14	a) Rates per million population from principal causes for boys and girls	DH2, Mortality – cause		Annual
	b) Also for each administrative and health area	DH5 fiche, Mortality – area		Annual
	c) Number and rates are published in more detail for deaths due to accidents and violence, e.g. accidents at home, road traffic accidents	DH4, Mortality – accidents and violence		Annual
	d) Detailed analysis of childhood deaths in terms of rates, SMRs and PMRs by parents' social class based on occupation, socio-economic group, and occupation order	DS no. 8 – Occupational Mortality, Childhood Supplement	1959–63	10–yearly
Glue sniffing deaths at ages: 10, 11, 12, 13, 14	Estimates of deaths to glue sniffing by sex	Series of reports from St George's Hospital Medical School	1971	Annual
Cancer registration rates for children aged under: 1, 1–4, 5–9, 10–14	Numbers and rates by sex and site	MB1 – general mortality	1962	Annual
	More details from the National Registry for Childhood Tumours	Series of publications and regular reports to DoH on incidence and survival	1962	Annual
Rare childhood disorders, e.g. AIDS, diabetes, galacto-saemia, drowning and near drowning, Reye's syndrome. Notifications of malformations identified in the first week of life or at stillbirth	Notification of specific diseases by paediatricians to the British Paediatric Surveillance Unit – follow-up for clinical and epidemiological study	BPSU annual reports	1986	Annual
	Rates per 10 000 births by condition, age of mother	MB3 – Congenital malformations	1964	Annual
Legal abortions due to fetal abnormalities	Numbers by condition	AB – Abortions	1968	Annual
Deliveries in NHS hospitals	Birthweight by maternal complications, outcome and parity. Anomalies and complications of babies by maternal age and parity, by birthweight, by mode of delivery, and by maternal complications	MB4 – Hospital In-patient Enquiry, maternity tables	1955	Annual to 1985
Discharges and deaths from NHS non-psychiatric hospitals in England for children aged 0–4, 5–9, 10–14	Deaths and discharges by ICD 3 digit codes: Operations and sex	MB4 – Hospital In-patient Enquiry	1955	Annual
Hospital cases treated for children 0–4, 5–14	HIPE data providing rates per 10 000 population	DH Statistical Bulletins	1949	Annual
Operations on children aged 0–4, 5–14	Operation rates per 10 000 by sex and operation code	DH Statistical Bulletins	1949	Annual
Admissions to mental illness, mental handicap hospitals and units for children aged 0–9, 10–14	Numbers by sex and diagnostic groups – from the Mental Health Enquiry	Booklets on Mental Health Statistics for England (DH)	1959	Annual
Day care facilities in child and adolescent psychiatry	Number of attenders	DH Summary (Form KH14)		

Notifications for food poisoning, malaria, measles, meningitis, tuberculosis, dysentery, infective jaundice, whooping cough, scarlet fever for children aged 0, 1, 2, 3, 4, 5–9, 10–14	Rates per 100 000 population by sex. Based on data supplied by the doctor in attendance to each local authority under the Public Health Acts and Infectious Disease Regulations Numbers for all notifiable diseases	MB2 – Communicable Disease Statistics		Annual
Home accidents to children aged 0–4, 5–15	Rate per 1000 population per year by sex. Based on GHS questions. Further details on type of injury and accident from DTI Home Accidents Surveillance System	GHS reports (OPCS) DTI HASS reports	1981 1976	3 yearly Annual
Episodes of illness presenting to GPs, detailed diagnosis for children aged 0–4, 5–14	Episode rates per 1000 persons at risk by sex, calculated from records of all consultations in a sample of practices during a one year period	MB5 – Morbidity statistics from general practice	1955/6	1971/2, 1981/2
Long standing illness at ages 0–4, 5–15	Proportions whose parents report long-standing illness by sex			
Limiting long-standing illness at ages 0–4, 5–15	Proportions whose parents report a long-standing illness that limits normal activity by sex	GHS Reports (OPCS)	1972	Annual
Restricted activity in the past two weeks at ages 0–4, 5–15	Proportions whose parents report limited activity due to illness or injury by sex			
Disability among children 0–4, 5–9, 10–15	Prevalence of disability assessed by detailed interviews with parents and classified by type of disability and severity	Prevalence of disability among children in Great Britain (OPCS)	1985	Ad hoc survey
Registrations of the blind and partially sighted aged 0–4, 5–15 Registrations of the deaf with speech, deaf without speech and hard of hearing aged 0–15 Registrations of the physically disabled aged 0–15	Local authorities keep registers of these three groups of disabled children. Since registration is voluntary they cannot be considered as reliable indicators of prevalence	DoH	1972	Trienially
Dental health at single years of age 5–15	Proportion of children with active decay, filled teeth, extractions, gum condition, crowding. Based on survey and dental examinations	Children's dental health in England and Wales 1973 and 1983, 1988 in preparation	1973	Repeated ad hoc survey
Dental treatments to children aged 0–4, 5–9, 10–14	Numbers provided from the General Dental Service and the Community dental service – covers fillings, extractions, etc	Dental practice board reports	1984	Annual
Prescriptions dispensed in general practice to children aged 0–15	Numbers from the Prescription Pricing Authority	Statistical Bulletin DoH	1977	Annual
Conceptions to girls aged under 14, 14, 15	Numbers and rates of conceptions and proportions ending in births and terminations	Birth statistics	1968	Annual

Live and still births to girls aged 11, 12, 13, 14, 15	Numbers of births	Birth statistics		Annual
Abortions to girls aged under 15, 15	Number of abortions	AB – Abortion statistics	1968	Annual
Children in need of protection	Numbers from local authority registers by age, sex, category of abuse, legal status, and whether in care	DoH publication	1987/88	Annual
Height, weight for children aged 10/11, 14/15	Mean heights and weights by age and sex	The diets of British schoolchildren, DHSS/OPCS	1983	Ad hoc survey
Height, weight, anthropometry for children aged 5–9	Means and distributions obtained from a large sample of schoolchildren followed up through primary school	St Thomas' survey of height and growth	1979	Annual/ continuous
Birthweight	See above			
Diets of schoolchildren aged 10/11, 14/15	Intakes of main nutrients by height, weight, age, sex, social class based on parents' occupation, family type	The diets of British school children, DHSS/OPCS	1983	Ad hoc survey
Infant feeding at ages up to nine months	Proportions of babies breast and/or bottle fed at different ages by age of mother, social class based on parents' occupation, education, region	Infant feeding reports 1975, 1980, 1985	1975	5-yearly surveys
Smoking among children aged 11, 12, 13, 14,15	Prevalence of different levels of smoking by sex	Smoking among secondary school children in 1982, 1984, 1986, 1988	1982	2-yearly surveys
Drinking among children aged 13, 14,15	Prevalence of different levels of drinking by sex	Adolescent drinking	1984	Ad hoc survey
		Smoking among secondary school children in England in 1988	1988	Repeated questions
Vaccination and immunisation for diphtheria, tetanus, polio, whooping cough, measles, mumps and rubella	Uptake rates for completed primary courses in different years of life	DoH Summaries (Form SBL607/KC51)	1950	Annual
Rubella immunisation for schoolgirls aged 10, 11, 12, 13, 14, 15	Uptake and cumulative uptake rate as a percentage of the schoolgirl population	DoH Summaries (Form SBL607/KC51)	1950	Annual
TB tests and BCG Vaccinations	Numbers tested, found positive and negative, and vaccinated	DoH Summaries (Form SBL655/KC50)	1971	Annual

Index

A

abuse *see* child abuse
Access to Health Records Act (1990) 88,
    118–19
accidents 237–48
  adolescents 434
  head injuries 245–6
  housing 247
  pollution 246–7
  prevention 241–4
  protection 240–41
  sites of 238–9
  statistics 35, 237
adolescents (young adults) 429–40
  growth 158
  health problems 434–6
  homeless 437–8
  learning disability 379
  nutrition 157–8
  services for 438–40
  sex education 439
  sexual activity 432–4
  teenage parents 233
  teenage pregnancies 35, 432–3
adoption 49–55
  adoption contact register 52
  health information 53–4
  HIV infection 55
  openness 54–5
  outcomes 55
  practice 50–52
  procedures 52–3
  and psychiatric disorders 215
  statistics 49–50
  transracial/inter-country 54, 215
adrenal disease 181
affection 229
age
  and accidents 239–40
  bone age 175
  and psychiatric disorders 208
aggression 402–3, 409–10
air pollution 246–7
alcohol abuse
  adolescents 434
  statistics 35
allergy, food 155–6, 392
allowances *see* benefits
anal dilatation 264–5
anal fissures 264

androgens 171, 181
anger 217, 409–10
anorexia nervosa 391
anxiety states 216–17, 407–8
aspirin 81
asthma
  prognosis 74
  at school 457
astigmatism 317
asymmetrical tonic neck reflex 187
attendance allowance (disability living
    allowance) 60–62, 65
attention control, poor 340–41, 356
attention-seeking 404
audiological assessment 325–30
audit 15, 18
autism 339

B

balance 187
Barnardo's 63
bathing aids 300
battered child syndrome 250
BCG vaccine 137
Beckwith's syndrome 340
bed wetting (enuresis) 395–400
behavioural problems 355–6, 386–406
  attention-seeking 404
  behaviour modification 198, 413–14
  children with learning disability 369–70
  difficult behaviour 402–3
  eating problems 390–92
  and food intolerance 156–7, 392
  habit training 387–9
  hyperactivity 156–7, 392, 401
  physically handicapped children 297
  school-based 404–6
  serious disturbance 386–7
  sleep problems 392–5
  tics 389–90
benefits 57–65
  homeless adolescents 437–8
  poverty traps 64–5
  stigma 64
  the system 63–5
  take-up levels 64
bereavement 212, 218–19, 291
birth records 79
bites 261
blindness 310–11, 319–22

see also vision
BLISS symbolics 304, 344
bonding 212
bone
    age measurement 175
    disorders, short stature 179–80
breast development 430
    isolated early (premature thelarche)
        181–2, 432
breastfeeding 141, 143–6
Bristol Child Development Programme
    233–4
bruising
    non-accidental 258–9
    perianal 264
bullying 405–6
burns 240
    non-accidental 260–61

C

cancer, nutrition 165
cannabis 436
cardiovascular disease 152, 461
care orders 44, 46, 69, 225
case conferences 272–3
case-control studies 81
caseload information 119
census data 79
central nervous system damage
    degenerating conditions 368–9
    speech disorders 339
cerebral palsy 304–6
    articulation disorders 340
    feeding 164–5
charities *see* voluntary organisations
child abuse
    Asian communities 274–5
    causation 254–7
    definitions 251, 252–3
    differential diagnosis 259–60
    disabled children 273–4
    emotional 253, 262–3
    enquiries 251–2
    fractures 260
    global view 251–2
    interventions 268–73
    and learning difficulties 356
    medical examination 263–6, 268, 271
    models 255, 256–7
    organised networks 250, 253
    physical (non-accidental injury) 250,
        258–62
    practice issues 275
    prediction 223
    procedures 269–71
    recognition 257–8
    risk factors 257–8
    ritualistic 250, 253
    sexual 250, 252, 263–6, 274–5
    victims 255
Child and Adolescent Psychiatry Service
    415
child assessment orders 70

child benefit 58
child development centres 15, 281
child health clinics 102–5
Child Health and Education Study 81, 224,
    231
child health services
    access 230
    aims and needs 8–9
    combined 8–9, 14–16
    history 1–5
    nursing services 16–17
    process 15–17
    structure 14–15
    support services 17
    see also health services; National Health
        Service
child health surveillance 4, 95–120
    child health clinics 102–7
    children in care 45–6
    children in daycare 44
    components 88
    computer systems 86
    ethnic minorities 101
    home visiting 105
    individual checks 97–9
    liaison functions 95
    neonatal examination 107–8
    pitfalls 100–102
    principles 95–7
    records 99, 116–19
    at school 105–6, 112–15
    timed routine checks 107–15
    see also screening
Child Poverty Action Group 63
child protection 69–70, 249–76
    Area Committees 250, 273
    case conferences 272–3
    history 249–50
    legal status of child 271–2
    registers 68, 258
Childline 269
childminders 42, 46–7
Children Act (1989) 21, 44, 66–72, 225
children in care 44–9
children in need 67–8, 284
Chlamydia trachomatis 267
chromosome disorders 445–7
    short stature 177–8
    see also genetics
Citizens' Advice Bureaux 63
cleft palate 340
clinics 102–7
clumsy children 358–61
cocaine 436
coeliac disease 165, 179
cohort studies 81
colic 151
colour vision testing 114, 316
communication
    computer-aided 304, 344
    deaf children 331–2
    physically handicapped children 296,
        302–4
    and psychiatric disorders 210

speech disorders 343–4
community mental handicap
    teams/nurses 379
community paediatricians 4
computers
    in child health 86–8
    communication aids 304, 344
concentration 340–41, 356
conduct disorders 355–6
conductive education 293
confidentiality 88, 99
consent to medical
            treatment/examination
    in child abuse cases 268
    children in care 46
    the law 70–71
constipation 151
consultations 97–9
contact orders 68–9
continence
    encopresis 395–6, 400–401
    enuresis 395–400
    physically handicapped children 296–7
    spina bifida 307
contraception 432
convulsions
    epilepsy 369, 459–60
    prognosis 74
Cope Street Centre, Nottingham 233
copper deficiency 260
cortisol 171
cost benefit analysis 76
cot deaths 458
counselling 418–28
    basic requirements 419–20
    characteristics 420
    first session 421–3
    genetic see genetic counselling
    health-related problems 39
    longer-term 418–19
    school nurse 39
    techniques 423–8
court orders 68–70
    care orders 44, 46, 69, 225
    checklist 67
Court Report (1976) 3–5
courts of law 71–2
crawling 187–8
crying 215–16
culture 228–9
    and language 350–51
    and learning difficulties 356–7
    see also ethnic minorities
cystic fibrosis 458
    carriers 444
    diet 161–2
    estimating risk 451
    genetics 449–50

D

Data Protection Act (1987) 88
day care facilities 42–3, 44
day nurseries 42–3

language development schemes 234, 302
    prevention of infection 123
    speech disorders 343
deafness see hearing loss
delinquency 437
dental care 295
dental caries 149, 150, 154
Denver Developmental Screening Test 204
Department for Education 20
depression
    childhood 217–18, 356, 411–12
    and housing 247
    maternal 214
deprivation see poverty
design safety 243
Desmopressin 400
development
    assessment scores 203–4
    clinical errors of judgement 100–101
    delayed 289
    emotional 197, 205–20
    intellectual 185–204
    motor skills 187–92, 195
    social 192–6
    and visual handicap 311, 320–21
diabetes mellitus 459
    diet 162–3
diarrhoea
    chronic, and short stature 179
    day nurseries 123
    short bowel syndrome 163–4
    toddlers 154–5
diet see feeding; nutrition
difficult child syndrome 207
diphtheria 138
disability, definition 68, 277
disability living allowance 60–62, 65
disability register 68
disabled children see handicap
discipline 403
Down's syndrome
    diagnosis 368
    genetics 445–6
    hearing loss 334
    Nottingham Down's Syndrome
        Children's Service 371–3
    obesity 183
    screening 76
    tongue abnormalities 340
drowning 240
drug abuse 35, 435, 436
Duchenne muscular dystrophy 307–8,
        444–5, 449
dyslexia 363–4

E

eating problems 390–92
    see also feeding; nutrition
eczema 459
education
    and accident prevention 244
    conductive 293
    deaf children 332–3

equal opportunities 31
funding 20, 22, 29–30
Local Education Authorities *see* Local
    Education Authorities
muscular dystrophy 308
parent power 30
physical handicap 24–7, 31, 282–4,
    292–3
pre-school 231, 232–3
segregated provision 31
services 20–32
special needs *see* special educational
    needs
special schools 21, 373–5
speech disorders 343–4
visual handicap 321–2
see also learning; schools
Education Act (1981) 282–4, 367
Education Reform Act (1988) 21, 22, 31
education supervision orders 69
Education Welfare Service 22
Educational Psychology Service 22
emergency protection orders 69–70
emotional abuse 253, 262–3
emotional development 197, 205–20
emotional problems 209–10, 407–17
    see also psychiatric disorders
employment of children 72, 354–5
encopresis 395–6, 400–401
enuresis 395–400
environment
    and infection 123
    and language development 339
    and well-being of children 227
epidemiology 73–94
    data 78–85
    health information systems 85–6
    incidence 77
    infection 121–2
    information sources 121–2, 466–9
    prevalence 77
    rates 76–8
    research 87
    screening 88–94
    uses 74–6
epilepsy 74, 369, 459–60
Erikson, Eric 198–201
erythema, perianal 264
ethnic minorities
    child health surveillance 101
    child sexual abuse 274–5
    children in care 48
    diet 166
    learning difficulties 350–51, 356–7
    learning disability 381
    planning 74
    well-being of children 228–9
examination, medical
    child abuse 263–6, 268, 271
    clumsy children 360
    consent to 268
    neonatal 107–8
    principles 98
    school entrants 105–6, 112–13

timed child health surveillance checks
    107–15
exercise 35

F

failure to thrive 155, 183–4, 230
    non-organic 262–3
families
    abusing and neglecting 254
    basic tasks 211
    birth of a child 214–15
    breakdown 211–12, 228
    disharmony 355
    homelessness 227
    income 228
    physically handicapped children 294
    single parent 213
    size and structure 212–13, 228, 380–81
    see also parents
family centres 43, 44, 231–2
family credit 58–60
family fund 63
family proceedings court 71
family therapy 413
fear 216–17
feeding
    aids 300
    cerebral palsy 164–5
    infants *see* infant feeding
    see also nutrition
first aid 242
fluoride 150
food *see* feeding; nutrition
foster care 44–6
fractures
    non-accidental 260
    spontaneous in infancy 260
fragile X syndrome 338, 349, 449
frozen watchfulness 262

G

Galant's reflex 186
General Household Survey 79–80
genetic counselling 450–51
    handicap 297–8
    hearing loss 324
    muscular dystrophy 308
genetics 441–55
    chromosome abnormalities 445–7
    clinical genetic services 452
    counselling *see* genetic counselling
    ethical issues 452–3
    genetic disorders 441–2
    genetic registers 452
    genetic screening 453
    and growth 168–9
    multifactorial disorders 447
    patterns of inheritance 442–5
    physically handicapped children 297–8
    and well-being of children 226
German measles 132–3, 324
Gesell, Arnold 197–8

gigantism 182
Gilles de la Tourette syndrome 389
glasses 318
glue ear 334
Goldenhar's syndrome 324
gonorrhoea 267
GP consultations 79
grasp reflex 187
grief 218–19
Griffith's scales 203
growth 167–84
  adolescent growth spurt 158
  advance 181–2
  delay 176–7, 230
  disorders 175–82
  genetic influences 168–9
  hormones 169–71, 178
  iatrogenic causes of suppression 179
  intrauterine retardation 177
  measurement 102, 171–6
  normal patterns 167–8
  and nutrition 169
  physically handicapped children 295
  recording 173–4
  short stature 176–80, 263
  and stress 169
  tall stature 180–82
  see also failure to thrive
guardian ad litem 70
gynaecomastia 431

H

habit training 387–9
haemoglobinopathies 460
haemophilia 460–61
Haemophilus influenzae 138–9, 324
hand function 294–5
handicap
  abuse 273–4
  assessment 293–4
  behavioural problems 297
  benefits 60–62, 65
  causes 278
  communication 296, 302–4
  continence 296–7
  definition 277
  dental care 295
  district handicap team 281–2
  education 24–7, 31, 282–4, 292–3
  epidemiology 291
  equipment 298–301
  language development programmes 302
  and learning 347–8
  leisure activities 298
  management 280–82, 293–4
  medical review 294–8
  mental see learning disability
  multidisciplinary assessment 281–2
  multiprofessional service 286
  multiple 368, 379
  physical 290–309
  prevalence 277–9
  reaction to 279–80

school leavers 284–5
social services 284–5
visual 310–11, 319–22, 448
hay fever 461
head circumference 173
head injuries 245–6
  child abuse 258
Heaf test 136
health education 36–9
  components 37
  drug abuse 436
  learning disability 380–84
  nutrition 158
  parent-held records as source 117
  and prevention of infection 123
  school health service 38–9
  schools 36–7
  sex education 37–9, 439
  see also health promotion
Health Education Authority 35
health information systems 85–6
Health of the Nation
  health promotion 33
  variations in health 7–8
health promotion 33–6
  see also health education
Health Service and Community Care Act
    (1991) 7
health services 6–19
  computerisation 87
  contacts in first year of life 96
  cost effectiveness 76
  initiating 13–14
  items of service 17–18
  levels 12–13
  needs and planning 74–5
  providers 11–13
  purchasers 11
  see also child health services; National
    Health Service
health visitors
  history 1–2
  role 16–17
  surveillance 97
  ten days check 108–9
hearing
  distraction test 75
  and learning difficulties 350
  physically handicapped children 295
hearing aids 330–31, 334
hearing loss 323–34
  audiological assessment 325–30
  causes 324
  communication 331–2
  conductive 324, 333–4
  education 332–3
  genetics 448
  incidence 323
  prevention 324
  screening 324, 325
  sensorineural 324, 330
  speech disorders 338–9
heart problems 152, 461
height

measuring 80, 172
  short stature 176–80, 263
  tall stature 180–82
  see also growth
hepatitis 139–40
herpes, genital 267
history taking 97–8
  child abuse 270
  counselling 421–2
HIV infection 267
  and adoption 55
home accidents 238
home visiting 105
homelessness
  adolescents 437–8
  families 227
hormones and growth 169–71, 178
hospital admissions data 80
housing 227, 247–8
hungry children 354
Hurler's syndrome 340
hydrocephalus 307
hymenal tissue 263–4, 265–6
hyperactivity 401
  and food additives 156–7, 392
hypermetropia 317
hypernatraemia 150
hypothyroidism 178–9

I

illegitimate children 228
illness
  and learning difficulties 351–4
  and psychiatric disorders 208–9
  sick role 352–3
immunisation 123, 124–40
  physically handicapped children 297
  programmes 125–7
  uptake 125, 127–8
immunity 124–5
immunoglobulins 125
impairment 277
income
  families 228
  and learning disability 380
income support 58
incontinence *see* continence
infant feeding 143–50
  problems 150–52
  surveys 80–81
infection 121–40
  epidemiology data 121–2
  morbidity 79, 122
  mortality 122
  notification 121–2
  prevention 123
  susceptibility 122–3
inflammatory bowel disease 179
information *see* epidemiology
influenza vaccine 140
intellectual development 185–204
intelligence
  bright children 358

and diet 230
intelligence quotient (IQ) 366
  limited and poor school progress 348–9
  and psychiatric disorders 208
  Wechsler scales 204
invalid care allowance 62
Inverse Care Law 224
iron deficiency 235
items of service 17–18

J

Jarman index 223
Jervell and Lange Neilsen syndrome 324

K

kidney disease
  diet 163
  short stature 179
Klinefelter's syndrome 182, 446
Korner Report 86, 93–4

L

Landau Kleffner syndrome 339
language 335–44
  comprehension 341–2
  and culture 350–51
  inner 341
  spoken, skills required 335–6
language development
  abnormal *see* speech disorders
  delayed 337, 338
  environment 339
  glue ear 334
  and learning difficulties 350–51
  normal 336–7
  schemes 234, 302
law 66–72
  child protection 271–2
  education services 21
lead poisoning 246
learning 345–65
  difficulties (poor progress at school)
    348–57
  disability (mental handicap) *see* learning
    disability
  theory 198
  see also education
learning disability (mental handicap) 366–
    85
  assessment 357
  behavioural problems 369–70
  care services 370–73
  characteristics 381–2
  community mental handicap
    nurses/teams 379
  diagnosis 368
  ethnic minorities 381
  genetics 448
  health care planning 378–9
  health education 36, 380–84
  moderate 367–8, 375–8

patterns of disadvantage 381
pre-school review 374
reports 357–8
and school staff 378
seriously ill children in school 378
severe 367, 373–5
sex education 38
socioeconomic factors 380–81, 382
special schools 21, 283–4, 373–5
young adults 379
left handedness 359
legislation see law
Lennox-Gastaut syndrome 369
leukaemia 461–2
lichen sclerosus et atrophicus 264
life events 230–31
enuresis 396
ligature marks 261
literacy 361–3
Local Education Authorities
central administration 23
funding 20, 22
future role 30–31
organisation structure 22–3
role in schools 23–4

M

magistrates 71
Makaton 303–4, 344
malnutrition see nutrition
management 9–11
Mantoux test 136
Marfan's syndrome 182, 442
masturbation 389
maternity benefits 58
measles 130–31
medical examination see examination,
medical
mental handicap see learning disability
milk 148–9
breast 143–4
breast milk substitutes 145–7
intolerance 151–2
nutritional content 154
pre-school children 153
minerals 158–9
mobility
allowance (disability living allowance)
60–62, 65
physically handicapped children 294,
300
spina bifida 307
morbidity data 79–80, 122
Moro reflex 186
mortality rates 78, 122
mother and toddler groups 43
motor skills 187–92, 195
clumsy children 358–61
mumps 131
hearing loss 324
Münchausen syndrome by proxy 261–2
muscular dystrophy 307–8, 444–5, 449
mutism, elective 339

myopia 317

N

nail-biting 388
National Child Development Study (1970)
74
National Health Service
aims and needs 8–9
costs 6–7
history 2–3
management 9–11
organisation 11–13
principles 6
structure 11
see also child health services; health
services
neglect 224–6, 254
definition 252
indicators 225–6
and learning 346–7
signs and conditions 262–3
neighbourhoods 227–8
neonates
audiological assessment 326
birth check 107–8
small-for-gestational age 177
non-accidental injury 250, 258–62
see also child abuse
Nottingham Down's Syndrome Children's
Service 371–3
nurseries 42–3
nursery nurses 42–3
nursing services 16–17
nurture 229
nutrition 141–66
adolescents 157–8
balanced diet 159–60
and behaviour 391–2
dietary reference values 142–3
in disease 160–66
eating disorders 390–92
ethnic minorities 166
fats 153, 159–60
fibre 153–4
food additives 155–6, 392
food allergies 155–7, 392
food fads 390–91
and growth 169
health education 158
hungry children 354
infants see infant feeding
and infection 123
iron deficiency 235
and learning difficulties 354
malabsorption 179
milk see milk
national advice 141–2
parenteral 164
physically handicapped children 295–6
and poverty 155, 230
pre-school children 141–2, 152–7
prescribed diets 165
problems 154–7

protein energy malnutrition 263
religion and diet 166
in school 157–8
see also feeding
nystagmus 320

O

obesity 390
causes 183
measurement 182–3
pre-school children 155
tall children 180
obsessional compulsive disorders 408
oestrogen 171
Office of Population Censuses and Surveys (OPCS) 81
ophthalmology services 311–12
opiates 436
orthoses 299
osteogenesis imperfecta 260
otitis media 324, 333–4
outcomes 18

P

Paget-Gorman sign language 304, 344
palmar grasp reflex 187
parachute reaction 187
parents
and child health surveillance 99, 100
depression 214
detecting hearing loss 326, 327
and education services 30
parent-held child health records 85, 116–18
parental responsibility 66–8
participation in case conferences 272–3
psychiatric illness 213–14
reaction to handicap 279–80
and sex education 38
single 213
teenage 233
see also families
Patient's Charter 8–9
Pendred syndrome 324
Perry Preschool Program 232–3
pertussis 133–4
pervasive habit training disorder 387–8
phenylketonuria 160–61
phobias 408
school phobia 406
photophobia 319–20
Piaget, Jean 201–3
Pierre Robin anomaly 324
play 192–6
physically handicapped children 298
playground accidents 239, 240
playgroups 43
pneumococcal vaccine 140
poliomyelitis 128–9
pollution 246–7
populations 73–4, 85
Portage scheme 234–5

post-traumatic stress disorder 409
posture 187–90
poverty 221–36
Child Poverty Action Group 63
deprivation dwarfism 263
deprivation measures 223–4
early intervention schemes 231–5
impact on child health 224
and learning 346–7
nutrition 155, 230
poverty traps 64–5
Prader-Willi syndrome 183
pre-school children
accidents 239–40
day care facilities 42–3
education 231, 232–3
nutrition 141–2, 152–7
obesity 155
severe learning disability 371–3
pregnancies, teenage 35, 432–3
prevention 88, 95
see also child health surveillance; screening
primary health care 12
psychiatric disorders 205–20
adopted children 215
aetiology 206–7
assessment 206–7
characteristics of the child 207–10
Child and Adolescent Psychiatry Service 415
definition 205–6
emotional problems 209–10, 407–17
and the family 211–15
in parents 213–14
social adversity 214
speech disorders 339
treatment 413–15
psychosis 356
puberty 430–32
delayed 431
precocious 181, 431

Q

quality management 17–18

R

Radford Family Centre 231–2
radiotherapy 179
reading difficulties 361–4
records 85–6
Access to Health Records Act (1990) 88, 118–19
birth 79
child health surveillance 99, 116–19
immunisation 128
linkage 87–8
parent-held 85, 116–18
reflex anal dilatation 265
reflexes 186–7
refractive error 317–18
religion and diet 166

renal disease *see* kidney disease
residence orders 68–9
residential care 48
respite care 15
    children with learning disability 370–71
Reye syndrome 81
rights of children 67
risk assessment 75
road traffic accidents 238, 240
rubella (German measles) 132–3, 324
Russell-Silver syndrome 177

S

---

sadness 217
scalds, non-accidental 260–61
school-based problems
    absence due to illness 351–2
    accidents 238–9
    asthma 457
    behavioural problems 404–6
    medication 352
    non-attendance (truancy) 355–6, 406, 437
    poor progress 348–57
    school phobia 406
    school refusal 355, 406
school health service
    adolescents 439
    child health surveillance 105–6, 112–15
    health education 38–9
    history 2
    learning disability 373–8
    role of 17
    sex education 38–9
school nurse 17, 105–6
    counselling 39
schools
    child health surveillance 105–6, 112–15
    community roles 30
    disabled pupils 24–7, 31, 282–4, 292–3
    expectations of children 28
    Governing Bodies 23–4, 30–31
    health education 36–7
    influence on learning 345–6
    management 23–4, 27–8, 30
    nutrition 157–8
    sex education 37–8
    special 21, 283–4, 373–5
    staff structure 24
    successful 27–8
    see also education
screening 88–94
    adequacy of cover 92–3
    congenital hearing loss 324, 325
    cost 92
    cost benefit analysis 76
    criteria 89
    genetic 453
    neonates 108
    predictive value 92
    programmes 75
    reliability 89
    sensitivity 89–90
    specificity 89–90

speech disorders 340–42
    variation 89
    vision 311, 314–16
    yield 92
    see also child health surveillance
secondary health care 12
self esteem 210
self harm 411–12
self help groups
    addresses 463–5
    benefits 62–3
    child protection 269
separation 218
sex education 37–9, 439
sexual abuse *see* child abuse
sexually transmissible diseases 266–7
short bowel syndrome 163–4
short stature 176–80, 263
sick role 352–3
sickle cell disease 74, 460
sign languages 303–4, 343–4
single parent families 213
sleep
    lack of 354
    problems 392–5
smacking 268–9
smiling 216
smoking
    adolescents 434–5
    passive 247
    specific enquiry 81–2
    statistics 35
    and temper tantrums 410
social class *see* socioeconomic factors
social development 192–6
social fund 60
Social Index 224
Social Security benefits *see* benefits
social services 41–56
    handicapped children 284–5
social workers, training 41
socioeconomic factors
    and accidents 242
    and learning 346–7
    learning disability 380–81, 382
    social class 221–3
soil pollution 247
solvent abuse 356, 435–6
Sotos syndrome (cerebral gigantism) 182
sources of information 466–9
    see also epidemiology
special educational needs 31, 277–89
    integration 353–4
    registers 119, 286–7
    resources 287–8
    statementing 283, 284
    teaching 22
    unnecessary exclusion 353–4
special schools 21, 373–5, 283–4
speech disorders 337–44
    articulation disorders 340, 342
    assessment 340–42
    deaf children 338–9
    differential diagnosis 338–9

education 343–4
epidemiology 335
management 342–4
see also language
speech therapy 302, 343
spina bifida 306–7
squint 313–14, 318–19
cohort study 81
stammering 338
standards 18
statementing 283, 284
stepping reflex 186
steroids 179
Stickler syndrome 324
stimulation 229
stress
and growth 169
and psychiatric disorders 209–10
suicide 412
supervision orders 69, 225
support organisations 463–5
surveillance *see* child health surveillance
syphilis 267

T

tall stature 180–82
teenage health clinics 439–40
teenage parents 233
teenage pregnancies 35, 432–3
temper tantrums 409–10
temperament 207, 231
termination of pregnancy 432–3
tertiary health care 12–13
testosterone 171
tetanus 137–8
thalassaemia 460
thelarche, premature 181–2, 432
thumb-sucking 388
thyroid hormone (thyroxine) 170–71
deficiency (hypothyroidism) 178–9
tics 389–90
toilet training 399–400
physically handicapped children 300–301
tongue abnormalities 340
travel abroad 140
Treacher Collins syndrome 324
Trichomonas vaginalis 267
truancy 355–6, 406, 437
tuberculosis 134–7
Turner's syndrome

genetics 446
short stature 177–8
tympanometry 329

U

Usher's syndrome 324, 448

V

vaccination *see* immunisation
vaginal injury 265–6
vaginosis, bacterial 267
varicella/zoster vaccine 140
vegetarianism 158
vision
binocular 313–14
colour vision testing 316
disordered 310–11, 319–22, 448
genetics 448
and learning difficulties 349
normal development 312–14
physically handicapped children 295
screening 311, 314–16
vitamins 149–50, 158–9
voluntary organisations
addresses 463–5
benefits 62–3
child protection 269
disabled children 285–6
speech disorders 344

W

Waardenburg's syndrome 324, 443
walking 187–9
warts, genital 266–7
waste disposal 247
water pollution 246
weaning 147–8
Wechsler Intelligence Scales 204
weight
measuring 80, 172
see also failure to thrive; growth; obesity
welfare of children 67
wheelchairs 300
whooping cough (pertussis) 133–4
writing difficulties 361–3

Y

young adults *see* adolescents